UNHEALTHY HEALTH POLICY

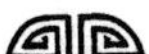

UNHEALTHY HEALTH POLICY

A Critical Anthropological Examination

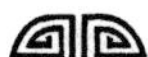

EDITED BY
ARACHU CASTRO AND MERRILL SINGER

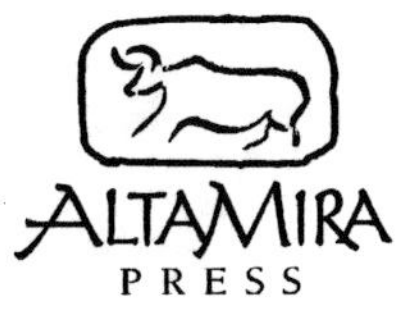

ALTAMIRA PRESS
A Division of Rowman & Littlefield Publishers, Inc.
Lanham • Boulder • New York • Toronto • Plymouth, UK

ALTAMIRA PRESS
A division of Rowman & Littlefield Publishers, Inc.
A wholly owned subsidiary of The Rowman & Littlefield Publishing Group, Inc.
4501 Forbes Boulevard, Suite 200
Lanham, MD 20706
www.altamirapress.com

Estover Road
Plymouth PL6 7PY
United Kingdom

British Library Cataloguing in Publication Information Available

Library of Congress Cataloging-in-Publication Data

Unhealthy health policy : a critical anthropological examination / edited by
Arachu Castro and Merrill Singer.
p. cm.
Includes bibliographical references and index.
ISBN 0-7591-0510-3 (hardcover : alk. paper) — ISBN 0-7591-0511-1 (pbk. : alk. paper)
1. Primary health care—Developing countries. 2. Medical policy—Developing countries. 3. Medical anthropology—Developing countries. 4. Social medicine—Developing countries. 5. Public health—Developing countries. I. Castro, Arachu, 1964– II. Singer, Merrill.

RA441.5.U556 2004
362.1'09172'4—dc22

2004004821

Printed in the United States of America

∞™ The paper used in this publication meets the minimum requirements of American National Standard for Information Sciences—Permanence of Paper for Printed Library Materials, ANSI/NISO Z39.48-1992.

To our respective children,
Diane and Naiara Appaix-Castro,
and Jacob and Elyse Singer,
who are our expressions of hope for a future
in which health policy might truly be healthy for all.

CONTENTS

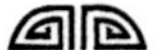

Introduction

Anthropology and Health Policy: A Critical Perspective

MERRILL SINGER AND ARACHU CASTRO

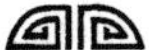

Policy is governed by entrenched myth.

—PETER MARRIS, 2003

IN RECENT YEARS, a number of anthropologists have argued that their field—which traditionally focused on detailed ethnographic description of the unique cultural patterns of small-scale societies around the globe—is at risk of becoming irrelevant in a changing and shrinking world unless its shifts direction and takes on new challenges. Central to this shift in thinking about the mission of anthropology has been a concern that the discipline be "inside the loop" and get invited to the table in public discourse on pressing health or social issues. As a counter to the fear that anthropology is becoming irrelevant in the contemporary world, some have called for the development of the discipline as a *policy science.* As defined by Van Willigen (1986), the purpose of a policy science "is to provide information to decision makers in support of the rational formation, and evaluation of policy" (p. 143).

The term "policy" is variously defined but generally is used to refer to the official guidelines implemented by a social institution intended to set direction for action. As used in this book, health policy refers to both codified guidelines relative to health (or policy with another purpose but nonetheless having a direct impact on health) or health-related programmatic actions that reflect either codified guidelines or what is sometimes referred to as "unstated policy." Since the nineteenth century, one of the defining features of the "modern" state (at the national, regional, and local levels) has been the implementation of policies and policy-guided programs to protect and promote the health of the body politic. Health-related policies are also formulated by international organizations, development organizations, and health care providers.

Given its usual public identity as an academic discipline, it is often overlooked that the first professional positions for anthropologists in the United States were not in universities, but in governmental policy research settings. Anthropological work at the Bureau of American Ethnology, for example, which was established 120 years ago, a decade before the first university department of anthropology in the United States, had the explicit goal of producing research findings that would have practical utility in the administration of Indian affairs. In this sense, in the United States and elsewhere, anthropology emerged as a policy-oriented field, most notably in the arena of colonial management of subjugated peoples. Despite this early, and indeed troubling, association of anthropology with one sector of the field of policy development and implementation, it was not until the World War II era that anthropological practitioners began to reflect extensively on their role in the policy arena. Numerous anthropologists found federal employment during the war, some in health policy-relevant institutions. Margaret Mead, for example, was very involved in diet and nutrition issues during this era. She served as head of the federal Committee on Food Habits, which developed policy recommendations on emergency feeding and food rationing. This involvement notwithstanding, anthropology did not readily develop an identity as an explicit policy science during the war.

In fact, the anthropological relationship with policy makers often has been conflicted. Most applied anthropologists have had firsthand experience with seeing their findings and recommendations largely ignored by policy makers because they did not match official truths and politically useful understandings. In the period after the war, a number of anthropologists left government employment with embittered feelings and with ambiguous attitudes about government service. This trend was enhanced during the baby boom era when the significant expansion in the number of academic jobs for anthropologists pulled people out of applied settings to teach a new generation of young adults entering the university. During this heyday of academic anthropology, teaching replaced applied work and social policy concerns for most people in the field. By the 1980s, however, the pendulum began to swing again in the opposite direction, as more and more newly graduated anthropologists were forced to find employment outside of the academy, sometimes in policy-relevant settings. As a result of this second shift, anthropological attention to significantly strengthening the role of the discipline in public policy debates while increasing the volume of the anthropological voice on issues of grave public concern has expanded anew in recent years. The contemporary focus on developing what has been called "a public interest anthropology" exemplifies part of this reinvigorated commitment to policy issues.

Actually, over the years there have been multiple applied roles that anthropologists and like-minded researchers have played relative to social policy beyond providing information to assist decision makers in developing guidelines, codes, laws, and other policy expressions, including going beyond merely providing findings to making specific recommendations for policy change. At times, although not commonly, anthropologists have themselves become health policy makers, as several anthropologists have either been elected to governmental office or been appointed to a decision-making role in a governmental or otherwise influential institution. In these instances, anthropologists in policy-making position have turned readily and often to their colleagues for anthropologically relevant insights on health and other issues. Anthropologists also have played roles in amending existing policy to be more effective (e.g., by using ethnographic data to demonstrate weaknesses of and needed adjustments to established guidelines) or in helping to draft new policies based on field-based experiences with pressing health and social issues.

This volume represents yet another role of anthropologists in the policy arena: using research to critically review the intended or unintended negative impact of policy on the lives and well-being of people targeted by social policies. Stated plainly, this alternative public role of anthropologists, the one developed in this book, is the informed critique of policy. Another way to think about these issues is to follow Van Willigen's (1986) differentiation (based on the work of Robert Strauss) between "anthropology in policy" and "anthropology of policy." The first of these terms refers to anthropological work designed to either provide information for utilization by policy makers or the development and implementation of interventions or other applications that stem from, and are supported by, existing health policy. For example, through the National Institutes on Health numerous anthropologists, including contributors to this volume, have worked on policy research and application initiatives targeted to a wide variety of health issues. By contrast, the anthropology of policy is concerned with studying and assessing the process of decision making, the actions of and influences on decision makers, and the impact of policy on human lives.

Unlike much policy-oriented anthropology, the chapters in this edited volume exemplify the "anthropology of policy." The underlying and shared assumption of the chapters that comprise this book, which it should be noted are not all written by anthropologists, is that health policies are shaped by a number of factors, only one of which (and sometimes the least of which) is concern with public health. Health policy formation and implementation unfold in a world of competitive social interest, opposed class agendas, unequal genders, and overt and covert power conflicts. Health policy may reproduce structural violence, defined as the set of large-scale social forces, such as racism, sexism, political violence, poverty, and other social inequalities, which are rooted in historical and economic processes. As a result, health-related policies, which have the ostensive goal of improving and protecting the health of the general public or sectors thereof, may, in their service of other masters, harm rather than enhance public health. Grounded in the field research of the respective authors, the chapters in this volume cast critical gazes on the actual nature of health-related policies in varied settings in both developed and developing countries around the globe.

Collectively, the chapters of this volume demonstrate the intricate understandings and keen insights gained through the application of a critical approach to knowledge generation. This approach, which seeks to locate health issues in the intersecting contexts of cultural heritage, human biology, and political economy, offers readers a sharply questioning and nonconventional vantage for thinking about public policy as a reflection of the reigning structure of social inequality.

The appraisals of policy that are presented in this volume are informed generally by the theoretical perspective known as critical medical anthropology (CMA) (Baer, Singer, and Susser 2003). This framework "emphasizes the importance of political and economic forces, including the exercise of power, in shaping health, disease, illness experience, and health care" (Singer and Baer 1995:5). The CMA perspective (1) recognizes that health itself is a profoundly political issue, one that often is contentious if not explosive; (2) is cognizant and critical of the colonial heritage of anthropology and the tendency of conventional medical anthropology to serve as a "handmaiden of biomedicine"; (3) balances concern for unbiased social science with an awareness of the sociohistoric origin and political nature of all scientific knowledge; (4) acknowledges the fundamental importance of class, racial, and sexual inequity in determining the distribution of health, disease, living and working conditions, and health care; (5) defines power as a fundamental variable in health-related research, policy, and programming; (6) avoids the artificial separation of local settings and micropopulations from their wider political-economic contexts; (7) asserts that its mission is emancipatory: it aims not simply to understand but also to change culturally inappropriate, oppressive, and exploitative patterns in the health arena and beyond; and (8) sees commitment to change as fundamental to the discipline.

As an expression of anthropology (as opposed to other approaches to the same issues), CMA does not view its subject matter from a narrow, top-down perspective (i.e., as the uniform enactment of power by dominant players and institutions and the obedient compliance of enfeebled subordinates). Rather, CMA in its approach to policy—which it sees as a conflicted expression of power (and, at times, becomes war by another means)—emphasizes the contested and particularistic nature of policy formation and enforcement. Policies, in short, are seen as reflecting a compromise between, and at the same time, the relative balance of power among conflicted forces (i.e., social groups with different and often opposed interests) at a particular time and in a particular place. While carefully exploring the undeniable importance of local and temporal conditions in policy, in its approach CMA is nonetheless centrally concerned with viewing unique actions and contexts from the perch of a more general political economic vista. From this standpoint, and as reflected in the chapters in this volume, there can be unhealthy health policies, including policies that cause tremendous social suffering and policies that can be seen as an expression of structural violence (Farmer 2003).

Anthropological concern with health issues generally dates to the early years of the discipline. Indeed, the first field expedition (a data-collection tour of the Torres Strait) driven by a distinctly anthropological mission was, in part, concerned with ethnomedical beliefs and practices. As a named subfield of the larger discipline, medical anthropology began to coalesce and develop a set of devoted adherents, specific academic courses and training programs, specialized subdisciplinary journals, and an organizational structure after World War II. Even prior to the emergence of medical anthropology, anthropologists had developed a long history of participation in national and international efforts to improve health. Anthropologists have worked with epidemiologists to explain disease patterns and have collaborated extensively with public health providers to promote successful, "appropriate," and "culturally sensitive" health interventions. But with few exceptions, anthropologists have focused most of their efforts on analyzing, improving, or evaluating specific problems within health programs, such as discrepancies of beliefs and values between implementers of health initiatives and their targeted recipients. Rarely have they stepped back to examine the wider socioeconomic constraints placed on those who control the budget strings of national and international health policies. Yet, if we are to get to the heart of why some health initiatives succeed in terms of improving health outcomes while others fail or even worsen health problems, we must also examine these constraints and the core principles and policies that guide national and international efforts to eradicate or control disease.

Are the principles guiding health policy based on beliefs in health as a human right and a public good? Are they tied to notions of health equity, with an ethical imperative to protect the poor and other vulnerable groups? Or are they driven more by fear and less benign ideological and geopolitical objectives? What are the implications for poor people of health policies generated from nonhealth concerns? Even when sound epidemiological findings, considerations of equity, and health as a fundamental human right form the core of national, bilateral, and international health policy, well-intentioned health efforts are often undermined at the implementation stage when the interests of capital and the interrelated trilogy of fear, ideology, and geopolitics come to take precedence over public health concerns (Castro and Millen 2001). This book offers multiple examples of how this trilogy comes into play and the consequences it produces.

Structure of the Book

This book is organized into three sections. Part I, "International Institutions and the Setting of Health Policies," demonstrates the distance between health policies that are conceptualized by international institutions and the reality of these policies on the ground, particularly throughout Latin America, Africa, and Asia. Often, these strategies reflect an ideology that does not necessarily respond to the needs of the people for whom they were designed. The chapters offer insightful perspectives on whose interests are served by current health priorities and policies. Chapter 1, by Paul Farmer and Arachu Castro, analyzes the increasingly disproportionate weight of economic arguments within the context of establishing priorities in the fight against AIDS. By examining the cases of two neighboring countries in the Caribbean—Haiti and Cuba—the authors demonstrate and analyze significant differences. In Haiti, a series of obstacles to the delivery of public health services can be attributed to the abuse and misuse of cost-effectiveness tools and to politicized arguments within the international community on the allocation of external resources to impoverished countries. Conversely, the Cuban case reflects self-determined health policies and resource allocation practices that generally follow and are shaped by the epidemiology of the disease. In chapter 2, Francisco Armada and Carles Muntaner analyze the role of international financial institutions in the reform and increased privatization of health systems in Latin America. The authors argue that this trend, part of the broader neoliberal agenda, primarily benefits national and transnational corporations, thereby reproducing and reinforcing already existing social inequalities. In chapter 3, James Pfeiffer explores the damaging fragmentation of health services in Mozambique, a direct consequence of structural adjustment policies set by multilateral and bilateral funding institutions. Joan Paluzzi, in chapter 4, reminds us of the 1978 Declaration of Alma Ata, which reinforced the importance of primary health care systems, and argues that international institutions continue to privilege restricted, vertical programs at the expense of primary programs. By exploring the Chilean case, Paluzzi demonstrates the interdependence that exists between these two health care delivery models.

In chapter 5, Fouzieyha Towghi analyzes the misguided attempts to integrate traditional midwives into primary health care in Pakistan, and the resulting devaluation of this human resource as a potential collaborator in the reduction of maternal mortality and morbidity. In chapter 6, Salmaan Keshavjee focuses on the implementation of a revolving medicinal drug fund in post-Soviet Tajikistan. Through the prioritization of privatization, the revolving drug fund has actually increased inequalities in access to medicines. In chapter 7, Alice Desclaux explores the impact of user fees on AIDS treatment in Senegal. In addition to the damaging impact on the financial capacity of households, user fees also have become an important factor in the pattern of decreasing drug adherence. In chapter 8, Arachu Castro analyzes the integration of reproductive health services in Mexico. Within the context of promoting contraceptive use as part of the routine birthing experience, health professionals often endorse broader, dominant population policies; as a result, some indigenous women are reluctant to deliver in hospital settings, thus increasing their risk for untreated obstetric complications. In chapter 9, Imrana Qadeer and Nalini Visvanathan examine some of the underlying issues that shape population policies in India, and link them to the trends toward the general privatization of health care and the marginalization of primary health care.

Part II, "National Health Policies and Social Exclusion," explores the impact of national health policies on the most disadvantaged people within countries in Latin America, Europe, and North America. Specifically, the chapters in this section reveal the ways in which health policies have contributed to the construction and maintenance of significant social inequality and related human suffering. Moreover, the chapters in this section call attention to health policies that can be beneficial for one group while punishing another—often less privileged—group within society. For this reason, and as documented by the chapters that follow, health policies can become intended or unintended implements of structural violence. Collectively, these chapters provide textured and historically rooted accounts of how health policies can create vulnerable social groups and put them in harm's way rather than protect the poor, women, or people of color. In chapter 10, César Abadía-Barrero analyzes the successful implementation of access to health care—including comprehensive AIDS care—education, and other social opportunities for children who live with HIV/AIDS in Brazil. Because poor children, many of them living on the streets, do not usually have access to these services, being HIV-positive has become a social advantage. Exemplary is Katherine Bliss's analysis, in chapter 11, of the gendered history of syphilis prophylaxis popularization in revolutionary Mexico, including the 1940 criminalization of infection transmitted through sexual contact. In chapter 12 Linda Whiteford and Graham Tobin, based on studying the lives of Ecuadorian people displaced by the eruption of a volcano, argue that emergency evacuation and resettlement policies have actually increased their risk of illness and disease. In chapter 13, Didier Fassin analyzes political choices that, despite the existence of a universal health system, contribute to the increase in health inequalities in France, predominantly among immigrant populations. In chapter 14, Kristen Jacklin and Wayne Warry explore Canadian policies that were designed to enhance self-determination in health care for First Nations peoples but that, in practice, have had very limited benefits for Aboriginal health. In chapter 15, Sarah Horton focuses on the attempts of the U.S. government to reduce the number of people without health insurance through managed care, and how these attempts actually decreased the number of Latinos eligible for federal health insurance in New Mexico. In chapter 16, Cathleen Willging, Howard Waitzkin, and William Wagner assess how other attempts at managed care to reform the provision of health services to the poor in the United States decreased access to mental health services in rural New Mexico. In chapter 17, Claudia Chaufan analyzes the social construction of the diabetes epidemic in the United States, and discusses how the commodification of health care and the impact of broader social inequalities have contributed to a failure to adequately respond to the needs of diabetics.

In chapter 18, David Buchanan, Merrill Singer, Susan Shaw, Wei Teng, Tom Stopka, Kaveh Khoshnood, and Robert Heimer examine the implications of policies on access to sterile syringes and how they can directly contribute to a decreased incidence of HIV among injecting drug users. The authors compare these policies between Connecticut, where a needle-exchange program exists, and the neighboring state of Massachusetts, where the difficulty of procuring a safe needle puts injecting drug users at a higher risk for HIV. In chapter 19, Merrill Singer reviews the U.S. War on Drugs, revealing thereby that in practice antidrug policies often serve to promote a war on young men of color while producing a number of "secondary benefits" for the dominant social class. In chapter 20, the final in part II, Philippe Bourgois demonstrates some of the ways in which the War on Drugs has backfired and helped to promote incipient inner-city apartheid.

The third and final part of the book, "Impact of Policy on the Practice of Medicine," focuses on the health care system and the role of policy makers in negatively shaping health care delivery. Chapter 21, by Hans Baer, examines the role of policy in the co-optation of alternative healing as a subordinate system to biomedicine. Chapter 22, by Robbie Davis-Floyd, focuses attention on the ways the health care industry is shaped by health policy, with special reference to recent trouble-filled and stressful interaction between health care providers and midwives. Chapter 23, the final chapter, asks why high-tech medical intervention rather than prevention is the focus of breast cancer policy in the United States. Ironically, the author, Catherine Hodge McCoid, notes that in treating rather than preventing breast cancer, industrial medicine profits from diseases caused by carcinogenic industries.

If, as Paul Farmer (1999:15) has argued, "inequality itself constitutes our modern plague," then health policy must be directed at outlawing inequality as a public health priority. This, however, has not been the case as documented by the chapters to follow. Indeed, the opposite has often been the case. Recognition of this fact provides direction for an anthropological role in health policy, namely contributing to the making of healthier societies through the making of healthier health policies, including policies that help to level an often very unleveled playing field. Rules and guidelines designed to equalize the quality of life across social strata and vulnerable subgroups improve access to quality health services for all, allow freedom from structural violence, and would aptly be titled healthy health policy (Wilkerson 2003).

We would like to thank our colleagues at Partners In Health and the Hispanic Health Council for their commitment and support. Both of these health and social justice organizations daily confront the damaging effects of unhealthy health policies and structures, and seek though their efforts to achieve a more just and healthier world for poor and oppressed populations. Special heartfelt thanks are extended to Joan Cruz of the Hispanic Health Council for her contribution toward the completion of this book, and to Grace Damio, Michael Duke, Susan Shaw, Anne Marie Nycolaysen, Claudia Santelices, Isabel Rodrigues, and Jeannette DeJesus for discussions on health disparities and advocacy. At Partners In Health, we are particularly grateful to our discussions on health policy with Ophelia Dahl, Loune Viaud, Paul Zintl, Joyce Millen, Mary Kay Smith Fawzi, Joia Mukherjee, Hamish Fraser, Heidi Behforouz, Jim Y. Kim, Yasmin Khawja, Mercedes Becerra, Salmaan Keshavjee, Nicole Gastineau, Michael Rich, Carole Mitnick, Jo Paluzzi, Jaime Bayona, Sarah Van Norden, Melissa Gillooly, Cynthia Rose, Alice Wilson, Margaret Paternek, Ed Nardell, Jen Furin, Sonya Shin, Tracy Kidder, and Howard Hiatt; a very special thank you goes to Paul Farmer. Lorena Barberia, Olivier Appaix, and Jesús M. de Miguel, and faculty in the Department of Social Medicine at Harvard Medical School, such as Byron Good, Mary-Jo Delvecchio Good, Leon Eisenberg, Arthur Kleinman, and Julius Richmond, were invaluable for their ongoing intellectual encouragement. We would also like to acknowledge the support of our friends in the Critical Anthropology of Health Caucus, a group that has helped to sustain the critical perspective expressed through the chapters of this book. Finally, we are most indebted to Pablo Guayasamín, from the Guayasamín Foundation, for granting us the use of the cover image, *Lágrimas de Sangre*, by Maestro Oswaldo Guayasamín, at no cost, and to Jaime Breilh for making it happen.

References

Baer, H., M. Singer, and I. Susser. (2003). *Medical Anthropology and the World System*, 2nd ed. Westport, CT: Praeger.

Castro, A., and J. V. Millen. (2001, January). "Praxis, Policy and the Poor: Critical Ethnography of International Health Policies." *Anthropology Newsletter*: 61.

Farmer, P. (1999). *Infections and Inequalities: The Modern Plagues*. Berkeley: University of California Press.

———. (2003). *Pathologies of Power: Health, Human Rights, and the New War on the Poor*. Berkeley: University of California Press.

Singer, M., and H. Baer. (1995). *Critical Medical Anthropology*. Amityville, NY: Baywood Publishing Co.

Van Willigen, J. (1986). *Applied Anthropology*. South Hadley, MA: Bergin and Garvey.

Wilkerson, J. (2003). "The Political Economy of Health in the United States." *Annual Review of Political Science* 6: 327–43.

I

INTERNATIONAL INSTITUTIONS AND THE SETTING OF HEALTH POLICIES

Pearls of the Antilles? Public Health in Haiti and Cuba

I

PAUL FARMER AND ARACHU CASTRO

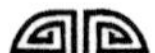

A DRAMATIC REDEFINITION OF HEALTH PRIORITIES now holds increasing sway in Latin America, where assessing public health has become a treacherous exercise. This is not because it is impossible to evaluate the state of the region's health, nor is it because the admittedly enormous variation, both across and within nations, leads to analytic impasse. To assess the health of a nation is treacherous because of the ideological minefields one now has to traverse when commenting on public health in Latin America.

In the past, such assessments may have been easier, and not because public health was then a more robust undertaking. Rather, there was previously a consensus that the health of the poor was a cardinal indicator of how well the stewards of the public's well-being were doing their job. At this point, however, it is unclear even who the stewards of public health really are. Rudolph Virchow has been called the father of social medicine, and it was he who dubbed doctors "the natural attorneys of the poor." Doctors were supposed to defend the poor because the impact of their social condition—poverty—was embodied as preventable or treatable sickness. Virchow also quantified this position in quite graphic modern-day epidemiological terms: "Medical statistics will be our standard of measurement; we will weigh life for life and see where the dead lie thicker, among the workers or among the privileged" (quoted in Rosen 1974:182, from Virchow's *Medicinische Reform*; see also Eisenberg 1984). In this chapter, we move from Virchow's insightful quantification to the critical examination of quantification of a different and even more troubling sort—the increasing weight assigned to economic arguments in assessing approaches to the AIDS pandemic—and the unhealthy outcomes that these arguments engender in poor countries. By exploring the AIDS trajectories in Haiti and Cuba, we analyze the impact of contrasting economic arguments and challenge some of the currently predominant ideologies in international public health.

Cost-Effectiveness and the Health of the Poor

As public health has become a larger enterprise, it has defined a turf of its own; as nation-states have come into being in Latin America, they have defined national public-health agendas, increasingly with the assistance of experts from international institutions. The "welfare state" that we think of as having been progressively built up, from the 1930s to the beginning of its decay in the 1980s, barely got a start in Latin America before debt, the cupidity of local strongmen, and the agenda setting of First World economic advisers attempted to terminate the welfare state as a public responsibility. The health of the poor is now deemed less important than the cost containment of public health services, and governments too often push to minimize the healthcare drain on national budgets increasingly dedicated to the supposedly higher goals of debt service and privatization (see Kim, Millen, Irwin, and Gershman 2000). Several recent years have noted the deadly consequences of the shift in priorities from the epidemiology of disease to economic arguments that promote the nonprovision of services termed "not cost-effective" without necessarily offering alternatives for those who need those services but are too poor to afford them (see Kim, Shakow, Castro, Vanderwerker, and Farmer 2003). We have been reminded by the World Health Organization (WHO 2001) that

> as with the economic well-being of individual households, good population health is a critical input into poverty reduction, economic growth, and long-term economic development at the scale of whole societies. This point is widely acknowledged by analysts and policy makers, but is greatly underestimated in its qualitative and quantitative significance, and in the investment allocations of many developing-country and donor governments (pp. 21–22).

It is precisely these national and international investment allocations, influenced by cost-effectiveness arguments, that have contributed to long delays in the provision of comprehensive AIDS programs, including highly active antiretroviral therapy (HAART). These delays have significantly amplified the magnitude of the AIDS pandemic.

Those struggling to promote the health of the poor are now in the defensive position of having to show that proposed interventions are both effective *and* inexpensive, regardless of the gravity of the health problem in question. Aside from local ministries of health, the largest financiers of public health in Latin America, except for Cuba, include the international financial institutions, such as the World Bank and, less directly, the International Monetary Fund (see case studies in Kim et al. 2000). In some regards, this makes sense, given the undeniable association between economics and health (United Nations Development Programme [UNDP] 1990; WHO 2001; Castro and Farmer 2004). But there is a dark side to the new accounting: such sources place funding for public health within a framework developed by economists working within a paradigm in which market forces alone are expected to solve health and social problems—a paradigm which is one of the ideological minefields. As efforts are made to determine whether or not an intervention is "cost-effective," the destitute sick are often left out altogether. In the highly contested WHO *World Health Report 2000,* we read that "cost-effectiveness by itself is relevant for achieving the best overall health, but not necessarily for the second health goal, that of reducing inequality" (WHO 2000:55). But, on the same page, an algorithm illustrates the "questions to ask in deciding what interventions to finance and provide." For example, if an intervention is a public good but is considered not cost-effective, the algorithm points us to "do not provide." If another intervention does not represent a public good (however defined), has significant externalities, adequate demand, and not a catastrophic cost, but the beneficiaries are poor and it is not cost-effective, we are again pointed to "do not provide" (WHO 2000:55, adapted from Musgrove 1999). Are these economic arguments, promoted by the highest international health authority, curtailing the provision of comprehensive health care to the poor?[1]

As time has gone by, certain trends in healthcare provision have become palpable within much of Latin America. Some have been favorable: vaccination and other interventions have lowered infant mortality. The Pan American Health Organization's (PAHO) regional report, *Health in the Americas 2002,* highlights some of the improving health indices in the region (PAHO 2002a). And that is the central irony of public health in Latin America: national statistics continue to suggest improvement, but the poor are not doing nearly as well as could be expected if the fruits of science and technology were used wisely and equitably (see Castro and Farmer 2003).

Even a cursory review of the *World Health Report 2002* reveals the wide gaps in health between countries in the region. Consider life expectancy, a standard assessment of a country's health and overall attainment. In 2001, Cuba boasted a life expectancy of 76.9 years; Haiti's populace, meanwhile, can expect to live only to age 50, down from 53 just one year earlier (WHO 2002:178–80). In addition, in most of Latin America, we see that a shrinking commitment to public financing of health care and a push for its privatization have led to a widening gap in access to quality health care (López-Acuña 2000). These trends are registered even as the fruits of science become ever more readily translated into effective therapies.

Since the 1980s in Latin America, many health system financing reforms that have been introduced aim to limit or reduce public spending to meet the requirements for fiscal adjustment, and to compensate for financial losses generated by adverse macroeconomic conditions, corruption, and mismanagement of local and national governments. Since many of the health sector reforms occurred as part of broader macroeconomic reforms, most of the changes were introduced without any assessment of their potential impact on access to health care or utilization of any of the current guiding principles of health sector reform (PAHO, UNDP, and CARICOM 1999). Instead, much of the health financing reforms focused on a shift to market-driven, managed care systems and an increased dependency on user fees, leaving informal sector workers and the unemployed without adequate access to health care and bearing all the financial risk of becoming sick (Russell and Gilson 1997). These market-inspired "innovations," eagerly adopted by policy makers as part of health care reforms (Iriart, Merhy, and Waitzkin 2001; Laurell 2001), have met with a groundswell of popular and political protest against privatization and other recently introduced market reforms (Rylko-Bauer and Farmer 2002).[2]

In this era of cost containment of public spending and health systems reform, providing adequate health services for the destitute sick may prove to be a true challenge, especially since the advent of AIDS in the 1980s has coincided with a reduction in social spending throughout Latin America (see Escobar 1995). With the transfer of the essential responsibilities of ministries of health to the private sector, many countries have documented a growing trend toward separating the functions of financing health care, covering health insurance, and delivering health services (PAHO 1996). The emergence of different public and private actors in health financing and service delivery, and greater demands for health care caused by emerging (such as AIDS or dengue) and persistent problems (such as tuberculosis and malaria) are presenting new challenges for health systems. These challenges, however, are compounded by longstanding problems that include institutional inefficiency in the health sector, persisting inequities in coverage and access, and rising costs and poor quality of services (Barberia et al. 2002).

In attempting to address the AIDS pandemic, the region of Latin America and the Caribbean now faces a formidable challenge (Castro et al. 2003). At this writing, 1.5 million people in Central and South America and at least 420,000 in the Caribbean are already living with HIV/AIDS (UNAIDS 2002a). The Caribbean, with an adult HIV prevalence of 2.2 percent (UNAIDS 2001), has the second-highest rate of HIV infection in the world (UNAIDS 2002a), second only to sub-Saharan Africa. Prevalence rates vary from country to country: in Haiti, adult prevalence of HIV exceeds 6 percent; in the Dominican Republic it is 2.5 percent; in Jamaica it is 1.2 percent; while in Cuba the prevalence is less than 0.05 percent (UNAIDS 2002b). The associated state of Puerto Rico has one of the highest AIDS prevalence rates in the United States (342.8 cases per 100,000), only after the District of Columbia and the State of New York, but has no data on prevalence of HIV (Centers for Disease Control and Prevention [CDC] 2002:23).

To date, the response of the affluent countries and their institutions to this crisis—from aid agencies, nongovernmental organizations (NGOs), and the pharmaceutical industry—has been insufficient. The death toll and increasing HIV incidence in countries highly dependent on foreign aid provide the most eloquent rebuke to economically driven assessments. Until the first disbursements were made by the Global Fund to Fight AIDS, Tuberculosis, and Malaria in 2003, the quasi-totality of AIDS assistance to the heavily burdened countries had consisted of the promotion of education and condom distribution to prevent HIV transmission.[3] Yet, many of those at greatest risk already know that HIV is a sexually transmitted pathogen and that condoms could prevent transmission. In Haiti, over 97 percent of the population knows of the existence of AIDS, and 62 percent of women and 81 percent of men know at least one way to prevent infection (Cayemittes, Placide, Barrère, Mariko, and Sévère 2001). Their risk stems less from ignorance and more from the structural violence that millions of people endure in Latin America as a result of historic, political, and economic processes (see Farmer 1999, 2003a; Castro 2003).

Aid agencies have increasingly relied on economic evaluation analyses to allocate resources. Current economic evaluation approaches to public health include cost-benefit and cost-effectiveness analyses, both of which rely more on projections of the outcomes derived from investments in specific health interventions than on empirical data. Still, they inform budgeting and financial planning, help assess the affordability of interventions, and help identify areas for improving efficiency of delivery of services and cost savings (Gold et al. 1996; Murray and Lopez 1996; Holtgrave 1998). Cost-benefit analyses measure the resources consumed by a particular intervention and only inputs are included in the equation. Most economic evaluations of health programs have relied on cost-effectiveness analyses (Holtgrave, Qualls, and Graham 1996), which not only account for inputs but also go a step further by including health outcomes in mathematical equations, measured in natural units such as "lives saved" or "infections averted." Cost-effectiveness allows for comparisons between interventions, as they estimate the cost per unit of outcome produced. A specific type of cost-effectiveness analysis is cost-utility analysis, in which outcomes are measured in "generic units" such as disability-adjusted life years saved (DALYs) (Murray and Lopez 1996) or quality-adjusted life years (QALYs) gained; the goal is to choose the outcome that produces the "most health" per dollar spent. This type of analysis has been deemed most appropriate when an intervention has the potential to affect both the quality and quantity of life—when it influences both morbidity and mortality.

There are a fair number of papers and articles asking and answering with confidence the question, "Is it cost-effective to treat AIDS in poor countries?" These cost-effectiveness exercises, which usually conclude that treating HIV disease in settings of great poverty is less cost-effective than preventing it, are based on scant data from the most affected continent. Our leading medical journals are devoid of reports of treatment projects in Africa, yet contain arguments pitting prevention against treatment: "Data on the cost-effectiveness of HIV prevention in sub-Saharan Africa and on highly active antiretroviral therapy indicate that prevention is at least 28 times more cost effective than HAART" (Marseille, Hofmann, and Kahn 2002:1851). Another self-proclaimed "systematic review of the evidence" concludes that the "most cost-effective interventions are for prevention of HIV/AIDS and treatment of tuberculosis, whereas HAART for adults, and home based care organised from health facilities, are the least cost effective" (Creese, Floyd, Alban, and Guinness 2002). Yet these conclusions are based not on real experience, but rather on other cost-effectiveness projections (see Freedberg and Yazdanpanah 2003). Finally, what are we to make of articles arguing that one intervention (prevention among commercial sex workers) is far more cost-effective than another (prevention of mother-to-child transmission or treatment) when such analyses are written as if Thailand and Tanzania, say, are experiencing comparable epidemics (Jha et al. 2001)? As it has been said, "In the absence of life, all other indicators are irrelevant" (Barnett and Whiteside 2002:282).

We argue that, with its many inherent underlying assumptions, the usefulness of economic analysis as a tool for policy makers and funders has been grossly overstated—creating another ideological minefield (see Moatti et al. 2003). By uncritically accepting that resources are limited—one of the fundamental assumptions of economics—and by advocating the use of decision tools designed to measure specific interventions rather than a comprehensive assessment of an entire health program, these approaches have curtailed potential investment in timely AIDS prevention and care in Haiti. Few economic evaluations have challenged current assumptions about wealth maldistribution (see Attaran and Sachs 2001). Even fewer have sought to move beyond a narrow definition of outcomes or to reformulate the mathematical equations to include other outcomes such as lower risk of transmission (Blower and Farmer 2003) or the social benefits derived from providing appropriate treatment to people living with HIV/AIDS, as it happens in Cuba. Such benefits have an impact at the household, community, and national level by helping patients resume work and take care of children and relatives.

The omission of these social variables should not be overlooked given the threat the AIDS pandemic poses to economic development. A study conducted by the United Nations Development Program found that, left unchecked, the rising incidence of the disease will lead to a fall in gross domestic product (GDP) and a decline in the level of domestic savings (Nicholls et al. 2001). But it wasn't until July 2003 that the World Bank warned that

> HIV/AIDS causes far greater long-term damage to national economies than *previously assumed*, for by killing mostly young adults, the disease is robbing the children of AIDS victims of one or both parents to love, raise and educate them, and so undermines the basis of economic growth over the long haul (World Bank 2003a, in reference to Bell, Devarajan, and Gersbach 2003; emphasis added).

Furthermore, AIDS in the Americas could result in the creation of a "missing generation," as has already occurred in parts of sub-Saharan Africa; in these areas, much of the middle- or working-age population has died or will die from the disease, leaving children (often orphans) and the elderly as survivors. Without the working-age population, there are fewer teachers, health workers, farmers, factory workers, and others to propel development of the most affected countries. We believe that, if the goal is to improve the public's health, the use of cost-effectiveness analysis has room for improvement. If social variables are taken into account in the cost-effectiveness analysis of health interventions, providing comprehensive AIDS treatment would be more "cost-effective" than current medical and public health literature suggests.

Other studies have pointed out a number of problems with the use of economic evaluation as a decision-making tool. These problems include the lack of reliable country-specific data, the lack of consistency in the methods used, the limitation in the extrapolation of results from one setting to another, and the inherent trade-off between efficiency and equity in resource allocation (Kumaranayake and Watts 2001; Kaplan and Merson 2002; Brock 2003). For example, most cost-effectiveness calculations have not been recalculated as the cost of antiretrovirals—the major culprit in the lack of affordability of comprehensive AIDS programs—began to drop (Farmer, Léandre, Mukherjee, Gupta, et al. 2001). All these combined factors have resulted in the failure to invest in comprehensive AIDS programs in a timely fashion.

Health in the Pearls of the Antilles

Neighboring islands Cuba and Haiti both claim to be "the Pearl of the Antilles," owing to the wealth they procured, under colonial rule, to Spain and France respectively. Yet, as Cuba's José Martí noted over a century ago, "Haiti is a land as peculiar as notable, and in its roots and constitution so different from Cuba, that only pure ignorance can find between them a reason for comparison, or argue with one with respect to the other" (1894:51). It is with fascination and a bit of dread that we turned to comparing public health and AIDS in these two countries, and the impact of the logic of cost-effectiveness in such diverse settings. We also explore the ideologies underpinning not only decisions taken locally, within Haiti and Cuba, but also external commentaries on these two countries and the health of their populations. The impact of neoliberal economic ideology on health policy is apparent in a number of rationing exercises, including those labeling certain interventions as not "cost-effective" and others as not "sustainable" or "appropriate" technology.

Haiti has the highest maternal mortality in the Americas; Cuba's is among the lowest. Haiti has the highest infant mortality rate in the Americas; Cuba, the lowest. The leading killers of young adults in Haiti are AIDS and tuberculosis; Cuba has the lowest prevalence of HIV in the Americas and remarkably little tuberculosis (PAHO 2002a). The *Human Development Index 2003* ranked Haiti 150 out of 175 countries; Cuba ranked 52 (UNDP 2003). Haiti is by all conventional criteria the poorest country in the Americas and one of the poorest in the world: per capita gross domestic product was US$460 in 2001 (UNDP 2003); 67 percent of the population lives in poverty (PAHO 2003), unemployment exceeds 70 percent, and fewer than one in 50 Haitians have regular employment (World Bank 1997). Political violence, among other afflictions of poverty, is endemic. Around 40 percent of the Haitian population has no access to health care; approximately 20 percent of the population uses the public sector, 20 percent the mixed public-private sector, and 20 percent the private sector (based on PAHO 2002a). In Cuba, in contrast, GDP per capita in 2000 was estimated at US$1,475 (PAHO 2002a:198), unemployment in 1998 at 7 percent (UNDP 2000), and access to public health care at 100 percent (PAHO 2002a).

The history of Haiti's impoverishment—how it was generated and sustained—is important, though often forgotten (for an overview of Haiti's turbulent history, see Farmer 2003b [1994]). Before the Haitian slave revolt of 1791, Haiti was Cuba's major competitor in the world sugar market. The success of the Haitian plantation-based sugar economy was dependent on fertile farmland, large French investments, and the abduction and importation of hundreds of thousands of slaves. The slave revolt led to independence in 1804 and secured freedom from an oppressive colonial system (Farmer 2003b [1994]). But tensions between elite Haitians who favored the production of commodities for the international market and peasants who preferred to grow their own piece of land reintroduced the inequalities of the colonial system (Mintz 1985b). In the meantime, the breakdown of sugar production in Haiti and in other French and British Caribbean colonies contributed to the rapid expansion of Cuba's market share, making it the world's leading producer (Ferrer 2000). In 1868, Cuban landowners, both frustrated by the repatriation of profits from the booming sugar industry to Spain, and fearing the violence and economic devastation witnessed in the Haitian slave revolt, began to see the potential benefits of abolishing slavery to unite Cuban *criollos* with slaves in a fight for independence (Portuondo and Pichardo 1974). Cuba managed to shift its source of labor from slavery to proletarian work (Mintz 1985a), obtain independence in 1898, and maintain its position as a leader in the world sugar market. Since 1902 in Cuba and 1915 in Haiti, both countries were occupied by the United States until 1934, after which they remained for several decades under the hegemony of their northern neighbor (Domínguez 1978). The search for national sovereignty was epitomized in Cuba by the 1959 revolution, two years after Haiti had started to endure the bloody rule of the Duvaliers.

Over the past four decades, their paths toward development have continued to diverge strikingly; this has been true of health care as well as economic and other social policies. While Cuba promoted the social and economic rights of its citizens, in particular the right to health care and education, Haiti succumbed to increased inequalities and foreign debt. After a short period of democratic rule in Haiti in 1991, yet another coup d'état worsened living conditions and sunk the country's already feeble economy. Although the international community promised a total estimated US$800 million to the restored democracy in 1994, most of this foreign aid has not reached Haiti's shores. In 2001, international financial institutions and major donor countries initiated a bilateral and multilateral aid embargo against the government of Haiti (Farmer 2003b; Farmer and Castro 2003). The deteriorating effect of the aid embargo on the health of Haiti's population and on the crumbling of its health system has been documented (Farmer, Smith-Fawzi, and Nevil 2003).

Health conditions in Haiti are among the worst in the world. All of Haiti's public health indices are poor, and it is not coincidental that Haiti has the highest incidence of HIV in the Americas. The impact of poverty on public health is evident at any health center. Patients are sicker; they fall ill with tuberculosis, hypertension, malaria, dysentery, and complications of HIV infection, all typically in an advanced state. The children are malnourished, and many of them will have severe protein-calorie malnutrition as well as an infection. Some will have typhoid, measles, tetanus, or diphtheria.[4] Some will have surgical emergencies: abscesses, infections in the chest cavity, fractures, and gunshot and machete wounds.

As elsewhere in the world, infant mortality rates in Haiti fell slowly but steadily over the course of the past few decades. More recently some of these trends have been reversed and infant mortality now stands at 80.3 per 1,000 live births. Infant mortality in Haiti has actually risen since 1996, when it was 73.8 per 1,000 live births; PAHO attributes this rise to increasing poverty, the deterioration of the health system, and AIDS (PAHO 2002a:338). Juvenile mortality rates, similarly, are the worst in the region, in large part because of malnutrition, low vaccination rates, and other by-blows of poverty. Maternal mortality rates are appalling. Even the low-end estimates (523 per 100,000 live births) are the worst in Latin America (PAHO 2002a), and the only community-based survey, conducted around the town of Jacmel in southern Haiti in the 1980s, pegged the figure at 1,400 per

100,000 live births (Jean-Louis 1989). During that same period, "official" statistics reported much lower rates for Haiti, ranging from a maternal mortality rate of between 230 and 340 for the years 1980–1987 (UNDP 1990) to a higher estimate in the years that followed, 1987–1992, of 600 maternal deaths per 100,000 live births (World Bank 1994). As for food and water, again the story is grim. According to the United Nations Food and Agriculture Organization (FAO), Haiti is the third hungriest country in the world (FAO 2000). The water story is even worse: in a recently developed "water poverty index," Haiti was ranked in 147th place out of 147 countries surveyed (Sullivan, Meigh, and Fediw 2002).

AIDS is a serious problem in Haiti. With an estimated 250,000 people living with HIV/AIDS (Global Fund 2002b), Haiti is perhaps the only country in the Americas in which AIDS stands as the number-one cause of all adult deaths (PAHO 2002a). Haiti was the first country after the United States to report AIDS cases. In the late 1970s, a number of previously healthy young Haitians presented with signs of immunosuppression, such as Kaposi's sarcoma and unusual opportunistic infections. In this Haitian "outbreak," 74 percent of the men with opportunistic infections lived in the urban area of Port-au-Prince, of which 33 percent lived in one particular suburb, Carrefour, which was the center for commercial sex workers (Pape et al. 1983; Pape 2000). Dispelling erroneous beliefs that Haitians had spread HIV from Africa to the United States, researchers discovered that none of these men had ever been to Africa, but had either traveled to the United States or had contact with American men. Amid a great deal of controversy over the origin of HIV in the Americas, researchers now believe that HIV spread to Haiti through contact with North Americans, and not vice versa. Male commercial sex workers, catering to a largely North American clientele, played a large role in the spread of HIV within Haiti and the rest of the Caribbean region (Farmer 1992).

The Haitian AIDS epidemic has been described as "generalized" since it affects women as much as or more than men (Pape 2000), is not confined to any clearly bounded groups, and has spread from urban areas to the farthest reaches of rural Haiti. HIV kills 30,000 Haitians each year, with an estimated cumulative number of 196,000 deaths and 200,000 orphans (UNAIDS 2002b; Global Fund 2002a). HIV has also aggravated an already severe tuberculosis epidemic. In one careful survey conducted in an urban slum in Port-au-Prince, fully 15 percent of all adults were found to be infected with HIV (Desormeaux et al. 1996; see also Farmer 1999). Stunningly, the rate of active and thus potentially infectious tuberculosis among these HIV-positive slum dwellers was 5,770 per 100,000 population. For Cuba, in 1999, the rate of active tuberculosis was 11 per 100,000 population (UNDP 2003). In Haiti, between 15 to 45 percent of hospitalized patients in urban areas are infected with HIV; in TB sanatoria, the proportion is more than 50 percent (Pape 2000). It is estimated that around 2,000 people with AIDS in Haiti are on HAART, both in rural Central Plateau and in Port-au-Prince; the number is expected to increase (Global Fund 2004b).

In 1989, soon after AIDS was declared a priority disease in Haiti, the National Commission to Fight AIDS was appointed, while the AIDS National Bureau was created with full-time personnel from the Ministry of Health (Global Fund 2002a). This bureau was operational until the coup d'état of 1991, when all foreign aid stopped (Pape 2000). While in 1991 the allocation of the Ministry of Health was US$6 million, after the resumption of foreign aid between the two embargoes the budget increased considerably, going up to US$57 million in 1999—which represents about 10.5 percent of the public budget and between 0.8 and 1 percent of the GDP. The majority of the budget of the Ministry of Health—69 percent in 1996–1997—depended largely on foreign aid (PAHO 2002a).

In 1998, the Haitian Ministry of Health recognized health as a fundamental human right, while acknowledging the difficulties with meeting that goal due to scarce human and financial resources (PAHO 2002a). Notwithstanding these constraints, the AIDS National Bureau was reorganized in 2001, when the president of Haiti launched the five-year National Strategic Plan exercise (Global Fund 2002a). One year earlier, the Bank of Haiti had estimated that the country produced the same amount of goods and services as it had in 1980, while the population had increased by 75 percent over the same period (Banque de la République d'Haïti 2000). With such a devolving economy, an international aid embargo, and the majority of international public health experts claiming that comprehensive AIDS care was unsustainable and not cost-effective in resource-poor settings, what was the government of Haiti left to do? Was the existing political will enough to woo external resources to fight AIDS?

Seeing the rest of Latin America through Haitian eyes is an instructive exercise. As in Haiti, the poor felt the impact of adverse trends before any others; their health suffered, often grievously. Haiti is often compared, unfavorably, to the Dominican Republic. Neither country has much to boast about in terms of public health. The Dominican Republic, sited on the other two-thirds of the island it shares with Haiti, has poor health indices, even if nowhere near as bad as those in Haiti. In 1999–2000, two-thirds of Haitians lived below the national poverty line; meanwhile, on the eastern two-thirds of the island (1998 data), 25.8 percent of Dominicans lived in poverty (PAHO 2002a).

But what about Haiti's second-closest neighbor, Cuba? One could not find a starker contrast within Latin America. There are some initial similarities: less than 100 miles apart, the two islands have identical climates. And like Haiti, Cuba has known major economic disruption in the past decade. In 1991, after losing 85 percent of its foreign trade as a result of the dismantling of the former Soviet Union (Economic Commission for Latin America and the Caribbean [ECLAC] 1997 [2000], 2001), Cuba entered an economic crisis, officially named the Special Period in the Time of Peace. The dependency on the Soviet Union had provided Cuba with a buffer against the U.S. economic blockade of the island that began in 1961. Although Cuba benefited greatly from its economic ties with the Soviet Union, this dependency proved disastrous starting in 1989; no longer able to import petroleum products, foodstuffs, or medicines and distribute them at heavily subsidized prices, Cuba's economy spiraled into crisis. In addition, in 1992, the U.S. Congress passed the Cuban Democracy Act, which restricts the sale of food, medicines, raw materials, and medical equipment to Cuba, and penalizes third countries that deliver drugs and other goods to this Caribbean island. These newly imposed restrictions and the loss of foreign currency resulted in significant shortages of drugs and medical equipment (Castro, Togores, and Barberia 2003).[5] This contraction was as severe as that faced by any Latin American economy.

So what about the impact of such seismic rumblings on the health of the Cuban poor? Was the story the same as in Haiti, where economic turmoil led inevitably to immediate and adverse impacts on the health of the most exposed part of the population? The short answer is no. In fact, although much is made of the harm done by the U.S. embargo to Cuban medicine, the Cuban people remain healthy. This is due in large part to the structure of Cuba's economic, social, and public health systems (see Feinsilver 1993; Chomsky 2000; Barberia and Castro 2003):

> Imagine a health care system that is universal, comprehensive, integrates alternative therapies, and provides care at no cost to the patient. Imagine that the practice of medicine does not involve a financial transaction between doctor and patient, hospital and patient, or clinic and patient. Imagine that medical training is free and that health care is not only considered a right, but a primary means of fostering the health and happiness of the community as a whole, as well as the individuals within it. This is medicine in Cuba (Beinfield 2001).

In addition, state control of the economy helped distribute the impact of the crisis far more equitably, preventing it from striking hardest at the poor—something that would have been impossible in what others would consider a "model," and therefore capitalist, developing country economy.

Indicators such as infant mortality have actually *continued* to decline: in 1985 infant mortality was 15 per 1,000 live births, in 1990 it was 10.7, in 1995 it was 9.4, and in 2000 it was 7.2 (Ministerio de Salud Pública [MINSAP] 2001). World Bank data records Cuba's infant mortality as 6 per 1,000 live births, far below the 27 per 1,000 live births registered for Latin America and the Caribbean

(World Bank 2003b). In fact, there was little impact on overall morbidity and mortality trends during the Special Period, except for a rise in infectious diseases that had been deemed under control, such as tuberculosis (Marrero, Caminero, Rodríguez, and Billo 2000).[6] One reason for such minimal effects—and there are no doubt several—is that health spending was increased during the economic crisis in order to shield the vulnerable from adverse health outcomes. Between 1990 and 1997, health spending rose in local currency in both absolute and relative terms, growing from 6.6 to 10.9 percent of federal outlays (Ministerio de Finanzas y Precios 1998). Spending in Cuban pesos increased despite the fact that medicines and other supplies cost significantly more than they had before the loss of Cuba's subsidized trade with the Soviet bloc (while those manufactured only in the United States are simply unavailable, such as certain cancer treatments or replacement parts for medical devices). While in the 1980s about US$227 million from imports were allocated to the Ministry of Public Health in addition to the national budget, between 1990 and 1995 the annual allocation from imports dropped to an average of US$80 million—and down to US$67 million in 1993 (MINSAP 1996).

Despite high prevalence rates of HIV in the Caribbean, as of the end of 2002, Cuba had registered 4,517 HIV-positive cases since the beginning of the pandemic—of the 3,413 alive, 928 had been diagnosed with AIDS at that date (Pérez-Ávila 2003)—and continues to boast an HIV-prevalence rate below 0.05 percent (UNAIDS 2002a). In 1983, although the etiology of the newly emerged disease was still unknown, Cuba created a National AIDS Commission, which recommended the costly destruction of its imported blood products and prohibited importation of new products. The National AIDS Commission, building on the already well-developed primary health care system, created an epidemiological surveillance system in each hospital to detect clinical manifestations of AIDS (Pérez-Ávila, Peña-Torres, Joanes-Fiol, Lantero-Abreu, and Arazoza-Rodríguez 1996).

At the end of 1985, the first Cuban HIV-positive case was diagnosed at the Institute of Tropical Medicine (IPK) in Havana. The patient had served as *internacionalista* (international aid worker) in Mozambique until 1977; his wife also tested positive. When the IPK reported these first two cases to the vice minister of epidemiology, the Cuban government assigned US$2 million to import 34 ELISA kits that would allow them to conduct 750,000 HIV tests—an average of 400,000 blood donations per year (Pérez-Ávila 2003, personal communication). The imported ELISA kits were distributed throughout all the blood banks and centers for hygiene and epidemiology of the country; by 1986, all blood donations were screened for HIV.[7]

In 1986, the sexual contacts of people diagnosed with HIV were enrolled in the Partner Notification Program and tested for HIV every three months for a period of one year after the last sexual contact with the HIV-positive patient (Hsieh, Chen, Lee, and de Arazoza 2001).[8] While from 1986 until 1993 Cuba relied on controversial HIV sanatoria to contain the epidemic, this strategy has shifted to a combination of in-patient and ambulatory care (Castro, Farmer, and Barberia 2002).[9] Cuba is one of the few developing countries to guarantee comprehensive health care and treatment for all people living with HIV/AIDS. Since 1997, pregnant women who have HIV receive AZT and breastmilk substitutes to prevent mother-to-child transmission of the virus (González-Núñez, Díaz-Jidy, and Pérez-Ávila 2000). Since 2001, all Cuban HIV-positive patients who meet certain clinical criteria are eligible for HAART, and, as of June 2004, there are 1,533 AIDS patients enrolled (Pérez-Ávila 2004, personal communication). Their treatment consists of three domestically produced generic antiretrovirals, which include several reverse transcriptase inhibitors and one protease inhibitor.[10] Since 2001, there has been a decrease in the number of deaths from AIDS and in the incidence of opportunistic infections related to HIV/AIDS. The number of patients hospitalized at the IPK has dropped—from 90 per month in 2000 to 12 per month in 2001—even though HIV incidence has increased (Pérez-Ávila 2002, personal communication).

Life and Death and the Logic of Cost-Effectiveness

What conclusions can be drawn from these comparisons? Aviva Chomsky minces no words in her commentary on Cuba's public health system and the "false assumptions" of economics and health it exposes:

> Where mainstream studies argue that "development" in standard terms—that is, an increasing GNP—is a prerequisite for improving the health status of a country's population, the Cuban example suggests that distribution of resources within a country is more important than the overall GNP in affecting health outcomes. Where mainstream approaches argue that *any* of the economic choices available to poor countries will require sacrifices in the area of health care for the poor, the Cuban example shows that in fact there are economic options that distribute the sacrifices differently (Chomsky 2000:332).[11]

Which countries, other than Cuba, would have invested US$2 million to contain the spread of HIV when only two cases had been diagnosed? The Cuban experience with AIDS is a rebuke to those who place overarching emphasis on cost-effectiveness in setting public health priorities. It also supports the compelling argument that comprehensive AIDS care is "sustainable" in the hardest-hit communities and demonstrates that care is "cost-effective" and a "ranking priority" in the face of other competing demands.

Some health economists suggest that a life-saving intervention that costs between two to three times the gross national product (GNP) per year-of-life saved represents a reasonable expenditure (Garber 2000). Even by this crude calculus (see Moatti et al. 2003:254–255 for its critique), a three-drug HAART regimen at generic prices would prove a sound investment by any criteria, even in Haiti, as long as drugs are used correctly. Still, when Partners In Health sought funding for expansion of a pilot project in rural Haiti (Farmer, Léandre, Mukherjee, Claude, et al. 2001) from a number of international agencies charged with responding to AIDS, all declined to support this effort on the grounds that the drug costs were too high to meet so-called sustainability criteria, given the profound poverty of Haiti. Pharmaceutical companies were approached for contributions or concessional prices, but they referred Partners In Health back to the same international agencies that had already termed the project unsustainable. Ironically, a survey conducted by the Pan American Health Organization in 2001 showed that some antiretrovirals were more expensive in Haiti than in the United States (PAHO 2002b).[12]

We argue that it is not the treatment of the destitute sick that is unsustainable, but rather the ever-widening global outcome gap that prohibits the fruits of science from reaching those most in need of them. The destitute sick remind us that sacrosanct market mechanisms will not serve the interests of global health equity.[13] It is difficult to support the assertion, widespread in international financial institutions, that the neoliberal economic policies now in favor will ever serve the interests of those living with HIV. If the goal is to heal or to ease the suffering of the poor, there are enormous obstacles erected in the way of financing what was once believed to be a public good (see Smith, Beaglehole, Woodward, and Drager 2003). We wonder if the neoliberal agenda of the international financial institutions might be driving up HIV risks while these institutions slap the hands of those who dare to treat the poor (Lurie, Hintzen, and Lowe 1995). As an example, on June 28, 2001, the World Bank approved $155 million to support programs to fight AIDS in the Caribbean. Although acknowledging that "the Dominican Republic and Haiti together account for 85 percent of the total number of HIV/AIDS cases in the Caribbean," Haiti was not included in this lending program (World Bank 2001). How can we envision an effective strategy against HIV when the rules of the game continue to be set by donor countries and their political and economic interests and institutions?

Although the ideological underpinnings of the various approaches to public health are the subject of medical anthropological inquiry, actual outcomes such as morbidity and mortality rates need to remain at the core of these analyses. Of course, the major debate in health and social policy is over which outcomes are most vital. For economists, such measures as GNP and external debt are key indices (which are ideologically freighted subjects in and of themselves). For education experts, literacy rates is a key measure. The human rights community, interestingly, almost always narrows its focus to privilege rights of expression and representation while excluding social and economic rights—an omission that should trouble physicians, who need supplies of tangible goods, the very tools of their trade, before they can go to work (Farmer 2003a). Unless the Latin American poor are accorded some right to health care, water, food, and education, their rights will be violated in precisely the ways manifest in Haiti: their lives will be short, desperate, and unfree.

And so we return, as always, to the health of the poor as the most telling social-policy outcome. Even as national economies and stock markets boom, the health of the Latin American poor remains abysmal by both absolute and relative criteria. The shiny towers of wealthy Latin American neighborhoods and dismal health statistics are of course related, since the privatization of health care occurs at the same time, and as part of the same policy environment, as do massive transfers of public wealth to private coffers (Kim et al. 2000).

Because we believe that assessing the health of the poor is the best way to assess public health in Latin America, we argue that it is wise to avoid confident claims regarding "cost-effectiveness" and "appropriate technology." Cuba has introduced sophisticated assays of viral load costing a small fraction of what tests cost in the United States; it has manufactured many antiretrovirals locally. "It is no accident that the country that disproves the assumptions behind the argument, Cuba, is virtually always left out of mainstream analyses that attempt to defend neoliberal reforms" (Chomsky 2000:332). Actually, Cuba's experience leads us to reconsider the economics of intervention in slowing the spread of HIV and reducing the death toll.

In Haiti, where AIDS is the reason for plummeting life expectancies and for increasing numbers of orphans, we discern fairly overt obstructionism to the use of HAART. Leaving aside all moral arguments, any economic logic that justifies as acceptable the orphaning of children is unlikely to be sound, since the long-term cost to society, though difficult to tabulate, is far higher than the cost of prolonging parents' lives so that they can raise their own children. Furthermore, AIDS treatment causes a dramatic drop not only in mortality (Marins et al. 2003) but also in the number of opportunistic infections and the consequent number of hospital admissions (Gebo, Chaisson, Folkemer, Bartlett, and Moore 1999). HAART has already been declared cost-effective in Europe, North America, and even Brazil, where HIV has become, for many, a chronic infection (Freedberg et al. 2000).

We keep hearing that we live in "a time of limited resources." But how often do anthropologists, physicians, or public health specialists challenge this slogan? The wealth of the world has not dried up; it has simply become unavailable to those who need it most. By questioning these unfounded economic assumptions, medical anthropologists can contribute to rethinking the long-standing public health paradigms that curtail access to health care for the poor. Alas, ethnographic inquiry is not often regarded, within public health, as a robust source of information. But the fetishism of numbers means that cost-effectiveness analysis holds sway among policy makers even when it is not underpinned by experience or empirical research.

What is to be done if we want to take stock of the health of Latin America's poor and act purposefully? Of course we need resources, and to be quite honest, resources should not be the problem. In this time of record profits for many industries—especially the research-based pharmaceutical industry—and dazzling individual fortunes, is it unthinkable that we should spread the wealth? Surely there is some way to redirect some part of the profit stream to take care of the destitute sick. Otherwise, doctors and public health experts will stand by, helpless, watching resources flow—along the gradient established for them by our policies, our choices, and our blind spots—to become ever more narrowly concentrated in the hands of a few. If the health of the poor is the yardstick by which our public health efforts in Latin America are judged, we will have a lot of explaining to do when history sits to consider our case.

Acknowledgments

We are grateful to Jen Singler and Theresa Liu for their research assistantship, to Lorena Barberia for our fruitful and ongoing discussions on the Cuban economy, and to James Pfeiffer, Debbie Sabin, and Nicole Gastineau for editing the manuscript. Jorge Pérez-Ávila was invaluable, as always, in sharing his knowledge on the Cuban health system and its National AIDS Program. The Ford Foundation, through a grant made to the David Rockefeller Center for Latin American Studies at Harvard University in January 2003 (grant number 1035-0359), helped us initiate our broader study on resource allocation practices for AIDS in the Caribbean, in collaboration with colleagues at the Pan American Health Organization.

Notes

1. It is worth noting that, on a more positive note, in a special session of the United Nations General Assembly on September 22, 2003, the World Health Organization declared a "treatment state of emergency" for the AIDS pandemic, putting forth an ambitious and necessary plan to provide HAART to 3 million people in poor countries by 2005.

2. It has been argued that as the U.S. market has become saturated, health care corporations have turned their attention to developing countries where they are exporting managed care programs that are coming under increasing scrutiny in the United States (Waitzkin and Iriart 2001).

3. Launched in January 2002, the Global Fund has approved projects for a total of US$2.06 billion and has disbursed US$285 million in grants to 227 programs in 122 countries in its first three round of grants, as of April 2004, and at this writing it is evaluating proposals submitted to the fourth round (Global Fund 2004a). The Global Fund was originally called for by United Nations Secretary-General Kofi Annan and authorized at the G8 summit in Genoa in July 2001. Regrettably, the Global Fund is facing a budget shortfall. Of the US$5.38 billion pledged, only US$2.38 billion have been disbursed to the Fund as of April 2004 (Global Fund 2004b).

4. Polio, which was announced eradicated from the Americas in 1994, resurfaced on the island in 2000 (CDC 1994, 2000). This unexpected resurgence occurred because of a sharp decline in vaccination rates under military rule. Haiti's self-appointed leaders had scant interest, it would seem, in public health. National vaccination rates for measles and polio reached their lowest point ever, with one PAHO survey suggesting that, in 1993, only 30 percent of Haitian children had been fully vaccinated for measles, polio, mumps, and rubella (PAHO 1993). It was only a matter of time—in this case, a few months to a few years—before these diseases came back. The measles epidemics came quickly, as we documented in central Haiti (Farmer 1996). But even polio, deemed vanquished forever, could and did return. The strain of polio that spread was actually derived from a vaccine: but it was a strain fully capable of causing paralysis and death, and able to spread only because so few children had been vaccinated during the early nineties (Kew et al. 2002).

5. But it also led to the growth of the local pharmaceutical industry, which by the mid-1990s was bringing Cuba some US$100 million a year in export earnings. In 2003, nearly 80 percent of the more than 800 essential medicines employed in Cuba are locally manufactured in 12 of the local factories. Nationally produced medicines are sold at heavily subsidized prices in the government network of neighborhood pharmacies (Castro, Togores, and Barberia 2003).

6. In 1998, Cuba's tuberculosis case notification rate was 11.7 per 100,000 population (although it was 3.8 in 1992 and had been steadily declining in the 1980s, averaging 6.9 during the decade, an incidence in fact lower than that reported for the United States). The rates, however, are still extremely low compared to other low-income countries, where between 45 and 59 percent of deaths are due to infectious disease (Gwatkin and Guillot 2000; WHO 1999).

7. A year later, Cuba manufactured its own HIV serologic test and, in 1988, a Cuban Western blot technique was available (Pérez-Ávila et al. 1996).

8. The screening progressively expanded to include, since 1987, specified risk groups: blood donors, pregnant women, adult in-patients, patients diagnosed with sexually transmitted infections, prisoners, army recruits, and those who have traveled abroad since 1975 or who have frequent contact with foreigners, among others.

9. The first AIDS sanatorium, in Santiago de la Vegas (near Havana), was opened on April 30, 1986.

10. Following the model of government production in countries such as Brazil, certain antiretrovirals (zidovudine [AZT], didanosine [DDI], lamivudine [3TC], stavudine [D4T], dioxicitidine [DDC], and indinavir [IDV]) to treat national cases of AIDS are

produced with imported raw materials at Novatec, a Cuban state-owned pharmaceutical industry (Castro et al. 2002).

11. In a 1992 article examining mortality rates in developed countries, Wilkinson argues that less inequality translates into better health outcomes:

> But the apparent effect of income distribution on health is too large to be explained by changes in the mortality of a poor group alone. If the United States or Britain were to adopt an income distribution more like that of Japan, Sweden, or Norway, the indications are it might add two years to average life expectancy. That is considerably more than would be gained even if the health detriment suffered by poor minorities were wholly overcome (Wilkinson 1992:1083).

He concludes: "Health inequalities result from the extent of relative deprivation in each society" (Wilkinson 1992:1084).

12. For example: indinavir (US$6.49 in Haiti and US$2.42 in the United States), efavirenz (US$4.84 and US$3.94), abacavir (US$8.45 and US$5.57), and lamivudine (US$5.43 and US$4.15) (PAHO 2002b).

13. The market fails when it comes to research and development—in the case of tuberculosis, for example, the last novel treatment was developed over 30 years ago (t'Hoen 2000). Over the past two decades (1975–1996), less than 1 percent of over 1,200 new molecular entities sold worldwide were earmarked for tropical diseases (Trouiller and Olliaro 1999)—despite the fact that infectious diseases remain a major cause of mortality throughout the world: in 1998, infectious diseases accounted for 25 percent of deaths worldwide and 45 percent of deaths in low-income countries (WHO 1999). One candid review of drug development notes that "few developments are need-driven"—the average cost of bringing a new drug to market is approximately $224 million, costs that pharmaceutical companies argue would not be recouped for diseases endemic in poor countries with few resources and no property rights laws to prohibit far cheaper generic products from entering the market (Trouiller and Olliaro 1999:164).

References

Attaran, A., and J. Sachs. (2001). "Defining and Refining International Donor Support for Combating the AIDS Pandemic. *Lancet* 357, no. 9249: 57–61.

Banque de la République d'Haïti. (2000). *Rapport Annuel.* Port au Prince, Haiti: Banque de la République d'Haïti.

Barberia, Lorena, and Arachu Castro, eds. (2003). *Seminar on Cuban Health System: Its Evolution, Accomplishments, and Challenges.* Working Papers on Latin America, Paper no. 02/03–4. Cambridge, MA: David Rockefeller Center for Latin American Studies at Harvard University.

Barberia, L., A. Castro, P. Farmer, C. Farmer, R. Gusmão, J. Y. Kim, E. Levcovitz, D. López-Acuña, K. Mate, P. Schroeder, G. Tambini, and E. Yen. (2002). *The Impact of Health Systems Reform on the Control and Prevention of Infectious Diseases in Latin America and the Caribbean.* Washington, DC: Pan American Health Organization and Partners In Health.

Barnett, T. and A. Whiteside. (2002). *AIDS in the Twenty-First Century: Disease and Globalization.* New York: Palgrave Macmillan, 416 pp.

Beinfield, H. (2001). "Dreaming with Two Feet on the Ground: Acupuncture in Cuba." *Clinical Acupuncture and Oriental Medicine Journal* 2, no. 2: 66–69. Retrieved April 17, 2004, from www.globalexchange.org/countries/cuba/sustainable/natTradMedicine/caomj0601.html.

Bell, C., S. Devarajan, and H. Gersbach. (2003). *The Long-run Economic Costs of AIDS: Theory and an Application to South Africa.* Washington, DC: World Bank. Retrieved April 17, 2004, from www1.worldbank.org/hiv_aids/docs/BeDeGe_BP_total2.pdf.

Blower, S., and P. Farmer. (2003). "Predicting the Public Health Impact of Antiretrovirals: Preventing HIV in Developing Countries." *AIDScience* 3, no. 11: 7 pp. Retrieved October 3, 2003, from www.aidscience.org/Articles/aidscience033.htm.

Brock, D. W. (2003). "Separate Spheres and Indirect Benefits." *Cost Effectiveness and Resource Allocation* 1: 4. Retrieved June 9, 2003, from www.resource-allocation.com/content/1/1/4.

Castro, A. (2003). "Determinantes socio-políticos de la infección por VIH: Violencia estructural y culpabilización de la víctima: Conferencia plenaria." [Sociopolitical determinants of HIV: Structural violence and the blaming of the victim: Plenary lecture]. In *2nd Latin American Forum on HIV/AIDS and STIs,* 22, Havana, Cuba. Retrieved April 17, 2004, from www.foro2003.sld.cu/conferencia/index_d.php?conferencia=2&lang=e.

Castro, A., and P. Farmer. (2003). "Infectious Disease in Haiti: HIV/AIDS, Tuberculosis, and Social Inequalities." *EMBO Reports* 4, no. 6s: S20–S23.

———. (2004). "Health and Economic Development." In *Encyclopedia of Medical Anthropology: Health and Illness in the World's Cultures,* edited by Carol R. Ember and Melvin Ember, 164–70. New York: Kluwer/Plenum.

Castro, A., P. Farmer, and L. Barberia. (2002). *Control of HIV/AIDS in Cuba: A Briefing Memo for President Carter's visit to Cuba.* Atlanta: Carter Center.

Castro, A., P. Farmer, J. Y. Kim, E. Levcovitz, D. López-Acuña, J. S. Mukherjee, P. Schroeder, and E. Yen. (2003). *Scaling up Health Systems to Respond to the Challenge of HIV/AIDS in Latin America and the Caribbean.* Special edition of the Health Sector Reform Initiative in Latin America and the Caribbean 8. Washington, DC: Pan American Health Organization, 100 pp.

Castro, A., V. Togores, and L. Barberia. (2003). *Access to Medicines in Cuba: The Hampering and Burgeoning Effects of the Economic Crisis.* Paper presented at the American Anthropological Association Annual Meeting, Chicago.

Cayemittes, M., M. F. Placide, B. Barrère, S. Mariko, and B. Sévère. (2001). *Enquête Mortalité, Morbidité et Utilisation des Services, Haïti 2000.* Calverton, MD: Ministère de la Santé Publique et de la Population, Institut Haïtien de l'Enfance, and ORC Macro.

Centers for Disease Control and Prevention (CDC). (1994). "International Notes Certification of Poliomyelitis Eradication—The Americas, 1994." *Morbidity and Mortality Weekly Report* 43, no. 39: 720–22.

———. (2002). "U.S. HIV and AIDS cases reported through December 2002," *HIV/AIDS Surveillance Report* 14. Retrieved April 17, 2004, from www.cdc.gov/hiv/stats/hasr1402/2002SurveillanceReport.pdf.

———. (2000). "Outbreak of Poliomyelitis—Dominican Republic and Haiti, 2000." *Morbidity and Mortality Weekly Report* 49, no. 48: 1094, 1103.

Chomsky, A. (2000.) "'The Threat of a Good Example': Health and Revolution in Cuba." In *Dying for Growth: Global Inequality and the Health of the Poor,* edited by J. Y. Kim, J. V. Millen, A. Irwin, and J. Gershman, pp. 331–57. Monroe, ME: Common Courage Press.

Creese, A., K. Floyd, A. Alban, and L. Guinness. (2002). "Cost-Effectiveness of HIV/AIDS Interventions in Africa: A Systematic Review of the Evidence." *Lancet* 359, no. 9318: 1635–42.

Desormeaux, J., M. P. Johnson, J. S. Coberly, et al. (1996). "Widespread HIV Counseling and Testing Linked to a Community-Based Tuberculosis Control Program in a High-Risk Population." *Bulletin of the Pan American Health Organization* 30, no. 1: 1–8.

Domínguez, J. I. (1978). *Cuba: Order and Revolution.* Cambridge, MA: Harvard University Press.

Economic Commission for Latin America and the Caribbean (ECLAC). (1997 [2000]). *La Economía Cubana: Reformas Estructurales y Desempeño en los '90.* Mexico: Fondo de Cultura Económica.

———. (2001). *Cuba: Evolución Económica durante 2000.* LC/MEX/L.465 Mexico: ECLAC.

Eisenberg, L. (1984). "Rudolf Ludwig Karl Virchow, Where Are You Now that We Need You?" *American Journal of Medicine* 77, no. 3: 524–32.

Escobar, A. (1995). *Encountering Development: The Making and Unmaking of The Third World.* Princeton, NJ: Princeton University Press.

Farmer, P. (1992). *AIDS and Accusation: Haiti and the Geography of Blame.* Berkeley: University of California Press.

———. (1996). "Haiti's Lost Years: Lessons for the Americas." *Current Issues in Public Health* 2, no. 3: 143–51.

———. (1999). *Infections and Inequalities: The Modern Plagues.* Berkeley: University of California Press.

———. (2003a). *Pathologies of Power: Health, Human Rights, and the New War on the Poor.* Berkeley: University of California Press.

———. (2003b [1994]). *The Uses of Haiti,* 2nd ed. Monroe, ME: Common Courage Press.

Farmer, P., and A. Castro. (2003). "Castigo a los más pobres de América: El embargo de la ayuda internacional crea una crisis humanitaria en Haití." *El País* (12 January): 8–9.

Farmer, P., M. C. Smith Fawzi, and P. Nevil. (2003). "Unjust Embargo of Aid for Haiti." *Lancet* 361, no. 9355: 420–23.

Farmer, P., F. Léandre, J. Mukherjee, M. Claude, P. Nevil, M. Smith-Fawzi, S. Koenig, A. Castro, M. Becerra, J. Sachs, A. Attaran, and J. Y. Kim. (2001). "Community-Based Approaches to HIV Treatment in Resource-Poor Settings." *Lancet* 358: 404–409.

Farmer, P., F. Léandre, J. Mukherjee, R. Gupta, L. Tarter, and J. Y. Kim. (2001). "Community-Based Treatment of Advanced HIV Disease: Introducing DOT-HAART (Directly Observed Therapy with Highly Active Antiretroviral Therapy)." *Bulletin of the World Health Organization* 79, no. 12: 1145–51.

Feinsilver, J. (1993). *Healing the Masses: Cuban Health Politics at Home and Abroad.* Berkeley: University of California Press.

Ferrer, A. (2000). *Thinking through Haiti: Cuban Slave Society and the Haitian Revolution.* Working document, New York University. Retrieved October 3, 2003, from www.princeton.edu/plasweb/news/Ferrer4-4.doc.

Freedberg, K. A., E. Losina, M. C. Weinstein, et al. (2000). "The Cost Effectiveness of Combination Antiretroviral Therapy for HIV Disease." *New England Journal of Medicine* 344, no. 11: 824–31.

Freedberg, K., and Y. Yazdanpanah. (2003). "Cost-effectiveness of HIV Therapies in Resource-Poor Settings." In *Economics of AIDS and Access to HIV/AIDS Care in Developing Countries. Issues and Challenges,* edited by J-P. Moatti, B. Coriat, Y. Souteyrand, T. Barnett, J. Dumoulin and Y-A. Flori. Paris: Agence Nationale de Recherches sur le Sida, 267–91.

Garber, A. M. (2000). "Advances in Cost-Effectiveness Analysis of Health Interventions." In *Handbook of Health Economics,* vol. 1, edited by A. J. Culyer and J. P. Newhouse, 182–221. Amsterdam: Elsevier Science.

Gebo, K. A., R. E. Chaisson, J. G. Folkemer, J. G. Bartlett, and R. D. Moore. (1999). "Costs of HIV Medical Care in the Era of Highly Active Antiretroviral Therapy." *AIDS* 13: 963–69.

Global Fund to Fight AIDS, Tuberculosis and Malaria. (2002a). *Haiti's Response to HIV/AIDS. Application to the Global Fund to Fight AIDS, Tuberculosis and Malaria.* Geneva: Global Fund to Fight AIDS, Tuberculosis and Malaria. Retrieved April 17, 2004, from www.theglobalfund.org/search/docs/1HTIH_483_29_full.pdf.

———. (2002b). *Global Fund Money to Scale Up AIDS Treatment and Prevention Efforts in Haiti.* Geneva: Global Fund to Fight AIDS, Tuberculosis and Malaria. Retrieved April 17, 2004, from www.theglobalfund.org/en/media_center/press/pr_021202.asp.

———. (2004a). *Current Grant Commitments and Disbursements.* Geneva: Global Fund to Fight AIDS, Tuberculosis and Malaria. Retrieved April 17, 2004, from www.theglobal fund.org/en/files/grantsstatusreport.xls.

———. (2004b). *Pledges and Contributions to the Global Fund.* Geneva: Global Fund to Fight AIDS, Tuberculosis and Malaria. Retrieved April 17, 2004, from www.theglobal fund.org/en/files/pledges&contributions.xls.

———. (2004c). *Coping with Chaos: How Haiti's AIDS Projects Are still Winning.* Geneva: Global Fund to Fight AIDS, Tuberculosis and Malaria. Retrieved April 17, 2004, from www.theglobalfund.org/en/media_center/press/pr_040305.asp.

Gold, M. R., J. E. Siegel, L. B. Russell, and M. C. Weinstein, eds. (1996). *Cost-Effectiveness in Health and Medicine: The Report of the Panel on Cost-Effectiveness in Health and Medicine.* New York: Oxford University Press.

González-Núñez, I., M. Díaz-Jidy, and J. Pérez-Ávila. (2000). "La transmisión materno infantil del VIH/SIDA en Cuba." *Revista Cubana de Medicina Tropical* 52, no. 3: 220–24.

Gwatkin, D. R., and M. Guillot. (2000). *The Burden of Disease Among the Global Poor: Current Situation, Future Trends, and Implications for Strategy.* Washington, DC: World Bank.

Holtgrave, D. R., ed. (1998). *Handbook of Economic Evaluation of HIV Prevention Programs.* New York: Plenum Press.

Holtgrave D. R., N. L. Qualls, and J. D. Graham. (1996). "Economic Evaluation of HIV Prevention Programs." *Annual Reviews of Public Health* 17: 467–88.

Hsieh, Y., C. Chen, S. Lee, and H. de Arazoza. (2001). "On the Recent Sharp Increase in HIV Detections in Cuba." *AIDS* 15, no. 3: 426–28.

Iriart, C., E. E. Merhy, and H. Waitzkin. (2001). "Managed Care in Latin America: The New Common Sense in Health Policy Reform." *Social Science and Medicine* 52, no. 8: 1243–53.

Jean-Louis, R. (1989). "Diagnostic de l'état de santé en Haïti." *Forum Libre (Santé, Médicine et Democratie en Haïti)* 1: 11–20.

Jha, P., N. J. D. Nagelkerke, E. N. Ngugi, et al. (2001). "Reducing HIV Transmission in Developing Countries." *Science* 292, no. 5515: 224–25.

Kaplan, E. H., and M. H. Merson. (2002). "Allocating HIV-Prevention Resource: Balancing Efficiency and Equity." *American Journal of Public Health* 92, no. 12: 1905–7.

Kew, O., V. Morris-Glasgow, M. Landaverde, et al. (2002). "Outbreak of Poliomyelitis in Hispaniola Associated with Circulating Type 1 Vaccine-Derived Poliovirus. *Science* 296, no. 5566: 269–70.

Kim, J. Y., J. V. Millen, A. Irwin, and J. Gershman, eds. (2000). *Dying for Growth: Global Inequality and the Health of the Poor.* Monroe, ME: Common Courage Press.

Kim, J. Y., A. Shakow, A. Castro, C. Vanderwarker, and P. Farmer. (2003). "Tuberculosis Control." In *Global Public Goods for Health: Health Economic and Public Health Perspectives*, edited by R. Smith, R. Beaglehole, D. Woodward, and N. Drager, 54–72. Oxford: Oxford University Press.

Kumaranayake, L., and C. Watts. (2001). "Resource Allocation and Priority Setting of HIV/AIDS Interventions: Addressing the Generalized Epidemic in Sub-Saharan Africa." *Journal of International Development* 13, no. 4: 451–66.

Laurell, A. C. (2001). "Health Reform in Mexico: The Promotion of Inequality." *International Journal of Health Services* 31, no. 2: 291–321.

López-Acuña, D. (2000). *La Naturaleza de las Reformas del Sector de la Salud en las Américas y su Importancia para la Cooperación Técnica de OPS.* Washington, DC: OPS/OMS/División de Desarrollo de Sistemas y Servicios de Salud.

Lurie, P., P. Hintzen, and R. A. Lowe. (1995). "Socioeconomic Obstacles to HIV Prevention and Treatment in Developing Countries: The Roles of the International Monetary Fund and the World Bank." *AIDS* 9, no. 6: 539–46.

Marins, J. R. P., L. F. Jamal, S. Y. Chen, M. B. Barros, E. S. Hudes, A. A. Barbosa, et al. (2003). "Dramatic Improvement in Survival among Adult Brazilian AIDS Patients." *AIDS* 17, no. 11: 1675–83.

Marrero, A., J. A. Caminero, R. Rodríguez, and N. E. Billo. (2000). "Towards Elimination of Tuberculosis in a Low Income Country: The Experience of Cuba, 1962–97." *Thorax* 55, no. 1: 39–45.

Marseille, E., P. B. Hofmann, and J. G. Kahn. (2002). "HIV Prevention before HAART in Sub-Saharan Africa." *Lancet* 359, no. 9320: 1851–56.

Martí, J. (1894[1959]). *La cuestión racial.* Havana: Lex.

Ministerio de Finanzas y Precios. (1998). *Políticas, estrategias y programas.* Havana: Ministry of Public Health. Retrieved April 17, 2004, from www.sld.cu/sistema_de_salud/estrategias.html.

Ministerio de Salud Pública (MINSAP). (2001). *Anuario Estadístico 2001*. Havana: Infomed, Red Telemática de Salud en Cuba. Retrieved September 20, 2003, from http://bvs.sld.cu/cgi-bin/wxis/anuario/?IsisScript=anuario/iah.xis&tag5001=mostrar^m694&tag5009=STANDARD&tag5008=10&tag5007=Y&tag5003=anuario&tag5021=e&tag5022=2001&tag5023=694.

———. (1996). Conferencia del Dr. Carlos Dotres, Ministro de Salud Pública, ofrecida el día 18 de julio 1996 en el teatro del MINREX. Havana: Infomed, Red Telemática de Salud en Cuba. Retrieved April 17, 2004, from www.infomed.sld.cu/discursos/minrex.html.

Mintz, S. (1985a). *Sweetness and Power: The Place of Sugar in Modern History*. New York: Penguin.

———. (1985b). "From Plantations to Peasantries in the Caribbean." In *Caribbean Contours*, edited by S. W. Mintz and S. Price, 127–53. Baltimore: Johns Hopkins University Press.

Moatti, J-P., T. Barnett, Y. Souteyrand, Y-A. Flori, J. Dumoulin, and B. Coriat. (2003). "Financing Efficient HIV Care and Antiretroviral Treatment to Mitigate the Impact of the AIDS Epidemic on Economic and Human Development." In *Economics of AIDS and Access to HIV/AIDS Care in Developing Countries. Issues and Challenges*, edited by J-P. Moatti, B. Coriat, Y. Souteyrand, T. Barnett, J. Dumoulin and Y-A. Flori. Paris: Agence Nationale de Recherches sur le Sida, 247–65.

Murray, C. J. L., and A. D. Lopez. (1996). *The Global Burden of Disease*. Geneva: World Health Organization, Harvard School of Public Health, World Bank.

Musgrove, P. (1999). "Public Spending on Health Care: How Are Different Criteria Related?" *Health Policy* 47, no. 3: 207–23.

Nicholls, S., R. McLean, K. Theodore, R. Henry, B. Camara, et al. (2001). "Modelling the Macroeconomic Impact of HIV/AIDS in the English Speaking Caribbean: The Case of Trinidad and Tobago and Jamaica," *Journal of South African Economics* 68, no. 5: 916–32.

Pan American Health Organization (PAHO). (1993). *Haiti—L'Aide d'Urgence en Santé*. Port-au-Prince: Pan American Health Organization.

———. (1996). "Progress of Activities in Health Sector Reform." Executive Committee of the Directing Council, 26th Meeting of the Subcommittee on Planning and Programming, SPP27/7 (in English), Washington, DC, March 25–27.

———. (2002a). *Health in the Americas 2002*. Washington, DC: Pan American Health Organization.

———. (2002b). "Average Prices of a One Year Treatment with Antiretrovirals in Countries of Latin America and the Caribbean." Washington, DC: Pan American Health Organization. Retrieved September 20, 2003, from www.paho.org/English/HCP/HCA/analysis.pdf.

———. (2003). "Country Profiles: Haiti," *Epidemiological Bulletin* 24:1, pp. 13–16. Retrieved April 17, 2004, from www.paho.org/english/dd/ais/EB_v24n1.pdf.

PAHO, UNDP, and CARICOM. (1999). *Implementing Decentralization and Financing Strategies while Protecting the Poor*. Washington, DC: Pan American Health Organization. Retrieved April 17, 2004, from www.paho.org/English/HDP/HDD/policygreeneonline.pdf.

Pape, J. W. (2000). "AIDS in Haiti: 1980–96." In *The Caribbean AIDS Epidemic*, edited by G. Howe and A. Cobley, 226–42. Kingston: University of the West Indies Press.

Pape, J. W., B. Liautaud, F. Thomas, J. R. Mathurin, M. M. St. Amand, M. Boncy, et al. (1983). "Characteristics of the Acquired Immunodeficiency Syndrome (AIDS) in Haiti." *New England Journal of Medicine* 309, no. 16: 945–50.

Pérez-Ávila, J. (2003). "Atención Integral y Tratamiento del VIH en Cuba." In *2nd Latin American Forum on HIV/AIDS and STIs*, Havana, Cuba.

Pérez-Ávila, J., R. Peña-Torres, J. Joanes-Fiol, M. Lantero-Abreu, and H. Arazoza-Rodríguez. (1996). "HIV Control in Cuba." *Biomedicine & Pharmacotherapy* 50, no. 5: 216–19.

Portuondo, Fernando, and Hortensia Pichardo. (1974). *Carlos Manuel de Céspedes: Escritos.* Havana: Editorial de Ciencias Sociales.

Rosen, G. (1974). *From Medical Police to Social Medicine: Essays on the History of Health Care.* New York: Neale Watson Academic Publications.

Russell, S., and L. Gilson. (1997). "User Fee Policies to Promote Health Service Access for the Poor: A Wolf in Sheep's Clothing?" *International Journal of Health Services* 27, no. 2: 359–79.

Rylko-Bauer, B., and P. Farmer. (2002). "Managed Care or Managed Inequality? A Call for Critiques of Market-Based Medicine." *Medical Anthropology Quarterly* 16, no. 4: 476–502.

Smith, R., R. Beaglehole, D. Woodward, and N. Drager, eds. (2003). *Global Public Goods for Health: Health Economic and Public Health Perspectives.* Oxford: Oxford University Press.

Sullivan, C. A., J. R. Meigh, and T. S. Fediw. (2002). *Derivation and Testing of the Water Poverty Index Phase I.* Wallingford, United Kingdom: Centre for Ecology and Hydrology. Retrieved April 17, 2004, from www.ciaonet.org/wps/suc01/suc01.pdf.

t'Hoen, E. (2000). "Statement from Médecins sans Frontières." Campaign for access to essential medicines at the Health Issues Group DG Trade, Brussels, 26 June.

Trouiller, P., and P. L. Olliaro. (1999). "Drug Development Output: What Proportion for Tropical Diseases?" *Lancet* 354, no. 9173: 164.

UNAIDS. (2001). *AIDS Epidemic Update.* Geneva: UNAIDS.

———. (2002a). *Epidemiological Fact Sheets on HIV/AIDS and Sexually Transmitted Infections: Haiti.* Retrieved April 17, 2004, from www.unaids.org/html/pub/publications/fact-sheets01/haiti_en_pdf.pdf.

———. (2002b). *Report on the HIV/AIDS Epidemic.* Geneva: UNAIDS.

United Nations Development Programme (UNDP). (1990). *Human Development Report 1990.* New York: Oxford University Press for UNDP.

———. (2000). *Human Development Report 2000.* New York: Oxford University Press for UNDP.

———. (2003). *Human Development Report 2003.* New York: Oxford University Press for UNDP. Retrieved April 17, 2004, from www.undp.org/hdr2003/.

United Nations Food and Agriculture Organization (FAO). (2000). *The State of Food Insecurity in the World.* Rome: FAO. Retrieved April 17, 2004, from www.fao.org/FOCUS/E/SOFI00/img/sofirep-e.pdf.

Waitzkin, H., and C. Iriart. (2001). "How the United States Exports Managed Care to Developing Countries." *International Journal of Health Services* 31, no. 3: 495–505.

Wilkinson, R. G. (1992). "National Mortality Rates: The Impact of Inequality?" *American Journal of Public Halth* 82, no. 8: 1082–84.

World Bank. (1994). *Social Indicators of Development.* Baltimore: Johns Hopkins University Press.

———. (1997). *Poverty Reduction and Human Development in the Caribbean: A Cross-Country Study.* World Bank Discussion Paper (WDP 366). Washington, DC: World Bank.

———. (2001). *HIV/AIDS in the Caribbean.* Retrieved September 19, 2003, from http://web.worldbank.org/WBSITE/EXTERNAL/NEWS/0,,contentMDK:20020360~menuPK:34457~pagePK:34370~piPK:34424,00.html.

———. (2003a). "Long Term Economic Impact of HIV/AIDS More Damaging than Previously Thought." World Bank press release, no. 2003/24/S. Retrieved September 19, 2003, from http://web.worldbank.org/WBSITE/EXTERNAL/NEWS/0,,contentMDK:20120894~menuPK:34463~pagePK:34370~piPK:34424~theSitePK:4607,00.html.

———. (2003b). *Cuba at a Glance.* Retrieved September 19, 2003, from www.worldbank.org/cgi-bin/sendoff.cgi?page=%2Fdata%2Fcountrydata%2Faag%2Fcub_aag.pdf.

World Health Organization (WHO). (1999). *Report on Infectious Diseases: Removing Obstacles to Healthy Development.* Geneva: World Health Organization.

———. (2000). *World Health Report 2000: Health Systems: Improving Performance.* Geneva: World Health Organization.

———. (2001). *Macroeconomics and Health: Investing in Health for Economic Development.* Geneva: Commission on Macroeconomics and Health.

———. (2002). *World Health Report 2002.* Geneva: World Health Organization.

The Visible Fist of the Market: Health Reforms in Latin America

2

FRANCISCO ARMADA AND CARLES MUNTANER

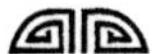

MOST LATIN AMERICAN COUNTRIES have implemented extensive reforms of their welfare states, reforms characterized by a shift from public to private sector in the delivery and financing of health and social services (e.g., old age and disability pensions, and workers' compensation). The rationale behind these changes is provided by the dominant neoliberal worldview that assigns to the private market the ability to best allocate and use social resources, even in the field of public health. The purpose of our study is to investigate the role of international financial institutions (IFIs)—the World Bank (WB), the International Monetary Fund (IMF), and the Inter-American Development Bank (IDB)—in current health policy reforms in Latin America, evaluate the assessment of such policies by the World Health Organization (WHO), and find out who directly benefits from these health policy reforms.

We begin by presenting the context in which health care reforms were implemented in Latin America as part of broader structural changes, and point out some of the main assumptions and inconsistencies of the neoliberal approach. We then examine IFI participation in health reforms, focusing on the World Bank and the position of the WHO as their de facto supporter, particularly in the key health policy goal of strengthening the role of the private sector in the financing and provision of health services. Next we show the economic benefits to private corporations resulting from these health policy reforms. Our analysis concludes with a discussion of several negative implications of neoliberal health policy reforms in Latin America, including rising social inequalities in health, and we comment on current encouraging alternatives to the dominant neoliberal trend.

Neoliberal Policies in Latin America

Neoliberal reforms in health services were implemented along with broader economic structural changes in most Latin American countries, beginning in the mid-1980s under strong pressure from IFIs. These policies were directed at stabilizing national economies, controlling inflation, reducing fiscal deficits, opening national economies to international trade, increasing the flexibility of labor markets, and reducing government intervention in the definition and implementation of public and economic policies (Lora 1997; Terris 1999). Although the ultimate goal of these measures is to promote economic growth, they also reflect IFI's goal to ensure that medium- and low-income countries pay their external debts (Petras 1999).

Navarro (1998) has identified several underlying hypotheses in neoliberal policies: (a) public deficits are intrinsically undesirable, (b) state regulation of the labor markets is also undesirable, (c) social protections guaranteed by the welfare state and their redistributive effects hinder economic growth, and (d) the state should not intervene in regulating foreign trade or international financial markets. The neoliberal principles behind these hypotheses are (a) the market is the best and most efficient way to create, produce, distribute, and allocate goods and services; (b) people follow rational choices mainly determined by their own individual (i.e., "selfish") interests; and (c) services provided by the welfare state, such as health care, are commodities.

The implementation of neoliberal reforms in Latin America has reached virtually every country in the region, although there is substantial cross-national variation in the timing, speed, extent, and other characteristics of the programs implemented (Torre 1997). Nevertheless, neoliberal reforms in Latin America as a whole have been growing since the 1980s. The scope of the neoliberal reforms in Latin America has been wide, covering virtually all economic sectors: the opening of trade and foreign exchange, tax reform, privatization of public enterprises, labor reform, health care reform, and pension reform (World Bank 1997, 1998a, 1999, 2000).

The social policy reforms promoted by IFIs were implemented despite lack of evidence on the benefits of "free market" reforms in health care, pensions, and other social services. A key assumption of these IFI-supported projects is that market forces make services more efficient because the private sector supposedly has an edge over the public sector—an assumption unsupported by evidence. In fact, studies of the U.S. health care model (in which market principles have been extensively applied) provide substantial evidence to the contrary. For instance, many studies show increased inequities resulting from the privatization of health services (e.g., Price 1988), higher administrative and overall costs among for-profit providers (Woolhandler and Himmelstein 1997), and worse health outcomes for patients receiving care in for-profit rather than not-for-profit institutions (Harrington et al. 2001, 2002). Moreover, user fees associated with neoliberal health policies effectively reduce consumers' available income and exacerbate health inequalities (Russell and Gilson 1997).

The World Bank, the International Monetary Fund, and the Inter-American Development Bank have directly intervened in policy making by dictating health reforms. Loans, their conditions, and external debt repayment negotiations have been the major tools of political leverage used by IFIs. A general objective of IFIs has been the alignment of health policies with comprehensive neoliberal changes (Sen and Koivusalo 1998). Thus, in the "letters of intent" that indebted Latin American countries are required to submit to the IMF, we can see evidence of how health reforms are embedded in major economic policies.

These letters of intent include a description of the policies that countries intend to implement or have already put in place in order to comply with IMF recommendations and obtain access to new loans. We obtained several examples of these letters that serve to illustrate the general point. For example, in 1998, Peru's minister of economy and finance and the president of Peru's Central Reserve Bank sent a letter of intent to the managing director of the IMF, in which they described "the policies that Peru intends to implement in the context of its request for financial support from the IMF." It included details of the necessary arrangements to maintain Peru's balance of payments regarding its external debt, further stating:

> The government will seek to complement its efforts in the education and health sectors by facilitating private investment in these areas. In 1997 the government issued a new law allowing private companies to provide health services within the social security system (Government of Peru 1998).

In addition, partnerships between the WB and international health agencies in need of funding have helped promote the WB's neoliberal policy agenda. The Pan American Health Organization (PAHO; 1998) reported that WB involvement in 30 health projects in 18 countries amounted to US$2.5 billion at the beginning of 1997; and participation of the IDB in 49 loans for the health sector totaled US$4.3 billion between 1992 and 1996. For instance, the U.S. Agency for International Development (USAID) has assigned several million dollars for health programs through the Child Survival and Disease Fund (U.S. Agency for International Development [USAID] 2000).

Unhealthy Reforms

Health care reforms in most Latin American countries (Bolivia, Brazil, Colombia, Dominican Republic, Jamaica, Mexico, Nicaragua, Peru, Panama, Trinidad and

Tobago, and Venezuela) have been supported by several WB and IDB loans. The stated objectives of these loans were to boost the financial sustainability, equity, efficiency, and quality of health services, as well as to extend coverage to the poor (World Bank 1997, 1999; Inter-American Development Bank [IDB] 1996). Ironically, in some cases the need to alleviate the social impact of economic reforms was also included among the goals of these loans (Government of Ecuador 2000). The activities financed by the WB and IDB include designing new health care systems, strengthening the agencies responsible for designing and regulating health policy, providing health care for low-income populations, decentralizing health services, and conducting research on health policy (De Beyer, Preker, and Feachem 2000). Regardless of the type of intervention, most loans favor the private financing and provision of health care over the former public financing and provision of such services that had predominated in most Latin American countries (Fiedler 1996; Kritzer 2000). The move from public to private represents a major shift in the financing, delivery, and ownership of health services.

Two closely related elements of health policy reforms led to the privatization of services: the separation of the financing and provision of health care, and the promotion of competition between providers. In contrast to the integrated functions of the traditional public sector, separation of financing from provision allows for the independent functioning of "buyers" and "sellers" of health services. The sellers must compete among themselves for the preference of buyers. This system promotes the creation of a market in the provision of health care services (Shackley and Healey 1993; Londoño and Frenk 1997).

The Colombian and Chilean models exemplify this approach (Bertranou 1999). In both instances, the separation between the provision and the financing of health care led to the emergence of new private providers financed through mandatory income transfers from the salaries of beneficiaries and through state subsidies. These new systems reinforced the already severe income-dependent differential access to health care in many Latin American countries.

Other explicit references to mechanisms for privatizing health care provision are often included in the descriptions of World Bank and IDB projects and loans. Some of these mechanisms include "cost recovery" in health care services (Lewis and Parker 1991), autonomous administration of hospitals and services, privatization of services, and reinforcement of private health insurance. For instance, the Ecuador Health Services Modernization Project (World Bank 1998b) included categorization of users according to income, development of a system of copayment and user charges, and formulation of a cost-recovery policy. Another example is found in Nicaragua (World Bank 1998c) in a proposed project for modernizing the health sector via the creation, in public hospitals, of private wards "catering to those able to pay" as a mechanism for cost recovery.

In addition to their participation in health care system privatization, the IFIs (and, in some cases, USAID) have also increased their influence in public health through the design and financing of specific interventions in Latin American countries (World Bank 1999; USAID 2000). For instance, health care agendas include care for the "vulnerable" sectors of the population such as mothers and young children (Dominican Republic, Ecuador, and Nicaragua) and the retired, disabled, and unemployed (Brazil); increased access to water supplies (Paraguay and Bolivia); measures to control the spread of HIV/AIDS (Argentina, Brazil, and Honduras); strengthening of national disease-surveillance programs (Brazil); and nutrition programs (Honduras). As admitted by a high-ranking WB officer, these interventions serve mostly as public relations efforts to counterbalance the public health effects of the privatization of health and social services (Coll personal communication).

Those that suffer most from the privatization of health services are the working class and the poor. They experience a severe reduction in their ability to purchase the goods and services that protect from disease and promote health (e.g., food, shelter, clothing, residential environment, and recreation) (Navarro 1997). Privatization also constitutes a draw on local and state public funds that reduces the amount of services provided to the population (e.g., unemployment benefits; social security; worker's compensation; social services for children, elderly, and people with disabilities; environmental protection; sanitation; garbage collection; security; parks; libraries; public transportation; road; and housing (Chomsky 1999). By generating a large pool of uninsured who cannot pay for private services, it increases the mortality rate among working class and poor citizens (Muntaner and Lynch 1999); lack of health care and uncertainty about ability to pay may produce anxiety, worry, and pain among those affected (Diala et al. 2000). Finally, the privatization of health services opens the door to other types of privatization such as pension and worker's compensation, or education.

The WHO View on Latin American Health Policy Reforms

The WHO and other intergovernmental institutions, such as the United Nations Development Program (UNDP), are converging with the IFIs in their health policy approach for Latin America: they all stress the importance of private participation in the financing and provision of health care. For instance, in a recent WHO report, the health systems of Colombia and Chile—which have undergone in-depth reforms favoring participation of the private sector in provision and financing—were ranked highest among the Latin American countries (WHO 2000). As it is derived from the report, the lesson to be learned by Latin

American countries is to strengthen the role of the private sector in financing and delivery of health care, a proposal sponsored by the World Bank since the 1980s (World Bank 1987, 1993). This alignment of financial institutions with international health and development agencies is another sign of the IFIs' influence on health policy. This explains why studies on the impact of neoliberal policies include policy recommendations that echo IFI's interests, even when conducted by independent intergovernmental agencies.

These associations between international health agencies and IFIs, apparently justified by budgetary deficits, not only reinforce the power of the IFIs in shaping health policy in Latin America but also jeopardize the independence of international agencies in policy evaluation and design, technical cooperation, research, and assessment of the social and health impact of economic policies.

A major consequence of these IFI-promoted and WHO-endorsed social and health policies is the overall growing "commodification" of social services in Latin American countries. Health care is managed as a commodity, and several companies profit from such business. Changes in the provision of services have mirrored and complemented the privatization of other public enterprises and services such as water, telephone, electricity, and airlines from which local and transnational ruling classes have benefited (Veltmeyer, Petras, and Vieux 1997).

The Beneficiaries of the "Commodification" of Health Care: Transnational and National Corporations[1]

The U.S. government, through its Departments of Commerce and State, has promoted the participation of the private sector in the economic liberalization of health and social services in Latin American countries. For instance, a telegraphic report from the American Embassy in Caracas (National Trade Data Bank 1995), in reference to the later-approved Health Sector Modernization Loan from the IDB, stated that a "significant part of the health care modernization project of government will be funded by IDB and the World Bank. In this regard, there is up to US$120 million in potential business to U.S. companies."

Several North American and European companies have entered or reinforced their participation in the health markets in the Americas (see Table 2.1). They belong to an extended network of companies that provide interrelated financial, banking, investment, and insurance services. Several businesses increased their share of the social services market in Chile in the 1980s, but it was mainly in the 1990s that most transnational companies intensified their presence in Latin American countries as providers of health care or pension management services. Most transnational corporations are North American or European.

Table 2.1. American Provision of Health Services in Latin America, 1999–2000

National Origin	*Services**	*Company*	*Companies and Countries of Investment*
United States	H, P	Aetna	**Argentina** (Asistencia Medica Social Argentina—Aetna, www.amsa.com.ar/), **Brazil** (SULAPREVI, www.sulaprevi.com.br/), **Chile** (Santa Maria, www.stamaria.cl), **Peru** (Novasalud EPS, www.novasalud.com.pe/, and **Integra Peru**, www.integra.com.pe/), **Mexico** (Bancomer, www.stamaria.cl/)
United States	P	Citicorp Group	**Chile** (Habitat, www.habitat.cl), **Uruguay** (Capital,www.capitalafap.com.uy/), **Peru** (Profuturo, www.profuturo.com.pe/), **Mexico** (Garante, www.garante.com.mx), **Colombia** (Colfondos, svrwebcol.colfondos.com.co/)
United States	H, P	Cigna	**Brazil** (AMICO Asistencia Medica, www.amico.com.br/, and Cigna, previdencia www.cigna.com.br), **Chile** (CIGNA Salud Isapre, www.cigna.cl/)
United States		Others	Bankboston: **Uruguay** (Union, www.unionafap.com.uy) Berkley Corporation: **Argentina** (BERKLEY, www.berkley.com.ar) Unum Corporation: **Argentina** (BOSTON, www.boston.com.ar) Pension Management Ltd.: **Argentina** (Siembra, www.siembra.com.ar/) Continental National American Group: **Argentina** (CNA Omega, www.omega-art.com.ar) General Electric Assurance Company: **Mexico** (Inbursa, www.gefinancialassurance.com) George Washington University: **Peru** (Novasalud EPS) Hartford Life Insurance: **Uruguay** (Union) Principal International Inc. Principal Financial Group: **Mexico** (Principal, www.principal.com.mx) Liberty: **Argentina** (Liberty) Inverlink Preferred Market: **Chile** (Magister, www.magister.cl) New York Life International Inc.: **Argentina** (Maxima)

* H = health; P = pensions.

Sources: Internet sites specified in the table and from the following national agencies: Argentina (www.srt.gov.ar/home.html), Chile (www.sisp.cl/), Colombia (www.superbancaria.gov.co/), El Salvador (www.spensiones.gob.sv), Mexico (www.consar.gob.mx), and Peru (www.safp.gob.pe/afp.htm and www.seps.gob.pe). All websites last accessed in 2001.

North American corporations participate significantly in the provision of social security services in Latin America. Stocker, Waitzkin, and Iriart (1999) have provided evidence of the activities of these corporations in a report on the export of managed care to Latin America. Whether using managed care or other approaches to health care, Aetna, CIGNA, AIG, and Citibank control large sectors of health care in several countries.

European companies have also entered the Latin American health and pension services market. Three Spanish companies dominate the scene: two huge financial groups, Banco Santander Central Hispano (BSCH) and Banco Bilbao Vizcaya (BBVA); and one insurance company, MAPFRE. These companies are present in several countries and are involved in pensions, health care, and workers' compensation, in addition to several other businesses. These three enterprises participate in a large network of institutions that provide diverse social security services in Latin America. As most of their reports indicate, these services create considerable profits, in addition to an opportunity to expand other financial, banking, and insurance businesses in Latin America (Banco Bilbao Vizcaya [BBVA] 1999; Banco Santander Central Hispano [BSCH] 1999).

Local companies have also benefited from the privatization of social security in Latin America. Joint ventures with foreign companies or the sale of national businesses to transnational corporations has been a common practice.

Lessons from Neoliberal Interventionism

We maintain that the implementation of neoliberal health and social policies in Latin America has reproduced already-existing social inequalities by promoting a transfer of resources from the majority of the population to large owners of capital at both the national and international levels. During the neoliberal reform of social security, the alliance between local and international large capitalist classes promoted and took advantage of the conversion of social security services to private commodities. Some scholars have suggested that neoliberal policies favored the transfer of resources from labor to capital within countries and from the peripheral to the core countries internationally (Vilas 1995). We differentiate three dimensions of such transfers. First, regardless of their labor conditions, all salaried workers are compelled to enroll in social security programs that require compulsory payroll taxes to finance the system, including a percentage for the profit of private fund managers. These reforms of social security have given place to the creation of private companies that profit with the management of the workers' resources; this constitutes a transfer from workers to capital. Second, the external debt, which played an important role in the implementation of neoliberal policies and explains the IFIs' further political and economic leverage over indebted countries for the last two decades (Lafay and Lecaillon 1993), is another ground for resource transfers from Latin American countries to core wealthy countries. Paradoxically, IFI loans to finance health reforms, including the transition from old to new social security schemes, and even special programs to alleviate the negative impact of neoliberalism, further increase or contribute to maintain the external debt already owed to them by Latin American countries. In addition, most of these loans generate service payments and fees for administration.

Finally, the impact of these reforms on health shows a different sphere of the transfers from labor to capital. Although several initiatives have been developed to evaluate health reforms in Latin America, there is still much controversy and lack of data on the effect of neoliberal reforms on population health. Furthermore, the impact of IFI-promoted health policies on the huge health disparities among and within Latin American countries is difficult to disentangle from the effects of other neoliberal measures. Regardless of the factors responsible for cross-national health disparities, the scant available evidence on the impact of neoliberal reforms suggests that these policies reinforce and maintain health inequalities (Fernández 1996).

Health policy reform as implemented in Latin American countries provides an example of welfare state dismantlement leading to a rise in health inequalities through the commodification of health services. This is just one of the mechanisms that have been suggested to explain the population health impact of neoliberal policies (e.g., Muntaner and Lynch 1999; Armada, Muntaner, and Navarro 2002).

Nevertheless, not all local capitalist classes have benefited, nor were all labor organizations hurt by health policy reforms. Local capitalist classes hold diverse and often contradictory interests and, depending on the source of their capital, have supported different positions on neoliberal policies. However, the core of this social class—that is, owners and managers of large corporations—benefits from and is supportive of neoliberal health policy reforms (Veltmeyer et al. 1997).

What Are the Alternatives?

There are calls for further neoliberal reforms of the remnants of several Latin American welfare states. There are also calls for strengthening ongoing reforms. Chilean and Colombian reforms are presented as an example for the rest of the region, underlining the idea that no other choices are possible for the world's welfare states and that national politics make little difference given this global trend.

However, implementation of IFI-sponsored reforms in Latin America has been closely related to national politics and occasionally has met with substantial popular resistance (e.g., in Brazil and Venezuela). The deepest privatization of social security was carried out in Chile under a repressive military regime that did not allow any political opposition (Richard 1996). Likewise, privatization in Peru was decreed under a regime that severely restricted political participation. On the other hand, the mixed (public and private) models that were developed in Argentina, Uruguay, and Mexico resulted from active opposition of political parties and organized labor to privatization (Cruz-Saco and Mesa-Lago 1998). And despite economic sanctions and a low level of development, Cuba succeeded during several years in developing a welfare state that produced some of the best health indicators in the region and lower health inequalities within the country (A. Chomsky 2000). Overall, this concurs with the evidence that countries where social democratic policies prevail are likely to be more successful in strengthening their welfare states, reducing inequalities, and improving population health status (Navarro 1992; Navarro and Shi 2001). In Latin America, Huber (1996) has shown that the development of social security was strongly influenced by the strength of the labor movement, and this also determines the extent to which neoliberal reforms are implemented.

Neoliberal reforms of the welfare states are not inevitable. There is room for national governments in Latin America to define and carry out redistributive, social-democratic policies and to strengthen their welfare states, as several international experiences confirm. From different political perspectives, countries such as Cuba and Costa Rica have maintained public universal systems of health under strong welfare states. In Venezuela, a 1998 law that decreed private sector participation in the health system following the Colombian model has been overruled by a new political constitution, which establishes health and social security as universal rights to be guaranteed by the state. It also sets up guidelines for creating a public and not-for-profit social security system, including a national health service that is based on public financing and provision of services and strengthens the principle of solidarity (República Bolivariana de Venezuela 1999). Electoral (The Worker's Party in Brazil) and nonelectoral popular movements, such as those of Chiapas in Mexico and the Landless Workers in Brazil, and the convergence between North and South labor and political organizations in opposing IFIs policies, provide room for the construction of alternatives to the neoliberal policies.

Final Remarks

Our analysis of the regional political economy of health care privatization in Latin America has several implications for future studies. Rather than analyzing one country at a time, we find what is common to the processes in the whole region. Such pattern forced us to focus on "North-South" or "Core-Semi Periphery" class relations that are necessary to understand the difficulty of social change in any single country (Muntaner and Lynch 1999). On the other hand, our systemic approach allows us to better understand the importance of local class politics by identifying exceptions (e.g., Venezuela). Thus, whereas wealthy countries show little political and economic variation with respect to health systems, medium-income and poor countries show greater variability in health systems and outcomes. This might be due to the relative political strength of alternatives to neoliberalism (H. J. Chung personal communication). A regional macro approach is also useful to complement the microanalyses of anthropological studies, as Paul Farmer (1999) and others (Kim, Millen, Irwin, and Gershman 2000) have shown recently.

Simultaneous analysis of multiple levels (international/regional, national, and local) with multiple methods (ecologic, survey, and qualitative), coupled with an interdisciplinary (e.g., political economy of population health) as well as multidisciplinary (e.g., sociology, anthropology, and public health) approach, seems to show most promise to understand inequalities in health and identify social policies that might reduce and eliminate them.

Acknowledgments

The authors are grateful to Pasqualina Curcio and Vicente Navarro for all their contributions to this chapter. Sections of this text are modified from F. Armada, C. Muntaner, and V. Navarro (2001), "Health and Social Security Reforms in Latin America: The Convergence of the World Health Organization, the World Bank, and Transnational Corporations," *Int J Health Serv.* 31, no. 4: 729–68.

Note

1. The main sources of information for this section, unless otherwise noted, are the home pages of the companies and agencies on the World Wide Web. We reviewed data from official publications and Web sites of the WB, the IDB, and the IMF to search for loans and projects in order to document the participation of these institutions in the processes of health policy reform. A review of the Web pages of the corporations and agencies involved in the regulation, provision, or financing of health and pension programs provided information on how these private parties have benefited from their participation in health policy reforms in Latin America.

References

Armada, F., C. Muntaner, and V. Navarro. (2001). "Health and Social Security Reforms in Latin America: The Convergence of the World Health Organization, the World Bank, and Transnational Corporations." *Int J Health Serv.* 31, no. 4: 729–68.

———. (2002). "Income Inequality and Population Health in Latin America and the Caribbean." *International Journal of Hispanic Health Care* 1: 42–55.

Banco Bilbao Vizcaya. (1999). *Annual Report.* Bilbao, Spain: Banco Bilbao Vizcaya.

Banco Santander Central Hispano. (1999). *Annual Report.* Santander, Spain: Banco Santander Central Hispano.

Bertranou, F. M. (1999). "Are Market-Oriented Health Insurance Reforms Possible in Latin America? The Cases of Argentina, Chile and Colombia." *Health Policy* 47, no. 1: 19–36.

Chomsky, A. (2000). "The Threat of a Good Example: Health and Revolution in Cuba." In *Dying for Growth,* edited by J. Kim, J. Millen, A. Irwin, and J. Gershman, 331–58. Monroe, ME: Common Courage Press.

Chomsky, N. (1999). *Latin America: From Colonization to Globalization.* New York: Ocean Press.

Cruz-Saco, M., and C. Mesa-Lago. (1998). "Conclusions: Conditioning Factors, Cross-Country Comparisons, and Recommendations." In *Do Options Exist? The Reform of Pension and Health Care Systems in Latin America,* edited by M. A. Cruz-Saco and C. Mesa-Lago, 377–428. Pittsburgh, PA: University of Pittsburgh Press.

De Beyer, J. A., A. S. Preker, and R. G. A. Feachem. (2000). "The Role of the World Bank in International Health: Renewed Commitment and Partnership." *Soc. Sci. Med.* 50: 169–76.

Diala, C., C. Muntaner, C. Walrath, K. J. Nickerson, T. A. LaVeist, and P. J. Leaf. (2000). "Racial Differences in Attitudes Toward Professional Mental Health Care and in the Use of Services." *Am J Orthopsychiatry* 70: 455–64.

Farmer, P. (1999). *Infections and Inequalities: The Modern Plagues.* Berkeley: University of California Press.

Fernández, A. (1996). "The Disruptions of Adjustment: Women in Nicaragua." *Latin Am. Perspect. Issues* 23: 49–66.

Fiedler, J. L. (1996). "The Privatization of Health Care in Three Latin American Social Security Systems." *Health Policy Planning* 11: 406–17

Government of Ecuador. (2000). Memorandum of Economic Policies of the Government of Ecuador for 2000 and Letter of Intent from Ecuadorian Minister of Finance and Public Credit Jorge Guzmán and Modesto Correa, president of the Board Central Bank of Ecuador, to IMF Acting Managing Director Stanley Fischer. Accessed at www.imf.org/external/np/loi/2000/ecu/01/index.htm, April 19, 2004.

Government of Peru. (1998). Letter of Intent from Peruvian Minister of Economy and Finance Jorge Camet and Germán Suárez, president of the Central Reserve Bank of Peru, to IMF Managing Director Michel Camdessus, Lima, Peru May 5, 1998. Accessed at www.imf.org/external/np/loi/050598.htm, April 19, 2004.

Harrington, C., S. Woolhandler, J. Mullan, H. Carrillo, and D. U. Himmelstein. (2001, September). "Does Investor Ownership of Nursing Homes Compromise the Quality of Care?" *Am J Public Health* 91, no. 9: 1452–55.

———. (2002). "Does Investor-Ownership of Nursing Homes Compromise the Quality of Care?" *Int J Health Serv.* 32, no. 2: 315–25.

Huber, E. (1996). "Options for Social Policy in Latin America: Neoliberal versus Social Democratic Models." In *Welfare States in Transition,* edited by G. Esping-Andersen, 141–91. Newbury Park, CA: Sage.

Inter-American Development Bank. (1996, August). *Supporting Reform in the Delivery of Social Services: A Strategy*. No. SOC–101. Washington, DC: Inter-American Development Bank.

Kim, J., J. Millen, A. Irwin, and J. Gershman, eds. (2000). *Dying for Growth: Global Inequality and the Health of the Poor*. Monroe, ME: Common Courage Press.

Kritzer, B. E. (2000). "Social Security Privatization in Latin America." *Soc Secur Bull* 63, no. 2: 17–37.

Lafay, J., and J. Lecaillon. (1993). *The Political Dimensions of Economic Adjustment*. Paris: Development Centre of Organisation for Economic Co-operation and Development.

Lewis, M. A., and C. Parker. (1991). "Policy and Implementation of User Fees in Jamaican Public Hospitals." *Health Policy* 18: 57–85.

Londoño, J. L., and J. Frenk. (1997, July). "Structured Pluralism: Towards an Innovative Model for Health System Reform in Latin America." *Health Policy* 41, no. 1: 1–36.

Lora, E. (1997). *A Decade of Structural Reforms in Latin America: What Has Been Reformed and How to Measure It*. Working Paper Green Series no. 348. Washington, DC: Inter-American Development Bank, Office of the Chief Economist.

Muntaner, C., and J. Lynch. (1999). "Income Inequality, Social Cohesion, and Class Relations: A Critique of Wilkinson's Neo-Durkheian Research Program." *Int. J. Health Serv.* 29: 59–81.

National Trade Data Bank. (1995, March 22). *Venezuela—Health Care Market Overview*. Washington, DC: National Trade Data Bank Market Reports.

Navarro, V. (1992). "Has Socialism Failed? An Analysis of Health Indicators under Socialism." *Int. J. Health Serv.* 22: 583–601.

———. (1997). *Bad for Your Health: Capitalism in Health Care*. New York: MRPress.

———. (1998). "Neoliberalism, 'Globalization,' Unemployment, Inequalities, and the Welfare State," *Int. J. Health Serv.* 28: 607–82.

Navarro, V., and L. Shi. (2001). "The Political Context of Social Inequalities and Health." *Soc. Sci Med.* 52, no. 3: 481–91.

Pan American Health Organization (PAHO). (1998). *Health in the Americas*. Scientific Publication no. 569. Washington, DC: PAHO.

Petras, J. (1999). *The Left Strikes Back: Class Conflict in Latin America in the Age of Neoliberalism*. Latin American Perspectives Series. Boulder, CO: Westview Press.

Price, M. (1988). "The Consequences of Health Service Privatisation for Equality and Equity in Health Care in South Africa," *Soc. Sci. Med.* 27: 703–16.

República Bolivariana de Venezuela. (1999). *Constitución Nacional*.

Richard, S. (1996). "Ideology Drives Health Care Reforms in Chile." *J Public Health Policy* 17, no. 1: 80–98.

Russell, S., and Gilson, L. (1997). "User Fee Policies to Promote Health Service Access for the Poor: A Wolf in Sheep's Clothing?" *Int. J Health Serv.* 27: 359–79.

Sen, K., and M. Koivusalo. (1998, July–September). "Health Care Reforms and Developing Countries—A Critical Overview." *Int J Health Plann Manage* 13, no. 3: 199–215.

Shackley, P., and A. Healey. (1993, September). "Creating a Market: An Economic Analysis of the Purchaser-Provider Model. *Health Policy* 25, nos. 1–2: 153–68.

Stocker, K., H. Waitzkin, and C. Iriart. (1999). "The Exportation of Managed Care to Latin America." *N. Engl. J. Med.*: 340.

Terris, M. (1999). "The Neoliberal Triad of Anti-Health Reforms: Government Budget Cutting, Deregulation, and Privatization." *J. Public Health Policy* 20: 149–67.

Torre, J. C. (1997). *Las Dimensiones Politicas e Institucionales de las Reformas Estructurales en America Latina. Serie Reformas de Politica Publica Comision Economica para America Latina y El Caribe (CEPAL/ECLatin American countries)*. Naciones Unidas.

U.S. Agency for International Development (USAID). (2000). "Latin American Countries Regional Summary Tables." Accessed at www.usaid.gov/country/lac/lac/lacreg_summtabs.html#pss, 2000.

Veltmeyer, H., J. Petras, and S. Vieux. (1997). *Neoliberalism and Class Conflict in Latin America*. New York: Macmillan.

Vilas, C. (1995). "Economic Restructuring, Neoliberal Reforms, and the Working Class in Latin America." In *Capital, Power, and Inequality in Latin America*, edited by S. Halebsky and R. Harris, 137–64. Boulder, CO: Westview Press.

Woolhandler, S., and D. U. Himmelstein. (1997). "Costs of Care and Administration at For-Profit and Other Hospitals in the United States." *N. Engl. J. Med.* 336: 769–74.

World Bank. (1987). *Financing Health Services in Developing Countries: An Agenda for Reform*. A World Bank Policy Study. Washington, DC: World Bank.

———. (1993). *World Development Report 1993: Investing in Health*. New York: Oxford University Press.

———. (1997). *Annual Report 1997*. Accessed at www.worldbank.org/html/extpb/annrep97/, April 19, 2004.

———. (1998a). *Annual Report 1998*. Accessed at www.worldbank.org/html/extpb/annrep98/, April 19, 2004.

———. (1998b). *Ecuador—Health Services Modernization*. Report no. 17326. Accessed at www-wds.worldbank.org/servlet/WDSContentServer/WDSP/IB/1998/05/20/000009265_3980625101542/Rendered/PDF/multi0page.pdf, April 19, 2004.

———. (1998c). *Project Appraisal Document on a Proposed Adaptable Program Credit in the Amount of SDR 17.9 Million (US$24 Million Equivalent) to the Republic Of Nicaragua for a Health Sector Modernization Project*. Report no: 17609 NI. Accessed at www-wds.worldbank.org/servlet/WDSContentServer/WDSP/IB/1999/06/03/000009265_3980630180502/Rendered/PDF/multi0page.pdf, April 19, 2004.

———. (1999). *Annual Report 1999*. Accessed at www.worldbank.org/html/extpb/annrep99/, April 19, 2004.

———. (2000). *Annual Report 2000*. Accessed at http://www.worldbank.org/html/extpb/annrep2000/, April 19, 2004.

World Health Organization (WHO). (2000). *World Health Report 2000: Health Systems Improving Performance*. Geneva: World Health Organization.

International NGOs in the Mozambique Health Sector: The "Velvet Glove" of Privatization

3

JAMES PFEIFFER

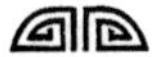

In May 2000, major international donors and agencies active in the Mozambique health sector met to discuss and sign a Ministry of Health (MoH) document entitled the Kaya Kwanga Code of Conduct (Mozambique Ministry of Health 2000). Signatories "pledged" to ensure that technical health assistance be "driven by MoH priorities" and that it clearly supports the institutional capacity of the MoH (2000:6). The agencies promised to "develop and maintain a climate of transparency, openness, accountability and honesty in all relations and transactions." The document asked that signatories "adhere to agreed national rates regarding remuneration and allowances for civil service employees, remuneration of consultants, payment for conferences, etc." and "avoid the departure of qualified personnel through contracting of civil servants for donor consultancies" (2000:3). Signatories included representatives from the U.S. Agency for International Development (USAID), the World Bank, key UN agencies, the European Commission, and most major Western European bilaterals active in Mozambique.

The appearance of the Code of Conduct begs several important questions. What *mis*conduct was going on to provoke such high-level action and self-policing? Were donors promoting programs that were *not* driven by MoH priorities and did *not* help build institutional capacity in one of the poorest countries in the world? Has there been, in fact, so much *dis*honesty and *lack* of accountability, transparency, and openness in foreign agency dealings with the health sector that top country representatives for major donors felt it necessary to meet and act?

The misconduct implied in the Kaya Kwanga document should be very troubling to those who assume that foreign health aid to the Third World is managed by well-meaning and committed professionals who work at great personal sacrifice to bring health care to the poor. However, to understand these disturbing dynamics it is necessary to look beyond individual ethical concerns, and even the resource management issues, to the broader policy environment that has recently transformed how aid from rich countries is transferred to poor countries. For the last two decades, the growing neoliberal emphasis on privatization of services promoted by major actors in international health, such as USAID and the World Bank, has resulted in the increased channeling of aid through international "nongovernmental organizations" (NGOs) rather than the public sectors of recipient nations (USAID 1995; World Bank 1993, 1997; Buse and Walt 1997; Green and Matthias 1997; De Beyer, Preker, and Feachem 2000). By 1999, 52 percent of World Bank–financed projects included NGOs, up from 20 percent in 1989 (World Bank 2000a). The major managers of foreign aid have argued that NGOs have a "comparative advantage" since they can allegedly reach poor communities more effectively, efficiently, and compassionately than public services (Edwards and Hulme 1996b; Green and Matthias 1997; World Bank 2000a; USAID 1995; Zaidi 1999; Turshen 1999). However, this policy shift has been ideologically driven, intimately bound up with the neoliberal emphasis on free markets and privatization couched in a new discourse that centers on an imagined "civil society" necessary for "sustainable development" (Edwards and Hulme 1996a; Powell and Seddon 1997; Turshen 1999; Stewart 1997; Hanlon 1996; Drabek 1987). As one USAID policy document states

> At all levels of development, a flourishing NGO community is essential to effective and efficient civil society. . . . Civil society organizes political participation just as markets organize economic participation in the society. . . . Sustainable development is likely to occur where both civil society and markets are free and open (1995:2).

Structural adjustment programs (SAPs) promoted by the World Bank and International Monetary Fund, which normally slash government health and education spending in developing countries saddled with foreign debt, are the key instruments in the push for privatization in this "New Policy Agenda" (Turshen 1999; Gary 1996; Edwards and Hulme 1996b; Laurell and Arellano 1996; Kim et al. 2000). International NGOs have been recruited by USAID (which calls them private voluntary organizations, or PVOs) and other major donors to substitute for shrinking state services in the provision of social safety nets for the poor as inequality has increased across the region (Anang 1994; Chabot, Harnmeijer, and Streefland 1996; Ndengwa 1996; Okuonzi and Macrae 1995; Mburu 1989). International NGOs have become the "velvet glove" of privatization.

However, based on findings from the following case study in Mozambique, where the health sector has been inundated by international NGOs and agencies since the late 1980s, it is argued here that channeling aid through NGOs has in fact harmed the delivery of primary health care (PHC). The flood of NGOs and their expatriate personnel has fragmented the health sector and contributed to intensifying social inequality in local communities with damaging effects on health care services for the poor majority. The emergence of the Kaya Kwanga document is an indicator of the degree to which NGO activity has disrupted health activities. The Mozambique experience described here challenges the assumption that NGOs are adequate substitutes for public services or contribute to an enhanced "civil society."

The global proliferation of NGOs is most visible in the capital cities of many developing nations, where agency offices and vehicles decorated with distinctive NGO logos are ubiquitous. An "unruly melange" (Buse and Walt 1997) of international health agencies, such as Doctors without Borders (*Médecins sans Frontières*), Save the Children, Africare, Care, World Vision, Oxfam, Concern, Food for the Hungry International, Family Health International, Pathfinder, Population Services International, and a range of others, has become a central feature of the neoliberal socioeconomic landscape of the Third World. This NGO phenomenon in the health sector has generated a significant literature over the past two decades (Green and Matthias 1997). A growing chorus of dissent argues that the flood of aid agencies into countries such as Mozambique may have had a negative impact on many local health systems (Cliff 1993; Pavignani and Durão 1999; Turshen 1999; Buse and Walt 1997). The overabundance of competing organizations that duplicate program support, create parallel projects, pull health service workers away from routine duties, and disrupt planning processes has fragmented health services and generated concern for both donors and recipients. The problem has provoked discussion among policy makers that focuses primarily on the dynamics of resource management at high levels in ministries of health and within agencies themselves (Gilson, Sen, Mohammed, and Mujinja 1994; Walt, Pavignani, Gilson, and Buse 1999; Buse and Walt 1996). I argue here, however, that an emphasis solely on the managerial aspects of aid coordination may distract attention from the greater structural transformation in local communities generated by the arrival of NGOs and other foreign agencies. The Mozambique case demonstrates that the fragmentation of primary health care is also the consequence of intensified local social inequality produced in part by foreign aid channeled through NGOs at the expense of the public sector.

Medical Anthropology, NGOs, and the Culture of Foreign Aid Workers

Expatriate NGO health workers can be found at all levels of many developing world health systems; from ministry of health offices in capital cities to remote villages where they are involved in health program implementation. These agencies' activities may be integrated into ministry programs or conducted completely outside the public system. The most direct confrontation between expatriate NGO aid workers and their target communities occurs outside capital cities, in the provinces where actual projects are implemented. This encounter constitutes an unusual social interface between highly educated technicians from rich countries and vulnerable communities in extreme poverty where relationships defined by inequalities in power and access to resources are enacted in ways that profoundly shape primary health care projects, programs, and policies. In these settings, the exertion of power by wealthy donors over their target populations, including local health workers, is laid bare, and the undermining of public sector services by international agencies is most visible.

Given how important these social dynamics are to the impact of foreign aid in the developing world, there is a surprising dearth of anthropological research on these relationships (see Fisher 1997). Ferguson (1994) and Escobar (1995) have provided broad critiques of the development enterprise and "discourse," and a small but growing body of ethnography of foreign aid and NGOs in local settings is finally appearing (see Crewe and Harrison 1998; Markowitz 2001; Grillo and Stirrat 1997). But medical anthropologists are especially underrepresented in the literature, having contributed relatively little to the study of social dynamics surrounding NGO activity in health, even though we are often very well positioned in the field to conduct the research. Medical anthropologists have made important contributions to the study of primary health care systems through research on the social world of national primary health care providers, and even the bureaucracies of international agencies (see Foster 1977; Coreil and Mull 1990; Justice 1987; Nichter 1996). However, little research on primary health care has examined the interface between expatriate foreign health agency workers in the field, their national counterparts, and the poor communities they are supposed to serve. Perhaps the inequalities of wealth and power are so obvious that they are taken for granted, or the presumed charitable good intentions and self-sacrifice of aid workers obscure the significance of these inequalities. Or, more cynically, perhaps social scientists are afraid to bite the feeding hand. As Peter Uvin states in his important analysis of the development industry in Rwanda before the 1994 genocide,

> To the extent that some people at some point do realize the political and social stakes and abuses that surround development aid and its projects, they often choose not to react. This has various causes, including fear of rocking the boat, of making enemies, of losing jobs (1998:156).

However, examination of these social processes is critical to understanding the development enterprise. As Uvin has shown in the Rwanda case, foreign aid can contribute to local processes of "exclusion" and "humiliation" that undermine equity-oriented efforts in development (1998). He writes:

> The development aid system contributes to processes of structural violence in many ways. It does so directly, through its own behavior, whether unintended (as in the case of growing income inequality and land concentration) or intended (as in its condescending attitude toward poor people). It also does so indirectly, by strengthening systems of exclusion and elite building through massive financial transfers, accompanied by self-imposed political and social blindness. . . . The material advantages accorded to a small group of people and the lifestyles of the foreigners living in Rwanda contribute to greater economic inequality and the devaluation of the life of the majority (143).

The quality and character of these social dynamics are not revealed in statistical data used by public health researchers, political scientists, or development experts. Nor do project evaluations, agency reports, or other detritus of the development industry honestly disclose these troubling aspects of many interventions. Participant observation and ethnographic research are the best tools for this kind of investigation, making it especially vital for medical anthropologists to redirect their gaze toward NGO activity in situ.

This chapter represents a modest attempt to provide an ethnographic sketch of the relationship between NGOs and the local community in two central provinces of Mozambique from 1993 to 1998. This brief vignette seeks to illustrate how the NGO model of technical assistance provision has intensified local social inequality, which has eroded the integrity of the primary health care system that serves the poor. The manner in which expatriate agency workers socially and financially engaged both their Mozambican counterparts, and the larger communities where they resided, had an enormous and often negative impact on many PHC community programs. These relationships were realized and enacted not only within formal work settings, but also in the daily life of the community where expatriates resided and conducted their social lives. While individual ethical choices and local administrative challenges contributed to PHC program difficulties, structural influences on expatriates and local health workers imposed by donor policies that favored NGOs over public services created the environment conducive to this dysfunction. The Mozambique experience throws into question the NGO model of foreign assistance to the health sector.

The findings reported here derive from nearly four years of fieldwork spread over two periods, from 1993 to 1998, when I was program coordinator and country representative for a U.S. health agency working in the health sector in two central Mozambican provinces. To obtain information on the social dynamics of international aid in the health sector, I conducted numerous formal and informal interviews with expatriates working for international agencies in the health sector, Mozambican workers in the national health system, and members of target communities. These interviews were complemented by participant observation throughout these periods, based on my involvement as an NGO coordinator working within both the provincial health directorate and the world of international agencies in the province. Neither the provinces where most of this information was collected nor the agencies discussed are identified by name.

An Ethnographic Profile

Over 90 percent of the population (surpassing 2 million) in the two provinces is engaged in the production of maize and sorghum staples on small parcels of land called *machambas*. Many men continue to migrate to Zimbabwe, to South Africa, and within Mozambique in search of waged work. The majority of the population in the provinces is very poor with an estimated annual per capita income under $200 at the time of this research (INE 1999). Health indicators reflect this impoverishment; cumulative under-five mortality is estimated at 150–200/1,000, while maternal mortality may be as high as 1,500/100,000 (Mozambique Ministry of Health 1997; UNDP 1998).

After independence from Portugal in 1975, Mozambique established a primary health care system that was eventually cited by the WHO as a model for other developing countries (Walt and Melamed 1983). The primary health care system was extended into isolated rural areas through construction of health posts and centers that offered basic maternal-child health, immunization, nutrition, first aid, and referral services. By the early 1980s, over 90 percent of the population had been vaccinated, 1,200 rural health posts constructed, and 8,000 midlevel health workers trained. About 11 percent of the government budget was committed to health care (Gloyd 1996). The war initiated by the Rhodesia and South Africa–backed rebels, known by their Portuguese acronym RENAMO, targeted infrastructure and personnel in the government health and education services from 1980 to 1992. By 1988, hundreds of health posts were ransacked and hundreds of health workers killed, injured, and terrorized. RENAMO-controlled areas (nearly 50 percent of the rural areas in some provinces) were devoid of any health services for many years. An estimated 1 million Mozambicans died as a result of the conflict. In 1987, Mozambique initiated an IMF-promoted structural adjustment program in which currency was devalued, government services cut back, prices increased, and a "free market" economy established. By 1990, state per capita spending on health was half of its 1980 level (Cliff 1993). In that year, the IMF pressed Mozambique to intensify economic reform and privatization (Hanlon 1996).

During the pre-SAP period, there were few, if any, NGOs operating in the country, and nearly all foreign aid was channeled through the National Health Service (NHS) at a national level. However, with the loss of aid from socialist countries and the government's turn to the IMF, increasing numbers of foreign aid agencies and NGOs began to descend on Mozambique in the late 1980s and early 1990s to tackle the humanitarian disaster created by RENAMO destabilization. By the late 1990s, the NHS received about 50 percent of recurrent expenditures and 90 percent of capital expenditures from international donors (Pavignani and Durão 1997). The state budget paid national staff salaries, while donors paid expatriates working within the NHS. Much of the foreign funding to the NHS came in the form of project aid directed toward specific donor-identified objectives. Nearly 100 agencies were spread throughout the country supporting the health sector by the early 1990s (Hanlon 1996). By 1996, there were 405 individual projects managed by these agencies within the NHS. As Wuyts points out (1996), most of these projects had high administrative costs (30–40 percent of project funds) and often failed to coordinate well with other donors. Even though some projects were integrated into NHS programs, Mozambicans often did not have actual control over budgets or project development (Cliff 1993). Some bilaterals such as USAID channeled the bulk of their health funding through NGOs that often operated quite independently of the NHS. By 1992, in the provinces where this research was conducted, there were ten foreign agencies supporting the health sector in one form or another, with foreign personnel and offices.

After several years of postwar rebuilding, each provincial health sector consists of nearly 70 rural health posts, and health worker staff of about 500, including ten Mozambican doctors and 200 nurses distributed throughout the districts. The Provincial Health Directorates, or DPS (*Direção Provincial de Saúde*), manage the health system from their offices in the provincial capitals. Each district has a health director who manages local programs with some limited autonomy in decision making. The provincial Department of Community Health (*Repartição de Saúde Comunitária*) within the DPS is structured to oversee maternal-child health, nutrition, health education, AIDS prevention, immunization (including mobile vaccination brigades), TB prevention and treatment, and a range of other community health programs implemented through the PHC network of health centers and posts. While efforts have been made to decentralize, by the mid-1990s the health system had a mix of national-, provincial-, and district-level control. Most major decisions were made at the national or provincial levels, but district directors were increasingly able to establish independent relationships with NGOs that pitched projects to them.

Arrival of the New Aid Set: "Pretoria" and "Soweto"

There have been two distinct periods of Western expatriate technical assistance to the health sector in postindependence Mozambique. In the early 1980s, hundreds of left-leaning Western health professionals came to support Mozambique's health system in the face of RENAMO's assault. Known as *cooperantes* in Portuguese, many worked within government health structures for local pay in difficult conditions. However, with the government's turn to the IMF and the flood of foreign agencies into Mozambique in the late 1980s, a new coterie of aid professionals appeared. Whereas the expatriates who had worked in Mozambique during the *cooperante* period tended to be idealists committed to supporting a public sector national health system, many of the new group were aid professionals who moved from contract to contract throughout the Third World and expressed no particular interest in Mozambique itself. Most of the new aid set were middle- or upper-middle-class Europeans and Americans with at least a college education, some with advanced degrees in medicine, public health, or international studies. Nearly all had career aspirations in international aid, academia, or public health, and many were working their way up the ladder in their respective organizations. Some were younger Europeans in their twenties who viewed their experiences in Africa as adventures that alleviated precareer ennui. A regular stream of European and American consultants also flowed through town to conduct baseline studies and program evaluations on short-term contracts.

International aid agencies arrived with large budgets and U.S. dollars. Several health organizations in the provinces where this research was conducted had budgets of over US$1 million to spend in the health sector per year, compared to the DPS budgets of only US$750,000. Dozens of expatriate health and development workers and their families set up their homes in the provincial capitals in the early 1990s. Two agencies built walled compounds for European staff, one with armed guards and a swimming pool, that soon became centers for expatriate social activity. Only a select few Mozambicans could make it past the armed guards at the gate. The construction of one of the compounds by a European agency to house its foreign staff generated great resentment among Mozambican health workers since the agency had also constructed several much smaller houses for higher-level nationals outside the compound walls. The Mozambicans jokingly referred to the walled-in European area as "Pretoria" and the Mozambican area as "Soweto." The compound provided the most prominent representation of the new environment of exclusion created by the arrival of aid in the province.

During this period, two new social figures emerged that were emblematic of the new aid culture. These were self-described "aid cowboys" and "aid mercenaries." The former term was often used to describe the foreign worker who derived a thrill from working in dangerous conditions and told aid "war stories" from places like Sudan, Cambodia, Angola, or Sierra Leone. Aid mercenaries, and there were several in the province who referred to themselves in these terms, admitted very frankly that their only real interest in working in Mozambique was the money. A majority of aid workers described themselves in discussions as nonideological technical specialists and professionals not particularly interested in Mozambican political history or culture, the context of international aid, or philosophical concerns with "development." Some privately expressed contempt for Mozambique and eagerly awaited their transfer out of the country. Many had little if any understanding of the recent conflict or colonial history of the country and simply wanted to fulfill their contracts and implement their projects. Their main concerns centered on perceived Mozambican ineptitude and the corruption of their counterparts in the government: corruption that had clearly been fed and nurtured by the arrival of loosely managed foreign aid. With the exception of two agencies, expatriates were paid from $1,000 to $6,000 per month, usually tax-free. Most agencies provided housing, private access to project cars, and funding for personal vacation or "R and R" time. One engineer working for a European agency calculated that at the end of his four-year contract, he would have saved nearly $300,000.

Many in the new aid set regularly left Mozambique on weekends for neighboring countries with better tourist infrastructures. For those who stayed, two local discos filled up on the weekends with aid workers back from the field and Mozambicans who could afford the stiff cover charge at the door. A growing sex work industry emerged around the city's nightspots. On any given weekend, one agency or another was hosting a party at their offices or homes. One particularly well-known European NGO gained a reputation for putting on the liveliest parties, and the sound of European techno dance music spread out over the poor barrios on many weekend nights. They were attended by other aid workers, and cadres of Mozambicans that had managed to ingratiate themselves into the European aid worker social scene. Some were NGO employees, while many others were members of an emergent middle class with higher educational levels, linguistic skills, and social talents. This new *comprador* group helped expatriates feel at ease within the Mozambican setting and became perhaps the primary Mozambican beneficiaries of the new aid dollars. Absent from most of these social functions were government health workers, the expatriates' poorly paid counterparts in the DPS.

The arrival of international agencies in the provinces coincided with the liberalization of the economy initiated by structural adjustment policies. The impact of these two connected factors on the economic and social life of the community was enormous. This international aid culture, with its "well-resourced" and driven foreign professional class, engaged a society experiencing its own rapid class formation in the privatizing economy. The new free market had stimulated the growth of the local merchant sector, and city stores began filling with gleaming commodities, in contrast to the years of war and socialism when consumer products were difficult to find. As one Mozambican put it, "During socialism we had money but nothing to buy, but now there's a lot to buy but we have no money." The rapid social differentiation was visible throughout the town. New cars here and there, fancier clothes and shoes on some, and roof tops in the cement city bristling with new TV antennae and satellite dishes where several years earlier there had been none. This contrasted with the deteriorating conditions in the poor barrios that ringed the city, where most of the population did not share in the new bounty. The removal of price subsidies had made it more difficult for many to obtain adequate food, and much of population remained in absolute poverty (UNDP 1998; Fauvet 2000; Hanlon 1996).

Health workers were among those whose incomes dropped drastically. From 1991 to 1996, nurses' monthly salaries dropped from $110 to less than $40, and doctors' salaries dropped from $350 to $100 (Hanlon 1996). Because of constraints on budget expenditures mandated by the SAP, staff salaries could not be increased with foreign aid. In spite of the influx of aid dollars, most of the funds were project-specific and were not used to increase staff salaries or benefits. Deteriorating work conditions contributed to a reportedly declining quality of health services in several ways. While hard data on changes in quality of service are not available for the province, widespread complaints of absenteeism, poor treatment, bribery, and illegal demands for payments for free services circulated in the community. The drop in salaries was matched by mounting material shortages, pharmaceutical deficits, equipment failures, and vehicle breakdowns in the midst of the millions of aid dollars that landed in the province. There were frequent reports that pharmaceuticals were being stolen from the health service and sold to market vendors or administered on a fee-for-service basis at the private homes of health service workers. For example, one survey of health post supplies conducted by my organization found that over half the health posts in one district had no chloroquin tablets for malaria treatment in spite of abundant supplies at the provincial level. Much of the chloroquin had been diverted to private practice or sold to private vendors in the open markets. Fuel shortages and lack of vehicle spare parts reduced the number of mobile motorcycle vaccination brigades into remote areas in some districts. These kinds of shortages fed the increasing frustration of health system workers. The drop in salaries and attendant demoralization amid a growing acquisitive and competitive culture in the towns made many health workers vulnerable to the financial temptations offered by the private sector and foreign agencies. By 1998, a private clinic had opened up in one city that provided fee-for-service treatment at prices that were unaffordable to the majority of the population. Health system workers, including some physicians and nurses, occasionally left their posts to treat patients at the clinic, or worked there during off-hours. It was widely reported that medical supplies were being diverted from the DPS to the clinic and to private practice in the homes of health staff.

Foreign workers confronted a different set of circumstances and challenges. Many hardworking and sincere foreign health professionals engaged in harmful organizational practices primarily because their positions demanded it. Appropriate planning, coordination, and concern for maintaining the integrity of existing public programs were generally not rewarded by the agencies and donors active in the province. In fact, adherence to the principles of good coordination and planning could potentially lead to poor evaluations and the loss of a job if project targets were not met as a result. In the prevailing aid culture, the tireless, dedicated, "results-oriented" project coordinator that stopped at nothing to meet his or her output objectives often produced uncompromising, short-term thinking and planning that undermined the broader goals of the health system. Many donors such as USAID, which funneled much of their aid to the health sector through grants to NGOs, increasingly emphasized the need to show short-term results; that is, measurable improvements in health outputs, such as under-five mortality or nutritional indicators, over short project periods (1–2 years in some cases). This directive was captured in the slogan "managing for results" promoted during annual meetings of USAID-funded NGOs in Maputo. The short-term orientation fit well with the general aid experience of most expatriates who moved from country to country and contract to contract. One European worker explained, "If you stay longer than two or three years people start wondering 'what's wrong with him?'" Mozambican counterparts in the health system were acutely aware that most expatriates had short-term contracts. One Mozambican planner remarked, "Just when they finally know how things work here, and they finally can speak Portuguese, they leave."

As a result of this orientation and professional imperative, the province was inundated with fast-moving project coordinators, most of whom worked 6–7 days per week setting up offices, administrative systems, baselines studies, interventions, and evaluations, and traveling around the province in newly arrived four-wheel-drive vehicles. To be successful in this world meant that coordinators had to be competitive and driven to promote both their own specific project goals and the public images of their organizations on the national stage. For many organizations it was important to become well known for work in a given area, such as nutrition, reproductive health, or AIDS prevention in order to attract further funding. This entrepreneurial and self-promotional ethos contributed to the notion among some expatriates that the government was an obstacle to their important, well-planned projects. Successful projects for many, usually measured by achievement of narrowly defined project outcomes, also meant the potential for promotion within their organizations. The frenetic pace of expatriate professional lives starkly contrasted with the inertia felt within provincial health offices where poorly paid health staff often found little motivation to show up, let alone invest significant energy in their work (although many did). Many expatriate workers expressed frustration at the perceived slower pace of their government counterparts who were seen as barriers to project success.

The Aid Patronage System: Coordinating Aid to the Health Sector

Because Mozambique had a relatively well-developed PHC network and set of community health programs, many foreign agencies sought to graft their projects onto the health system. Others created parallel projects outside the health system. The most popular of the government programs chosen for support were those in maternal-child health such as traditional birth attendant (TBA) trainings and prenatal care, mobile immunization brigades, nutrition and growth monitoring, AIDS prevention, and health education. In order to manage the confusing array of aid program interests in the province, one provincial health directorate called an annual meeting each January of all foreign agencies with interests in funding specific programs, usually primary health care–oriented, in the province's annual plan. Most foreign agencies arrived at the meeting with programs and pet projects approved by their donors or head offices, with very specific objectives and targets that would be evaluated to ensure their own continued funding. Most expatriate program coordinators were under pressure to meet their individual targets before their next formal evaluations conducted by their individual donors. This pressure drove individual coordinators, including me, to promote their own agendas and interventions, whether or not they made sense in the overall provincial plan.

The special annual meeting with NGOs and agencies provided an opportunity for all the provincial players in the health sector to sort out who would support which programs. For example, if several NGOs wanted to support mobile vaccination brigades, which was often the case, their support could be rationally allocated during the meeting to different districts to avoid overlap. However, in practice, behind-the-scenes deal making and turf struggles among foreign agencies actually dominated the coordination process. The deal making nearly always hinged on the provision of extra financial benefits to health service workers in a new aid-specific patronage system. These strategies were generally considered temporary alternative ways to augment salaries that nearly everyone in the aid community and the health system acknowledged were far too low. However, these special benefits were also used to sway DPS program heads to support one NGO's program over another in turf conflicts. These conflicts were frequent and disruptive, and in spite of the ritual calls for better NGO coordination during the annual meeting, nearly everything about the circumstances produced less coordination. DPS workers could play NGOs off one another and bargain for better deals, while NGO coordinators placed greater emphasis on achieving their program targets than supporting vaguely defined ideals of agency coordination.

The process of deal making, patronage, and foreign agency influence hinged on the use of several key incentives: per diems, seminar trainings with per diems attached, extra contracts for work tasks such as surveys conducted during off-hours, temporary topping off of salaries, and special travel opportunities for higher level staff to neighboring African countries and even to Europe. These direct incentives were often complemented by smaller favors, such as rides to work provided by foreign agency vehicles, and support for personal home construction. Many of these favors and benefits were provided by foreign workers in a spirit of support and compassion for Mozambican colleagues who could barely feed their families on their formal salaries. However, such favors were also frequently used for gaining support for agency programs and securing positive responses from health workers when projects were evaluated by donors.

Per diems, virtually never used during the earlier years of the national health system, gradually became necessary components of all field-based project work. Competition among agencies for access to health system workers contributed to inflationary pressures on the per diem rates. From 1992 to 1998, the average overnight per diem increased from about US$3 to nearly US$15 for midlevel health workers where one week of per diems, on average, yielded higher pay than a month's salary for many workers. Government and agency regulation was weak, and per diems thus became the best way for government health workers to augment their salaries in the face of government spending caps. As community health plans were developed each year, projects with per diems for numerous field visits away from home were often favored.

The per diem phenomenon had immediate detrimental effects on some routine community health programs. In the early postindependence period, mobile vaccination brigades initially relied on local communities to provide food and lodging to visiting vaccination teams. However, by the early 1990s, as salaries plummeted, large per diems were routinely paid to the mobile brigades. Foreign agencies vied for the opportunity to provide the brigades with funding for gasoline and per diems so that immunization coverage could be added to individual project achievements in selected districts. However, at times shortfalls led to some districts receiving insufficient funds for per diems, gasoline, or motorcycle repair, and mobile brigades would stop altogether. Health workers often refused to make trips without per diem payments, and unneeded personnel often accompanied brigades in order to receive the payments. The provincial head of immunizations became exasperated: "Nothing gets done without per diems anymore. People won't even show up for a training at their own health post if there isn't a per diem attached."

The per diem problem was intensified by a proliferation of seminars and training for health workers in the annual provincial plan; training was usually designed to upgrade skills for involvement in foreign agency projects. Health workers eagerly supported seminars because they often involved one- to two-week periods away from home for which per diems would be paid. As mentioned earlier, for most pay levels in the system, one week of per diems was worth more than a month's salary. This proliferation of seminars was jokingly referred to by planners as *seminarite* in Portuguese (i.e., seminaritis). Seminars allowed agencies to claim that they were "capacity building" and training local workers, while the training per diems provided crucial salary augmentation for local workers, so there was little incentive by either side to reduce the number of trainings. The seminars also pulled workers away from their routine duties leading to major gaps in key activities such as patient consultation, data collection, supervision visits, and reporting.

Most foreign projects included baseline studies, surveys of target communities, evaluations, and additional project activities outside the scope of normal health worker duties. Foreign agencies regularly hired key health system staff to work on these extra activities offering lucrative contracts. A standard payment in 1998 for one day's work on a survey was US$25, almost equivalent to half an entire month's salary for midlevel workers. The contracts could provide valuable training to the workers, but they also drew health staff away from their routine duties.

One organization that worked within the DPS in one province made additional contributions to the salaries of higher level health workers, ostensibly to compensate them for the extra work they would have to do to participate in the foreign agency's activities. An agency also provided travel to Europe for top provincial personnel to visit the home offices of the donor organization. Travel opportunities outside the province or to neighboring African countries, ostensibly for work purposes, were extended to higher level provincial personnel who could accumulate significant per diem income from the trips. Such favors and incentives could be seen as providing valuable experiences and important salary supports. But in the context of foreign agency competition and health worker competition for benefits, these practices were often part of endless negotiations and power plays around health project promotion. And as Pavignani and Durão state,

> The variety of topping-up, subsidies, incentives, part-time private practice, grants, per diems has reached enormous proportions, and one may wonder if the global cost of these transactions is not approaching, even surpassing, the bill that would be paid by the treasury if the salary levels were adjusted to acceptable levels. (1999:12).

As a result of participation in NGO-sponsored seminars, travel, surveys, evaluations, and other activities, the DPS offices began to empty out. By 1998, there were weeks in which no community health program heads conducted routine health system work; all were either conducting NGO sponsored surveys or attending training seminars put on by NGOs to prepare for NGO projects.

Some Mozambican health workers in the province were lured out of the DPS by high salaries to work for NGOs. NGO salaries for trained health professionals ranged from US$500 to US$1,500 per month, compared to the US$50 monthly wage for midlevel staff in the NHS. In one year of work for an NGO, one could potentially earn the equivalent of 20 years' salary in the NHS, so retirement benefits and job security in the NHS could not motivate workers to stay. Jealousy and conflict within the DPS surrounded any speculation that a DPS worker was being wooed for an NGO position. I was contacted discreetly on many occasions by counterparts in the DPS seeking work. Careers in the NHS paled in comparison to a professional life within the well-maintained offices, new cars, high salaries, and social status associated with NGO positions.

Health Outcomes in the NGO Era

Measuring the impact of this NGO model on actual health outcomes and indicators is extremely difficult. The period of greatest NGO support to the health sector corresponded with the end of the war and the reconstruction of the health infrastructure in formerly RENAMO-held areas throughout the country. Access to health services increased across the country because these areas became accessible, workers were redeployed, and health posts rebuilt, so estimates of health care utilization, coverage, and some health indicators improved as would be expected in a period of recovery from war (Mozambique Ministry of Health 1997). Unquestionably, the funds and resources that flowed into the province had many positive effects on the system. However, the more appropriate question becomes: if the millions of aid dollars had been provided directly to the NHS to increase salaries, improve health worker conditions, strengthen systems of accountability, and more rationally allocate resources, would there have been even better coverage, service quality, and health outcomes? Disentangling the effects of poor coordination and fragmentation caused by foreign agencies on health outcomes from the range of other factors influencing health during this period of sweeping change is a difficult, if not impossible, challenge. There is, however, so much qualitative evidence and general agreement among veterans of the NHS that it is difficult to dispute that the fragmentation caused by disjointed aid projects had a lasting impact on health service effectiveness. In the short term, reduced mobile vaccination brigades, poorer treatment of patients by demoralized health workers, pharmaceutical shortages, loss of skilled personnel, under-the-table payments for free services, absenteeism from regular duties, and a host of other systemic dysfunctions have clearly undermined NHS effectiveness in ways that may have offset the positive impact of foreign aid.

Discussion

The Kaya Kwanga Code of Conduct agreement signals a recognition among the major actors in international health of the confusion, corruption, and fragmentation of health services fomented by the flood of foreign NGOs and agencies into Mozambique. However, the actual intent of the donors in signing on is difficult to interpret. Is the nonbinding code an empty strategic gesture to stave off the considerable criticism of foreign aid activity in Mozambique that has mounted in recent years? Or is it the product of compromise among the various international actors whose ideological positions on privatization range from social democratic support for state services among Scandinavian donors to the free market extremism of USAID? If taken at face value, the Kaya Kwanga document appears to be a significant attempt to rein in foreign agencies and strengthen the state sector by addressing the kinds of abuses outlined in the preceding vignette. Indeed, the World Bank has recently retreated somewhat in its advocacy of private sector health services and has proposed modest increases in state health budgets, often linked to debt forgiveness strategies (World Bank 1997, 2000a, 2000b). Mozambique has been allowed to gradually redirect more resources to the NHS since 1996 (Fauvet 2000).

While the change in rhetoric in the Code of Conduct is welcome, one may remain skeptical whether the new commitments are sincere or will even be implemented. The ongoing promotion of privatization both within the health sector and, more generally, the economy will further reinforce a two-tiered provision of health care that siphons off resources and personnel from the public system and thus undermines morale, commitment, and organizational capacity. The current World Bank position proposes that free or low-cost public sector services be provided only to the poorest "vulnerable" populations, while private sector services should be available to those who are able to pay. NGOs continue to figure prominently in the bank's "public-private partnership" discourse. Since the Code of Conduct document is nonbinding and a great deal of funding will still be channeled through NGOs without any means of "code" enforcement, the same structural incentives for expatriates to engage in aid abuses in the field will outweigh any costs to violating these new rules. In interviews, several veterans of the NHS expressed skepticism that the code will change behavior, arguing that too much damage has already been done to the health system's autonomy and integrity through loss of key personnel, morale, and feelings of loyalty. The intervention may be too little, too late.

The Kaya Kwanga agreement developed out of a broader ongoing planning process that seeks to better coordinate aid projects in the health sector through what is known as the Sector Wide Approach to Programming (SWAp) (Walt et al. 1999). However, a closer look at the Mozambican experience suggests that better coordination schemes, while urgently needed, will only have limited impact on the fragmentation of primary health care. The source of the dysfunctions lies deeper in the social structure of international aid itself in poor countries: that is, multiple competing private entities (i.e., NGOs), managed by ambitious expatriate coordinators with large budgets, working alongside underpaid demoralized public sector counterparts in local environments of intensifying social inequality, exclusion, and poverty. Rather than contributing to "civil society," these circumstances have lead to decidedly uncivil behavior.

Since the seminal 1978 Alma Ata Health for All conference, medical anthropologists have worked extensively within international aid agencies, including NGOs, to help build primary health care programs. But most applied research has focused on the culture and behavior of poor target populations, rather than the behavior and beliefs of providers. But now with equity-oriented PHC systems unraveling in the push for privatization, the role of NGOs demands more critical scrutiny that medical anthropologists can best provide. Positioned as culture brokers in the world of international aid, anthropologists can systematically examine firsthand the social and health impact of NGO activity in specific settings. They may find that in many cases, NGOs and their expatriate managers have not brought health care more efficiently and effectively to poor communities. And hopefully they will vigorously advocate for a rechanneling of aid to equity-oriented public sector health care in desperate need of a lifeline.

References

Anang, F. T. (1994). "Evaluating the Role and Impact of Foreign NGOs in Ghana." In *The Changing Politics of Non-Governmental Organizations and African States*, edited by E. Sandberg, 101–20. Westport, CT: Praeger.

Buse, K., and G. Walt (1996). "Aid Coordination for Health Sector Reform: A Conceptual Framework for Analysis and Assessment. *Health Policy* 38: 173–87.

———. (1997). "An Unruly Melange? Coordinating External Resources to the Health Sector: A Review." *Social Science & Medicine* 45, no. 3: 449–63.

Chabot, J., J. W. Harnmeijer, and P. H. Streefland. (1996). *African Primary Health Care in Times of Turbulence*. Amsterdam, the Netherlands: Royal Tropical Institute.

Cliff, J. (1993). "Donor Dependence or Donor Control? The Case of Mozambique." *Community Development Journal* 28, no. 3: 237–44.

Coreil, J., and Mull, D. (1990). *Anthropology and Primary Health Care.* Boulder, CO: Westview.

Crewe, E., and E. Harrison. 1998. *Whose Development? An Ethnography of Aid.* London: Zed Books.

De Beyer, J. A., A. S. Preker, and R. G. Feachem. (2000). "The Role of the World Bank in International Health: Renewed Commitment and Partnership." *Social Science & Medicine* 50, no. 2: 169–76.

Drabek, A. G. (1987). "Development Alternatives: The Challenge for NGOs—An Overview of the Issues." *World Development* 15, supplement: ix–xv.

Edwards, M., and Hulme, D. (1996a). "Too Close for Comfort? The Impact of Official Aid on Non-Governmental Organizations." *World Development* 24, no. 6: 961–73.

———. (1996b). "Introduction." In *Beyond the Magic Bullet: NGO Performance and Accountability in the Post-Cold War World,* edited by M. Edwards and D. Hulme, 1–22. West Hartford, CT: Kumarian.

Escobar, A. (1995). *Encountering Development: The Making and Unmaking of the Third World.* Princeton, NJ: Princeton University Press.

Fauvet, P. (2000). "Mozambique: Growth with Poverty, a Difficult Transition from Prolonged War to Peace and Development." *Africa Recovery* 14, no. 3: 12–19.

Ferguson, J. (1994). *The Anti-Politics Machine: Development, Depoliticization, and Bureaucratic Power in Lesotho.* Minneapolis: University of Minnesota Press.

Fisher, W. (1997). "Doing Good? The Politics and Antipolitics of NGO Practices." *Annual Reviews in Anthropology* 26: 439–64.

Foster, G. (1977). "Medical Anthropology and International Health Planning." *Social Science & Medicine* 11: 527–34.

Gary, I. (1996). "Confrontation, Co-operation or Co-optation: NGOs and the Ghanaian State during Structural Adjustment." *Review of African Political Economy* 68: 149–68.

Gilson, L. P., D. Sen, S. Mohammed, and P. Mujinja. (1994). "The Potential of Health Sector Non-Governmental Organizations: Policy Options." *Health Policy and Planning* 9, no. 1: 14–24.

Gloyd, S. (1996, Spring). "NGOs and the 'SAP'ing of Health Care in Rural Mozambique. *Hesperian Foundation News*: 1.

Green, A., and Matthias, A. (1997). *Non-Governmental Organizations and Health in Developing Countries.* New York: St. Martin's.

Grillo, R., and R. Stirrat, eds. (1997). *Discourses of Development: Anthropological Perspectives.* Oxford: Berg.

Hanlon, J. (1996). *Peace without Profit: How the IMF Blocks Rebuilding in Mozambique.* Portsmouth, NH: Heinemann.

INE (Instituto Nacional de Estatistica). (1999). *II Recenseamento Geral da População e Habitação, 1997: Provincia de Manica (Second General Census: Manica Province).* Maputo: Government of Mozambique.

Justice, J. (1987). "The Bureaucratic Context of International Health: A Social Scientist's View." *Social Science & Medicine* 25, no. 12: 1301–1306.

Kim, J. Y., J. V. Millen, A. Irwin, J. Gershman, eds. (2000). *Dying for Growth: Global Inequality and the Health of the Poor.* Monroe, ME: Common Courage Press.

Laurell, A. C., and O. L. Arellano. (1996). "Market Commodities and Poor Relief: The World Bank Proposal for Health." *International Journal of Health Services* 26, no. 1: 1–18.

Markowitz, L. (2001). "Finding the Field: Notes on the Ethnography of NGOs." *Human Organization* 60, no. 1: 40–46.

Mburu, F. M. (1989). "Non-Government Organizations in the Health Field: Collaboration, Integration, and Contrasting Aims in Africa." *Social Science & Medicine* 29, no. 5: 591–97.

Mozambique Ministry of Health. (1997). *Mozambique Demographic and Health Survey*. Maputo: Mozambique Ministry of Health and Macro International.

———. (2000). *The Kaya Kwanga Commitment: A Code of Conduct to Guide the Partnership for Health Development in Mozambique*. Maputo: Mozambique Ministry of Health.

Ndengwa, S. N. (1996). *The Two Faces of Civil Society: NGOs and Politics in Africa*. West Hartford, CT: Kumarian.

Nichter, M. (1996). "The Primary Health Care System as a Social System: Primary Health Care, Social Status, and the Issue of Team-Work in South Asia." In *Anthropology and International Health: Asian Case Studies*, edited by M. Nichter and M. Nichter, 367–92. Amsterdam: Gordon and Breach.

Okuonzi, S., and Macrae, J. (1995). "Whose Policy Is It Anyway? International and National Influences on Health Policy Development in Uganda." *Health Policy and Planning* 10, no. 2: 122–32.

Pavignani, E., and J. R. Durão. (1999). "Managing External Resources in Mozambique: Building New Aid Relationships on Shifting Sands?" *Health Policy and Planning* 14, no. 3: 243–53.

Powell, M., and D. Seddon. (1997). "NGOs and the Development Industry." *Review of African Political Economy* 71: 3–10.

Stewart, S. (1997). "Happy Ever After in the Market Place: Non-Government Organizations and Uncivil Society." *Review of African Political Economy* 71: 11–34.

Turshen, M. (1999). *Privatizing Health Services in Africa*. New Brunswick, NJ: Rutgers.

United Nations Development Programme (UNDP). (1998). *National Human Development Report on Mozambique*. Oxford: Oxford University Press.

U.S. Agency for International Development (USAID). (1995). *Policy Guidance: USAID–U.S. PVO Partnership*. Washington, DC: USAID.

Uvin, P. (1998). *Aiding Violence: The Development Enterprise in Rwanda*. West Hartford, CT: Kumarian.

Walt, G., and A. Melamed. (1983). *Toward a People's Health Service*. London: Zed Books.

Walt, G., E. Pavignani, L. Gilson, and K. Buse. (1999). "Managing External Resources in the Health Sector: Are There Lessons for SWAPs?" *Health Policy and Planning* 14, no. 3: 273–84.

World Bank. (1993). *World Development Report: Investing in Health*. Washington, DC: World Bank.

———. (1997). *Health, Nutrition, and Population Sector Strategy Paper*. Washington, DC: World Bank.

———. (2000a). *The World Bank–Civil Society Relations: Fiscal 1999 Progress Report.* Washington, DC: World Bank.

———. (2000b). *World Development Report 2000/2001.* Oxford: Oxford University Press.

Wuyts, M. (1996). "Foreign Aid, Structural Adjustment, and Public Management: The Mozambican Experience." *Development and Change* 27: 717–49.

Zaidi, S. A. (1999). "NGO Failure and the Need to Bring Back the State." *Journal of International Development* 11: 259–71.

Primary Health Care since Alma Ata: Lost in the Bretton Woods?

4

JOAN E. PALUZZI

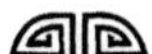

Governments have a responsibility for the health of their people which can be fulfilled only by the provision of adequate health and social measures. A main social target of governments, international organizations and the whole world community in the coming decades should be the attainment by all peoples of the world by the year 2000 of a level of health that will permit them to lead a socially and economically productive life. Primary health care is the key to attaining this target as part of development in the spirit of social justice.

—DECLARATION OF ALMA ATA, SEPTEMBER 12, 1978[1]

ENDORSED BY THE WORLD HEALTH ORGANIZATION (WHO) Executive Board in 1979, the Member States of the World Health Assembly ratified the Declaration of Alma Ata as a foundation for the formulation of national health strategies based on systems of primary health care (PHC). In the 25 years since the declaration, health system design and management has continued to evolve, but we are, in many ways, at an even greater distance from the realization of the goals envisioned by the 1978 slogan, "Health for All by 2000."

Since the formation of the World Bank (WB) and the International Monetary Fund (IMF) at the Bretton Woods Summit in 1944, donors and lenders have continued to wield increasing power in the international community. In a world where the survival of impoverished countries and their governments is almost universally defined at the international level by their ability to enter into and participate in global markets, the power of donors/lenders (who define the parameters of market participation and debt management) is felt at every level.

Notably, since the 1970s, the impact of multilateral funding agencies such as the WB, the IMF, and bilateral donors such as the U.S. Agency for International Development (USAID) on international public health policy has moved beyond the arena of influence to one of domination. Now controlled to a significant degree by economists, private insurers, and bankers, it should come as no surprise that health care and, consequently, health itself have become commodified. Through the reproduction of larger, dominant socioeconomic hierarchies within the health sector, the ability to obtain and mobilize fiscal resources has become a key determinant of the ability of individuals, communities, and countries to obtain the essential services and goods needed to maintain health and to treat disease or injury.

Understanding the ways in which critical health care policy continues to be driven by financial institutions with larger, market-based, reform agendas (rather than by physicians, public health personnel, nurses, and other health care experts) permits a clearer understanding of the ways in which dominant global health policy can often become more of an obstacle than a facilitator of good health.

After a brief summary of the historical impact and consequences of the global monetary institutions on health policies in selected regions, an examination of vertical and integrated (also referred to as primary system) approaches to health care will serve as an effective lens through which to examine the current state of international health care. While often presented as an "either/or" dichotomy, the reality is that there is interdependency between the two models as well as great promise in the promotion of their collaboration and partnership.

Situating Health Care within Neoliberal Reform: A Procrustean Sick Bed

The utilization of neoliberal policies and economic reforms, known since the 1980s as structural adjustment policies (SAPs)—and most recently reincarnated as poverty reduction strategies—occurs throughout all sectors of societies, including health care systems. As is the case in the larger socioeconomic context, neoliberal policies within the health sector almost inevitably increase the hardship experienced by the most disadvantaged members of societies (Kim et al. 2000; Field, David, Kotz, and Bukhman 2000).

The designers of SAPs readily admitted from the onset that there would be some initial negative impact ("belt-tightening") as the result of adjustment, but few spoke openly that this negative impact could last for decades. By 1995, none of the 88 countries that adopted adjustment as the condition for their ability to obtain loans was on the WB's projected schedule (Abbasi 1999).

Two of the most pervasive trends within the context of structural adjustment health-sector reform have been toward the privatization of health services and the institution of fee-for-service policies in public sectors. The damaging impact of these policies has been repeatedly documented: during a Structural Adjustment Participatory Review Initiative (SAPRI) conference, the representatives from Ghana reported, "The poor are simply being priced out of hospital care, and a two-tiered health-care system now exists, with better facilities for those who can afford to pay. Once again, women often bear the brunt of these policies" (Ghana 1998). The 1999 SAPRI conference to review the impact of reform in Zimbabwe was harsh in its assessment of the consequences of structural adjustment:

> The World Bank acknowledged that structural adjustment has failed to achieve macroeconomic stability in Zimbabwe and has resulted in a falling standard of living for many, particularly members of urban households. The percentage of those households classified as poor rose from 40 percent in 1991 to 60 percent in 1995, and average consumption levels dropped by 25 percent. Cutbacks in public expenditures have also negated achievements in health and education made during the first decade of independence (before the implementation of structural adjustment), according to the Bank (Zimbabwe 1999).

David Simmons (2002), in his ethnographic examination of the extent and consequences of structural adjustment policies on health and health services in Zimbabwe, details examples of public hospitals unable to supply critically needed services and medications; of overworked, poorly compensated physicians and nurses leaving the country to work elsewhere; and of changing patterns of health care–seeking behaviors, including the correlation of decreased visits by women and their children, with the introduction of user fees. This overall degradation in health services was accompanied by increasing rates and levels of malnutrition, increasing unemployment, and crowded, deficient housing, and has led to the embodiment of structural adjustment and its consequences "as a biological event" (Simmons 2002:94).

User fees and general privatization trends are not the only apparent neoliberal influences within the healthcare sector. For example, Waitzkin (2003) maintains that, through its advocacy of vertical programs, WHO "has diverted attention from its priority of encouraging more responsive national systems. In particular, WHO's goal of 'health for all' has given way to advocacy of narrower interventions envisioned as effective in contributing to economic growth" (1478). The global funding spotlight is firmly fixed on the vertical model of health care provision, and its glare threatens to render invisible other critical issues, particularly the universal need for sound primary health care systems.

Vertical Programs

Vertical programs are narrowly focused, centrally administered, and usually "top-down" in the development of protocols and policies. The programs are typically designed around the treatment and prevention of one specific disease, such as HIV/AIDS or tuberculosis (TB), or around a specialized health issue (for example, reproductive counseling and services). There is little room for modifications or local adaptations in the program regimens. One of the most widely used examples of this type of program is directly observed treatment, short-course (DOTS), which is utilized throughout much of the world for the treatment of tuberculosis.

Vertical programs are attractive to donors; they are clearly delimited, well defined, and the results are amenable to quantification. Most vertical programs can predict with accuracy the cost per patient (or "unit" cost) of treatment, which in turn facilitates budgetary planning, funding, and accountability. Program outcomes can also be relatively easy to quantify. Staff members are supposedly highly specialized and the programs are thought to be effective precisely because their narrow focus permits concentrated resources and attention to a single, targeted problem. However, the reality is that in most low-resource settings, both facilities and personnel must be utilized for a wide variety of health issues, including (but certainly not limited to) the concurrent administration of multiple vertical programs. The lack of formal recognition of this fact by the international agencies that design and implement vertical programs prevents the development of practical, reality-based assistance and support to these overextended health care providers.

Treatment provision that emerges from direct experience and operational research inevitably reflects the need for integration: for example, in rural Haiti, components of the directly observed therapy model developed for the treatment of TB have been successfully implemented in this resource-poor setting for the complex treatment of multidrug-resistant tuberculosis (MDR-TB); (Farmer, Kim, Mitnick, and Timperi 1999; Mitnick et al. 2003). Continuing to expand services in response to the needs of the same communities, the practical experience and operational elements utilized in the treatment of TB and MDR-TB were incorporated into the treatment of AIDS (Farmer, Léandre, Mukherjee, Claude, et al. 2001). Rather than separate, vertical programs, these are critically important elements of the wide-ranging health services that are now available to individuals on the Central Plateau of Haiti. Major infectious diseases, as well as the myriad other diseases, illnesses, and injuries that can be directly correlated to the conditions of poverty, are fully integrated into the lives of individuals, families, and communities. The response to these threats must be equally integrated.

With the creation of initiatives, such as the Global Fund to Fight AIDS, Tuberculosis and Malaria, the narrow, vertical treatment paradigm will be increasingly rewarded as funding to implement programs for these diseases will now be more accessible to many low-income settings. However, with the inflow of resources for the treatment of these diseases into the parts of the world suffering the highest burden of diseases and poverty, there is also an unprecedented opportunity to combine administrative and infrastructure costs and to cross-train (and adequately compensate) health workers—in other words, to use vertical treatment programs to "seed" the development, expansion, and support of comprehensive, primary health systems.

Integrated (Primary Health Care) Systems

Integrated approaches are best understood as comprehensive or primary health care (PHC) systems. Pushing the treatment boundaries outward while still maintaining the focused intervention associated with a vertical program for the treatment of AIDS in rural Haiti has demonstrated the importance of approaches that are both integrated and comprehensive.

> The rapid spread of HIV demands a comprehensive global AIDS strategy that includes prevention, testing, and counseling, the treatment of opportunistic infections, and the use of HAART. Social assistance to families and communities affected by HIV is also critical. For most of the hardest hit communities, AIDS is the latest in a long line of health threats. The greatest of these are poverty and inequality, both of which are co-factors for and consequences of HIV transmission. If HIV reveals a lack of basic primary care services for the poor, an aggressive response to this comparatively new disease may help to solve a host of old problems (Farmer, Léandre, Mukherjee, Gupta, et al. 2001 :1149).

In the midst of the HIV/AIDS and tuberculosis pandemics and the impetus to deal with the crises they have engendered, the fact that these diseases are just two of the many health issues confronting people living in developing countries has frequently been lost from the larger view. Integrated systems provide a broad range of health care services, oriented not only to the treatment of acute and chronic illnesses, but also to the provision of education and prevention programs. These are the types of programs that address broader issues such as nutrition, hygiene, and maternal and well-child care. The Alma Ata Declaration extensively detailed the essentials of an integrated health system that included elements that were politically, economically, and culturally appropriate to their respective communities and based on current scientific research and experience. Other critical aspects of an integrated primary system include the utilization and development of local human resources and the appropriate interface with "related societal sectors such as agricultural, animal husbandry, food, education, housing, public works, and communications" (World Health Organization 1978).

Connecting Vertical/Horizontal Programs: The Chilean Case

The symbiotic relationship between vertical and horizontal approaches to health care was demonstrated during fieldwork conducted on the experience of individuals who were diagnosed with TB in Southern Chile during the year 2000 (Paluzzi 2002). By the early 1970s, Chile (along with Cuba and Uruguay) was one of the first countries in the world to adopt the strategy that would later become known as DOTS for the treatment of tuberculosis on a national level. Developed from the "best practice" experiences and research in countries such as India and later refined by Dr. Karel Styblo in Tanzania, ten other African countries, and Nicaragua during the 1960s and 1970s, DOTS was formally adopted by WHO as a global treatment strategy in the early 1990s.

The history of TB in latter twentieth-century Chile is a story of remarkable success. However, early in the first half of the century, the country had the highest reported incidence of TB-related deaths in the world. In this pre-antibiotic era, the official estimate of deaths from TB (for the year 1938) was reported to be 248 per 100,000. Dr. Salvador Allende, later president of Chile and, during this era, minister of health, estimated that only about half of the deaths were actually reported. In the far southern and northern regions of the country, characterized by extreme climates and overwhelming poverty, the numbers of reported deaths due to TB were even higher, ranging from 475 to 535 per 100,000 (Allende 1999). Even before the widespread introduction of antibiotics, some inroads in reducing the toll from the disease were made with the introduction of progressive social reforms that addressed the conditions of poverty within which much of Chile's emerging urban working class struggled (Magallanes 1935; Marín Rojas 1934). With the discovery of streptomycin in 1943 and the rapid developments of biomedical science, the mainstream medical vision increased in depth, but its breadth was diminished as large-scale social reform was not seen as part of the mainstream biomedical agenda.

By the mid-1950s, the death rate from TB began to decrease dramatically; by 1960, the mortality incidence was reported to be 53.2 per 100,000 (Ministerio de Salud 1996). Some dedicated facilities, including a few Andean mountain sanatoriums, existed in the pre-antibiotics/DOTS era; but with the founding of the Chilean National Health System (NHS) in 1952, TB treatment was integrated into the NHS by utilizing existing hospitals, rural posts, and urban clinics for inpatient care and subsequently for outpatient treatment. However, it remained a centrally regulated program with detailed, standardized treatment and reporting as well as dedicated staff and treatment areas.

Unlike most of the industrialized world, including the United States, Chile did not experience a resurgence in TB cases during the late 1980s and early 1990s. There were several factors to account for this, not the least of which was a well-established TB treatment program whose committed advocates in the Ministry of Health had managed to keep the program going—throughout this tumultuous time in Chile's history—even as the NHS became increasingly threatened due to privatization and its impact on public health funding. Prior to the neoliberal economic reforms initiated by the military dictatorship after the coup of 1973, the NHS was supported largely through a universal 7 percent tax on formal-sector earnings. Since the mid-1980s, the Chilean health system has witnessed a dramatic increase in privatization. With the advent of private health insurers that function similar to HMOs in the United States, working Chileans are given the option of allocating their 7 percent to a private health plan. Most of the highest wage earners have opted into the private system, and the result has been what one Chilean health worker referred to as "our 15-year crisis."

Over 70 percent of Chileans still continue to rely upon the NHS that has now been stripped of the health-tax contribution from the highest wage earners (ISAPRE 2000). Additionally, a system of weighted (based on income) user fees was instituted within the NHS. Indigent individuals and those in the lowest (i.e., less than US$200 per month) economic strata were not required to pay the fees. However, the 10 percent charge for services levied on individuals making from US$200 to 300 per month and the 20 percent co-payment for anyone earning more than US$300 per month often represents a genuine hardship for many of these individuals.

The interdependency between the vertical nationalized treatment program and primary care within the NHS was evident during interviews conducted with 59 patients currently enrolled in the NTP in the Ninth Region of southern Chile. Because of the consistency of the NTP and the relatively low rate of abandonment in this region of the country, antecedent histories (the history of the illness prior to its diagnosis as TB) were obtained as a way of exploring differential attitudes, outcomes, or both. Relevant to this discussion were the frequencies of delays in diagnosis. People with symptoms that were ultimately diagnosed as tuberculosis were dependent upon the primary health care system for initial diagnosis and referral into the NTP. However, 41 percent of the patients interviewed who presented to clinics, hospitals, and emergency rooms within the NHS with respiratory symptoms of at least three weeks' duration experienced delays in testing for and diagnosis of their TB. The delays ranged from four to twenty-four weeks, with an average delay of around twelve weeks.

Many of them described multiple and repeated visits to the overcrowded public clinic, where they were seen and given antibiotics to treat "a cold," then sent home without any diagnostic tests. Segundo, a 55-year-old carpenter, related his experience in the primary system:

> I started to cough in May. It was terrible, I would cough, cough, cough and I had this pain in my back. . . . I saw a doctor in the *comuna* where I was working in early June, he gave me some pills and said I had a bad cold. But I continued to feel very bad. . . . I was finally too sick to work. I went to the *consultorio* three more times. The doctor would examine my back and take my blood pressure and give me more medicine, but nothing worked. On the second visit, they told me to get a chest x-ray but I could never get a number at the hospital so they told me to go to the private hospital . . . a private hospital that costs money. So there I am trying to fill out all of the paper work to get approval for the x-ray and all the time I was feeling sicker and sicker. I never did get an x-ray until after they finally ordered a sputum test in August. I got a message to return to the *consultorio* immediately, this time, another doctor examined me and I knew it was something serious because he walked in wearing a face mask.

Don Segundo's history highlights the consequences of the inevitable intersection between a faltering primary health care system and an effective (vertical) treatment program. He continued returning to the clinic long after the time when his persisting respiratory symptoms and weight loss should have been a red flag that signaled the need to do a sputum smear. He was finally referred into the TB treatment program, and within three weeks of initiating treatment he reported that he had begun to gain weight and felt "like myself again."

Just as the primary health system relies upon the NTP to maintain high standards of specialized care for individuals diagnosed with TB, without active case finding, the TB program remains dependent upon the frequently overwhelmed primary system to diagnosis and refer infected individuals into the treatment program. Obstacles and deficiencies in one of the systems will become related obstacles and deficiencies within the other.

"Planting" Vertical Programs within Primary Health Care

Chile's wider experience is illustrative of the damaging impact of privatization on a functioning primary health care system. But in much of the developing world, the issue is that primary health care is not available in any form to millions of individuals. The recent increases in funding for vertical interventions, targeted specifically at the "big" infectious diseases such as HIV/AIDS, TB, and malaria in the world's poorest countries, provide us with an unprecedented opportunity to use these programs as the cores around which primary systems can be developed and sustained. The integration of HIV/AIDS with other health system elements, including TB programs, has become an increasing focus of attention (Castro et al. 2003; Hirschel 2001).

With the increasing attention to the need to integrate vertical programs, there has been a renewed focus on the lessons of the past. For example, Céline Gounder (1998) notes that a 1950s global initiative that eventually failed (the Malaria Eradication Program) was characterized by a separate, exclusively dedicated health infrastructure rather than any effort to integrate it into existing primary systems. This creation of parallel, separate systems created serious problems when it later became apparent that cooperation across health care sectors would be necessary (Gounder 1998). Further, careful planning is essential in any effort to integrate vertical programs lest the characteristics and quality controls responsible for the programs' successes become lost during the process.

In terms of providing treatment and follow-up for chronic and acute injuries and health problems, preventative modalities, emergency services, and educational programs, a functioning primary health system is clearly the superior model. In addition to its general and wide-ranging health care services, a PHC system could incorporate a vertical program into its existing structure; the same cannot be said of a vertical program that, by definition, cannot incorporate comprehensive primary health care services into its narrow treatment strategy.

Briggs, Capdegelle, and Garner (2003) undertook a review seeking to elaborate, among other issues, the factors that made integration successful (or not). They note the paucity of large, high-quality studies that have compared the efficacy of vertical or integrated approaches to health services in middle- and low-income countries. None of the studies they reviewed met all criteria in terms of randomization, generalizability, or consistent inclusion of data: all of which were seen by the reviewers as essential in making any definitive determination. Of the four studies they reviewed, there was "no consistent pattern of benefit"; for example, one study demonstrated a clear benefit to integration (mainly in terms of cost savings), whereas another compared integration unfavorably with vertical programs. Clearly, more work is ahead of us on this critically important topic.

Obstacles and Challenges: The HIV/AIDS Pandemic

One of the most profound obstacles to the implementation and development of universal primary health care has been the HIV/AIDS pandemic. But it is also seen as an opportunity to strengthen health systems (Castro et al. 2003). The epidemic in developing countries has overwhelmed existing health care systems with the sheer number of those infected and the severity of their illnesses, including its deadly synergy with tuberculosis. In many of the countries most affected, there are neither the resources necessary to provide treatment for opportunistic infections nor for the antiretroviral drugs needed to treat AIDS. It has cut a wide swath through the African sub-Saharan region, lowering national life expectancies, leaving millions of orphans, and pushing existing health systems well beyond their limits. The disease continues to take a wide toll on the human and economic resources necessary to build and support social systems, including primary care services, throughout these societies (Wehrwein 2000).

Both primary care systems and vertical programs have suffered from a profound shortage of human resources that can also be attributed, in part, to the AIDS epidemic. In the countries with the highest rates of infection and death, there has been the loss of doctors, nurses, and other health workers to the plague (Atulomah and Oladepo 2002; Gounden and Moodley 2000). Other factors that contribute to this shortage include the emigration of physicians and nurses from developing countries to the United States, Canada, and Europe, often as a response to inadequate wages and the deterioration of health services and infrastructures. In the Eastern Cape Province of South Africa, a 1997 report detailed a doctor-patient ratio of 1:40,000 in the rural areas of that province (Channel Africa 1997).

Defining and Guarding the "Territory"

Although less marked in the social sciences than in medicine, there is a tendency to reify the current global epidemics as if they were isolated islands of human tragedy amid the day-to-day existence of people living within the "real" world. This demarcation of the international health "territory" is evident in the paucity of crosscutting conferences and symposia; the clearly defined, and at times vociferously protected, territorialism of many of the largest international agencies; and the apparent blind spot that permits duplication of administrative, physical, and personnel infrastructures.

The incidence of infectious diseases of all kinds, euphemistically referred to as "tropical diseases," strongly correlates to the conditions of poverty, not just in terms of the ability to obtain treatment, but also in its higher occurrence in individuals who are increasingly vulnerable to infection because of their poverty. These diseases typically take their greatest toll among individuals in their prime, economically productive, and childbearing years, contributing to impoverishment not just of individuals and their families but also of communities and ultimately, in the most affected regions, to entire countries (Whiteside 2001).

In this age of widespread neoliberal reform, the correlation between the socioeconomic profiles of countries and the health and social features that describe the experience of its citizens is now an ubiquitous feature of the international public health discourse (see Table 4.1).

Table 4.1. Life Expectancy and Mortality Rates, by Country Development Category (1995–2000)

Development Category	*Population 1999 (Millions)*	*Annual Average Income (U.S. Dollars)*	*Life Expectancy at Birth*	*Infant Mortality < Age 1 per 1,000 Live Births*	*Under 5 Mortality Deaths before Age 5 per 1,000 Live Births*
Least Developed Countries	643	296	51	100	159
Other Low-Income Countries	1,777	538	59	80	120
Lower-Middle-Income Countries	2,094	1,200	70	35	39
Upper-Middle-Income Countries	573	4,900	71	26	35
High-Income Countries	891	25,730	78	6	6

Source: J. D. Sachs (2001), *Macroeconomics and Health: Investing in Health for Economic Development,* Report of the Commission on Macroeconomics and Health. Originally from UNDP, *Human Development Report 2001,* Table 8, and CMH calculations using World Development Indicators of the World Bank, 2001.

As egregious as these numbers are in their portrayal of world inequalities, the standard classifications of countries by annual average incomes render large numbers of the world's poorest individuals virtually invisible. Not evident in the global picture demonstrated in Table 4.1 are the intranational economic class disparities. For example, 88 countries out of 184 are classified by the World Bank as "upper- or lower-middle income," and these countries are frequently excluded from studies seeking to quantify the impact of poverty in the world. Three of these countries are Brazil, Venezuela, and Mexico. Table 4.2 details the income gaps of these countries.

Over 52 million people living in extreme poverty in these three countries alone will encounter the same higher health risks conditioned by their poverty as individuals living in "low-income" countries. The question remains whether their citizenship in a "middle income" country will mitigate the impact of poverty through the provision of a social "safety net" including the provision of primary care for the treatment of illness and injury. The very existence of such large numbers of people in extreme poverty would seemingly argue against the existence of an effective social welfare network. Here again, we see the intersections between health and recent international economic trends:

> Neo-liberals, I contend, are not particularly concerned about inequality or regard it either as a positive virtue or as inevitable or necessary. . . . The welfare state, in the neo-liberal view interferes with the "normal" functioning of the market (Coburn 2000:138).

Table 4.2. Income Gap and Profound Poverty in Countries Classified as "Upper and Lower Middle Income Economies" (1998)

Country (1998 Population[1])	*% Income Share Held by Highest 10%[1]*	*% Income Share Held by Lowest 20%[1]*	*Number of People in Lowest 20%[1]*	*People Subsisting on One Dollar[2] a Day[3]*
Brazil (165,926,200)	47	0.55	33,185,240	19,911,144
Mexico (95,222,340)	42	3.94	19,044,468	15,235,574
Venezuela (23,242,000)	36	2.98	4,648,400	5,345,660
Totals			56,878,108	40,492,378

1. Figures from World Bank (1998), *World Development Indicators* http://devdata.worldbank.org.ezp2.harvard.edu/dataonline (accessed April 12, 2004).
2. The value of "one dollar a day" as a realistic indicator of actual hardship continues to be criticized for, among other factors, its inability to measure depth of poverty as well as the general recognition that, in many urban areas, even two or three dollars a day is not sufficient to purchase essential goods and services.
3. Figures from the United Nations Department of Economic and Social Affairs, *Millennium Indicators Data Base,* http://unstats.un.org/unsd/ (accessed April 12, 2004).

Moving toward Solutions

The advantages of an integrated health system can be summarized as follows: it provides health care to all of the adults and children in a region, not simply those people suffering from a specific, life-threatening disease; it emerges from within communities and is therefore responsive to local health issues; it provides a permanent base from which treatment and prevention services can be maintained; and it optimizes the utilization of scarce human and fiscal resources by consolidating and cross-training. A well-functioning primary system also becomes the core of coordinated educational and disease-prevention outreach programs.

Vertical programs were in existence long before the arrival of SAPs on the international scene. They are highly effective within narrowly focused health contexts. But they cannot (and were never designed to) take the place of primary health care systems; rather, these systems should exist concurrently as mutually supportive, complementary models of health care delivery.

In its 2001 Health Sector Strategic Plan, Uganda joined a small but growing number of African countries that are seeking to revise policies that were implemented indiscriminately in an attempt to meet the conditions imposed by lending institutions: "As part of the Financing Strategy, the Government will also implement a revised fee-for-services policy which will seek to provide revenue for improving services whilst exempting poor and vulnerable groups" (Republic of Uganda 2001:93).

Because reform often originates on the national level as a response to pressure from lending and donor agencies, general efforts to counter the negative impact of these reforms will need to begin at that level as well. However, the importance of grassroots movements to pressure governments to be more responsive to the needs of its citizens will be vitally important. Further, there must be reform among the reformers: for example, economist Ozay Mehmet (1999) criticizes the continued imposition of Eurocentric models in developing countries:

> Sound theories of economic development need to be grounded in culture-specific reality, just as an infant learning to walk must have its feet on the ground. Such theories need to be constructed endogenously, inductively, rather than deductively, with open minds to learn about cross-cultural values, institutions and environments before prescribing policy interventions. In particular, economists must be willing to learn from past mistakes (5).

Creative, innovative solutions that address immediate health care needs, as well as the larger societal context in which they are occurring, must be sought. Funding for these interventions and health systems cannot realistically come from within deeply impoverished countries. As it stands now, the management of punishing national debt amounts to the imposition of a model analogous to the debtor's prisons of the past, creating cycles of dependency and hardship. Consistent support for initiatives such as the Global Fund and similar multinational initiatives is a promising start, as are the private/public partnerships that have emerged in recent years. But we do not have the luxury of time to move slowly toward the discovery of solutions:

> The choice before us is stark. We can accept a world of radical polarization between haves and have-nots, in which the calculus of cost-effectiveness determines that poor people must die of diseases for which the affluent are successfully treated as a matter of course. Or we can work for a world of solidarity, in which people from different backgrounds cooperate to mobilize resources and build the foundations of a dignified life for all, prioritizing the needs of the most vulnerable (Farmer 2003:xxiii).

Health care and health cannot be isolated from the larger socioeconomic context in which they occur: poverty both contributes to and is caused by poor health. Structural adjustment and neoliberal policies have worsened the quality of life among the world's poorest people and increased the number of people living in poverty. The long-term resolution of global inequalities will require fundamental, profound, and massive changes in policy at both national and international levels. One of the most profound legacies of Bretton Woods is our inability to see the trees in this forest: as we work toward finding the big solutions to the underlying socioeconomic issues, we must remain cognizant of the opportunities before us today to improve the quality of life for millions of individuals through the provision of primary health care and, ultimately, health for all.

Note

1. Accessed at www.who.int/hpr/NPH/docs/declaration_almaata.pdf (April 12, 2004).

References

Abbasi, K. (1999). "The World Bank and World Health: Under Fire." *British Medical Journal* 318, no. 7189: 1003–1006.

Allende Gossens, S. (1999). *La Realidad Médico-Social Chilena,* 2nd ed. Santiago de Chile: Editorial Cuarto Propio. (Originally published in 1939).

Atulomah, N. O., and O. Oladepo. (2002). "Knowledge, Perception and Practice with Regards to Occupational Risks of HIV/AIDS among Nursing and Midwifery Students in Ibadan, Nigeria." *African Journal of Medicine & Medical Sciences* 31, no. 3: 223–27.

Briggs, C. J., P. Capdegelle, and P. Garner. (2003). "Strategies for Integrating Primary Health Services in Middle- and Low-Income Countries." *Cochrane Database of Systematic Reviews* 1.

Castro, A., P. Farmer, J. Y. Kim, E. Levcovitz, D. López-Acuña, J. S. Mukherjee, et al. (2003). *Scaling Up Health Systems to Respond to the Challenge of HIV/AIDS in Latin America and the Caribbean.* Special Edition of the Health Sector Reform Initiative in Latin America and the Caribbean 8. Washington, DC: Pan American Health Organization, 100 pp.

Channel Africa. (1997). *Channel Africa News Service.* Accessed at www.sabc.co.za/units/chanafr/news/971013.htm.

Coburn, D. (2000). "Income Inequality, Social Cohesion, and the Health Status of Populations: The Role of Neo-Liberalism. *Social Science and Medicine* 51: 135–46.

Farmer, P. (2003). "Introduction." In *Global AIDS: Myths and Facts: Tools for Fighting the AIDS Pandemic,* edited by A. Irwin, J. Millen, and D. Fallows, xvii–xxiii. Cambridge: South End Press.

Farmer, P. E., J. Y. Kim, C. Mitnick, and R. Timperi. (1999). "Responding to Outbreaks of Multidrug-Resistant Tuberculosis: Introducing 'DOTS-Plus.'" In *Tuberculosis: A Comprehensive International Approach,* 2nd ed., edited by L. B. Reichman and E. S. Hershfield, 447–69. New York: Marcel Dekker.

Farmer, P., F. Léandre, J. S. Mukherjee, M. S. Claude, P. Nevil, M. C. Smith-Fawzi, et al. (2001). "Community-Based Approaches to HIV Treatment in Resource-Poor Settings." *Lancet* 358: 404–409.

Farmer, P., F. Léandre, J. S. Mukherjee, R. Gupta, L. Tarter, and J. Y. Kim. (2001). "Community-Based Treatment of Advanced HIV Disease: Introducing DOT-HAART (Directly Observed Therapy with Highly Active Antiretroviral Therapy." *Bulletin of the World Health Organization* 79, no. 12: 1145–51.

Field, M., G. David, M. Kotz, and G. Bukhman. (2000). "Neoliberal Economic Policy, 'State Desertion' and the Russian Health Crisis." In *Dying for Growth,* edited by J. Y. Kim, J. V. Millen, A. Irwin, and J. Gershman, 155–76. Monroe, ME: Common Courage Press.

Ghana. (1998). "Civil Society Perspectives on Structural Adjustment Policies." Accessed at www.saprin.org/ghana/ghana_forum1.htm, April 12, 2004.

Gounden, Y. P., and J. Moodley. (2000, June). "Exposure to Human Immunodeficiency Virus among Healthcare Workers in South Africa." *International Journal of Gynaecology & Obstetrics* 69, no. 3: 265–70.

Gounder, C. (1998). "The Progress of the Polio Eradication Initiative: What Prospects for Eradicating Measles?" *Health Policy and Planning* 13, no. 3: 212–33.

Hirschel, B. (2001, April 9–11). "Reason Why Treatment of TB Must Be Combined with HAART." Paper presented during the first meeting of the Global TB/HIV working group, Geneva. Geneva: World Health Organization.

ISAPRE. (2000). *Boletín Estadística: Enero-Junio 2000.* Superintendencia de ISAPRES. Santiago: Government of Chile.

Kim, J. Y., A. Shakow, J. Bayona, J. Rhatigan, and E. L. Rubin de Celis. (2000). "Sickness amidst Recovery: Public Debt and Private Suffering in Peru." In *Dying for Growth*, edited by J. Y. Kim, J. V., Millen, A. Irwin, and J. Gershman, 127–54. Monroe, ME: Common Courage Press.

Magallanes. (1935). *La Liga Antituberculosa de Magallanes y Sus Fines.* Pamphlet no. 1. From the archives of the Biblioteca Nacional, Santiago.

Marín Rojas, M. (1934). *El Problema Social de Tuberculosis (Trabajo de Divulgación).* Temuco, Chile. From the archives of the Biblioteca Nacional, Santiago.

Mehmet, O. (1999). *Westernizing the Third World: The Eurocentricity of Economic Development Theories.* New York: Routledge.

Ministerio de Salud. (1996). *Programa Nacional de Control de la Tuberculosis: Actualizaciónde Normas Técnicas.* Ministerio de Salud: Santiago de Chile.

Mitnick, C., J. Bayona, E. Palacios, S. Shin, J. Furin, F. Alcántara, et al. (2003). "Community-Based Therapy for Multidrug-Resistant Tuberculosis in Lima, Peru." *New England Journal of Medicine* 348, no. 2: 119–28.

Paluzzi, J. E. (2002). *The Road to Health: The Experience of Tuberculosis in Southern Chile.* Ph.D. diss., University of Pittsburgh.

Republic of Uganda, Ministry of Health. (2001). *Health Sector Strategic Plan: 2000/01–2004/05.* Accessed at www.health.go.ug/docs/HSSPfinalEdition.pdf, April 12, 2004.

Sachs, J. D., chair. (2001). "Macroeconomics and Health: Investing in Health for Economic Development." Report of the Commission on Macroeconomics and Health. Geneva: World Health Organization.

Simmons, D. S. (2002). *Managing Misfortune: HIV/AIDS, Health Development, and Traditional Healers in Zimbabwe.* Unpublished Ph.D. diss., Michigan State University.

UNDP. (2001). *Human Development Report 2001: Making New Technologies Work for Human Development.* New York: Oxford University Press.

Waitzkin, H. (2003). "Correspondence: Report of the WHO Commission on Macroeconomics and Health." *The Lancet* 361, no. 9367: 1477–78.

Wehrwein, P. (2000). "The Economic Impact of AIDS in Africa." *Harvard AIDS Review* 12–4 (winter).

Whiteside, A. (2001). "Demography and Economics of HIV/AIDS." *British Medical Bulletin* 58: 73–88.

World Health Organization (WHO). (1978). *Declaration of Alma Ata.* Accessed at www.who.dk/eprise/main/WHO/AboutWHO/Policy/20010827_1, April 12, 2004.

Zimbabwe. (1999). *Civil Society Perspectives on Structural Adjustment Policies.* Accessed at www.saprin.org/zimbabwe/zimbabwe_forum1.htm, April 12, 2004.

Shifting Policies toward Traditional Midwives: Implications for Reproductive Health Care in Pakistan 5

FOUZIEYHA TOWGHI

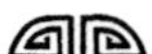

Economic growth, improvement in education, growth in medical technologies, and public spending on health are necessary but not sufficient conditions for improving health status. It is how governments implement national health policy that has impact on improving health status.

—PEABODY ET AL., 1999

PAKISTAN IS ANOTHER POSTCOLONIAL COUNTRY where the scientific progress of the recent decades and the biomedical technology innovations do not benefit the majority of the people. The most recent internationally imposed and state-mandated structural adjustment strategies of Pakistan pose increasing difficulty for any objective of national self-reliance.[1]

To understand the implications on the people for whom policies are designed, it is important to question how, when, and why health policies are implemented. An examination of the shifting national policies can unravel the underlying reasons for human subjects becoming targets of achieving particular health outcomes. In Pakistan, an ethnically diverse nation, policies concerning *dais* (or traditional midwives), whom I prefer to call local community midwives, have not been guided by the knowledge of their full complexity and worth. Neither have the attempts to integrate them in health care promotion been primarily for the needs of women.

This chapter outlines Pakistan's strategies to incorporate the local community midwives in the national health care policies since the Declaration of Alma Ata of 1978. Pakistani health policies have been driven by international trends and donor priorities. Assessments of available resources were required for every new trend in health care strategy, from primary health care (PHC), child survival, family planning, and safe motherhood to reproductive health care. An examination of health policies shows that *dais,* commonly known as traditional birth attendants (TBAs), have been largely used in short-term, vertical, and target-oriented health care programs (e.g., in increasing child immunization and contraceptive rates), at the expense of the *dais'* unique and complex roles and women's varied health needs. Such improvised use of *dais* perpetuates an incomplete understanding not only of their work and their relationship with the women they serve, but also of the prevailing social-economic context.

Despite regional variations in social and economic status, local community midwives are called to assist in more than labor, delivery, and prenatal and postpartum care. They provide massage for the newborn and the mother, handle childhood illnesses, and address women's infertility problems. They also advise on the use of herbal and allopathic-based contraceptive methods, support and assist women in performing abortions, and address gynecological and other female health-related problems for which they then recommend herbs (El Hakim 1981; MacCormack 1982; Van der Most 1982; Nieof 1988, 1992; Mangay-Maglacas and Pizurki 1981; Mongay-Maglacas and Simon 1986; Mothercare 1993). To date, there are no ethnographic studies of local community midwives in Pakistan. Anthropological conceptions of Pakistani *dais* are particularly influenced by what is written about South Asian *dais* in India, Bangladesh, and Nepal (Rozario 1998; Jeffery and Jeffery 1993; Jeffery 1988).[2] These studies have emphasized the *dais'* low social status, their role in "birth pollution," and their handling of the vulnerability of the mother and child to spirits at the time of childbirth. They allege the *dais'* lack of expertise and minimal involvement in antenatal and postpartum care of women. However, there is no evidence suggesting that these are dominant attributes of *dais* in Pakistan. Rather, what we found is that even among the economically disadvantaged, where allopathic services are scarce, a *dai* is called based on her reputation as a competent and dependable midwife at all stages of the reproductive processes.[3] Considering the diversity of roles, practices, and social status of local midwives in the Third World, generalizations that posit TBAs to be substandard, superstitious, and incapable of doing complex tasks (Browere et al. 1998) are dangerous. So for example, in Pakistan, while some of the generalizations about Indic cultural zones of South Asia may apply to northeastern parts of Punjab and Mohajir populations, they would not necessarily apply to Balochs. Finally, when we also consider the political economy of health care, the implications of Pakistani national health policies upon midwives' existing and potential contribution in women's reproductive health care of women become clearer.

Locating *Dais* for Primary Health Care

The Pakistani state bureaucracy has repeatedly called upon the *dai* to assist with national health improvement. The targeting of *dais* to serve state interests began in the late colonial period (Arnold 1993:259). Since then, the national health establishment has been keen to elicit and utilize the "natural" connection that *dais* are perceived to have with their communities, and to use them for infant and child health, family planning, and maternal health care programs. While the integration of *dais* in the health care system was considered crucial in accessing communities, the conceptions of her value in health care have shifted over time. A *dai* during the colonial period was considered to be "uneducated and dangerous," needing to be replaced by Western midwives (Arnold 1993:259); in the postwar period, as one in need of hygiene training and being useful for linking the clinic and community; and in the last ten years, as one seen to add to the risks associated with maternal death (Browere et al. 1998). British colonial policy in Asia aimed at eradicating "traditional" midwives. When this was found to be impossible, there was a reversal of policy to feature government-sponsored training for the midwives to improve child-delivery practices (Rogers and Solomon 1975). When the World Health Organization (WHO) first promoted the systematic training, encouraging countries to incorporate them into the health care delivery system based on the Declaration of Alma Ata of 1978, the theoretical case for training them was that they were numerous, they attended 60 to 90 percent of births in their respective countries, and they functioned as the primary-care providers for many who otherwise had none or very little access to health care. So, in sheer numerical terms, local midwives became a means to speedily introduce some family health care to large numbers of people relatively cheaply. Consequently, there have been more Third World health projects that used local community midwives than any other traditional practitioner. An estimated 60,000 women were recruited for PHC in Pakistan to address international and nation-state concern with family planning and child survival (Phillips, Simmons, Chkaraborty, and Chowdhury 1984).

PHC was readily adopted, but it was implemented with varying degrees of success (Mosley 1983). Efforts to improve maternal and child health (MCH), in particular, did not achieve the envisioned level of success. Underutilization of health centers was identified as a major weakness of the PHC strategy. Recognition of this led to a reorientation of policies so that the assessment of community needs and their mobilization became a core strategy and a prerequisite for future intervention plans. It is in this context that WHO recognized the need to recruit traditional health practitioners, particularly local midwives, as a *resource* in the overall strategy of orienting "all" health programs to the needs of the people (WHO 1978). Pakistan, like many other countries, agreed to train TBAs to bridge the gap until all women could have access to professional and modern health care services. The perception of the benefit of including TBAs in PHC prevailed up to the mid-1980s. They were identified and used as a unified group by the tasks they performed, such as assisting in the delivery of a high proportion of births, and because of their close contact with and received respect from the communities (Heggenhougen and Shore 1986). However, in Pakistan local midwives were at first recruited to promote family planning to meet contraceptive targets long before the state-sanctioned PHC agenda was initiated for national health care.

Using *Dais* in Family Planning Programs

Family planning was first initiated in 1953 in the private sector. In the First Plan (1955–1960), the Pakistani government allocated a grant of 5 million rupees (US$1.06 million) to the Family Planning Association of Pakistan (FPAP) to provide contraceptive services. The existing government-based Population Welfare Program began with the second Five-Year Plan (1960–1965; Pakistan, Federal Bureau of Statistics 1998). These efforts received support by nearly all of the major international donors[4] involved in international fertility reduction activities (Robinson, Makhdoom, and Nasra 1981).

Since local midwives were attending nearly two-thirds of all births in the world, they became ideal subjects in promoting family planning, especially in rural areas (WHO 1979, 1986; Piper 1997). WHO and UNICEF policies encouraged using them as agents to promote contraceptive use and a large number of Third World countries made concerted efforts to recruit and train selected TBAs (Rogers and Solomon 1975). Governments had a similar underlying rationale in TBA recruitment strategies, namely that because TBAs were influential in their communities, their participation would lessen the burden on the rural professional medical staff.

Experimenting with four approaches in family planning programs (target-oriented approach, 1965–1969; continuous motivation system, 1970–1973; contraceptive inundation, 1970–1973; and integration, 1978–present), Pakistan was the first country to use local midwives as the main field workers for family planning. The first program strategy "was based on a large, complex bureaucratic structure at the center, and was supported in the provinces and districts by an extensive publicity campaign" (Robinson, Makhdoom, and Nasra 1981:86). Annual targets were set to achieve acceptors of contraceptives and to reduce the birthrate from 50 to 40 per 1,000 in five years. The overall national targets were divided into provincial and subsequently into district-level targets. The plan called for employing 20,000 *dais,* each of whom was to cover a population of two villages in rural areas, or 2,000 people in urban areas. In 1969 approximately 50,000 *dais* had been trained to supply contraceptives to women (Zeichner 1988). The supplies could also be accessed through village shops, stores, pharmacies, and other public and private outlets. The Union Council Secretariats were to provide the vital link between the family planning officers (FPOs), full-time employees of the program, and the *dais*, who were paid part-time wages. A *dai* was to receive a referral fee for each acceptor she referred for IUD insertion or sterilization. Besides enrolling doctors to insert IUDs to make up for the shortage of trained medical personnel, a special cadre of paramedical personnel (Lady Family Planning Visitors) were trained and employed to do IUD insertion. The *dais*, however, were not provided any technical training about contraceptives (Zeichner 1988).

The target approach for promoting family planning was terminated when the results of national impact survey (1968–1969) showed that fewer than 6 percent of married women of reproductive age were using contraception. Gardezi and Inayatullah (1969) found that initially *dais* were unwilling to provide information on family planning. In the same study, they found that about one-third of the *dais* saw family planning as being against their profession, and only one-seventh believed that modern contraceptives effectively prevented pregnancy. It is unclear why Pakistani *dais* held the former view. Rogers and Solomon (1975) suggested that in Java and Bali, midwives' resistance may have been more to do with their hostility toward the health establishment rather than their views about family planning.

In Pakistan, Robinson et al. (1981) found that the activities emphasized for *dais*, distributing devices and getting new acceptors, were not equivalent to providing continuous, effective contraceptive protection for motivated couples. That is, the focus was on methods rather than clients. The state-mandated strategy contradicted the preexisting relations that the *dais* and women would have had—that is, knowing one another as whole persons, possibly on an everyday basis, and having kinship ties. The decision to recruit midwives for family planning failed to consider the potential conflicts this may have created within *dais* as well as the expectations community members had of them. The government blamed *dais* for program failures, calling them "unreliable" family planning workers. Literate male-female teams, who would be paid competitive wages, replaced the *dais*. But it became impossible to recruit married couples for this, so the focus turned to the recruitment of young unmarried women from nearby urban areas. Still, all the posts could not be filled. While the *dais* had enjoyed the confidence of the village women, the young "educated" women were often not trusted by the older women whom they were assigned to serve. Still, the latter strategy was considered to have more impact than the target-oriented approach that had relied upon *dais* (Robinson et al. 1981).

In Pakistan, just as in India (Mani 1980) and Bangladesh, the national focus on population and family planning detracted from the local midwives' potential in the provision of maternal and child health as a whole. Due to the perceived ineffectiveness of midwives, in the mid-1970s the Bangladesh government, for example, discontinued the training of local community midwives and replaced them with family welfare visitors. This was done to prioritize the promotion of contraception at the community level and consequently caused the provision of maternity care to be compromised (Simmons, Koenig, and Zahidul Huque 1990).

Remembering the "M" in Maternal and Child Health Care: Recalling the *Dai*

Financial limitations and the lack of allopathic trained professionals were impetuses for recruiting local midwives for maternal and child health care programs. In this seemingly pragmatic decision, midwives were initially recruited and trained to help avert neonatal deaths and postpartum tetanus, considered to be the result of unhygienic delivery practices (WHO 1979, 1986). Later, the focus turned to including midwives as part of the government health personnel (Awan 1987). Others saw them as important for linking women to health facilities for antenatal care (Favin, Bradford, and Cebula 1984; Viegas, Singh, and Ratman 1987).

However, concerns about maternal health became a policy focus only after Safe Motherhood was initiated by a World Bank–supported conference in February 1987 in Nairobi, Kenya. Between 1987 and 1988, 12 conferences on safe motherhood in Africa, Asia, Latin America, and the Middle East were funded by international agencies (WHO, UNDP, UNICEF, the World Bank, and the Ford Foundation). The slogan of these programs "putting the M back in MCH" reflected the grassroots push for recognizing how women were largely ignored in favor of children in PHC programs (Justice 2000), coupled by an increasing awareness of the biological as well as socioeconomic bases of the intimate connection between women's health and that of their infants.

Although implementation of safe motherhood programs began only in the 1990s, in the very same decade researchers began to question the necessity of training midwives for reducing maternal mortality. In a collaborative pre-Congress workshop attended by International Confederation of Midwives (ICM), WHO, and UNICEF members to formalize professional midwifery, a document was devised that explicitly questioned the continued investment in TBA training programs. The decision to decrease support of TBA trainings was based on the conclusion that TBA trainings had not had any notable improvement in outcomes for newborns and women. The document projected the need to promote midwifery skill to "modern" educated women in place of TBA training rather than in addition to it (WHO 1997).

Questioning the Value of Training TBAs and the Risks of Devaluing Them

While earlier evaluations focused on the training programs designed for TBAs (Parra 1993), researchers increasingly began to question their "usefulness" in the safe motherhood strategy as a whole. Brouwere, Tonglet, and Lerberghe (1998) criticized the training programs' role in reducing maternal mortality. They argued that it is an illusion to suppose that a course of training alone, "even when given added status by the gift of a case of instruments and a few pharmaceutical products," can have any effect on maternal mortality. What they overlooked, however, is that most trainings only emphasized prenatal care, and the referral of women with obstetric complications, without teaching midwives basic life-saving skills that would buy time while waiting for the transport necessary to move the ailing woman to an equipped health facility (Lefeber 1994; Jordan 1993; WHO 1986). Studies show that the families' perceptions of illness, including that of the woman with the complication, her husband, and her mother-in-law, influence when a midwife is contacted (Fawcus, Mbizvo, Lindmark, and Nystrom 1996; Wall 1998, Prevention of Maternal Mortality Network 1992; Midhet and Towghi 1999).

Blaming the midwife for when women and their families seek "modern" health care is not new. Midwives were once considered the cause of the delay in women's decisions to seek antenatal care (Nomboze qtd. in Brouwere et al. 1998). The argument assumes that antenatal care exists and is accessible to all women who decide to seek the services. Studies, however, show that local midwives are one part of a complex set of circumstances and family/community decision-making dynamics that influence women's desire and social and economic ability to access the medical facilities for antenatal care as well as for emergency obstetric care (Midhet, Becker, and Heinz 1998). A study in Pakistan that reviewed 118 pregnant cases who had been brought dead to a major hospital in Karachi between 1981 and 1990 found that all women were poor and had been looked after by a *dai*, family members, or small maternity homes, and all of them had died of a major complication. When their families were interviewed about the delay to reach the hospital, half of them mentioned economic constraints, and the other half spoke of social and cultural constraints such as disapproval from the husband or uncertainty about the nature of the complication (MacCormack 1994). Women's need for permission from male members to attend health centers (social), having a low income and the convenience of home care (economic), and the distance to a health center (physical) are all factors impacting women's ability to access health services (Asian Development Bank [ADB] 1997). In Balochistan, for example, the average distance to a Family Welfare Center is 47.5 km (Tinker 1996). In Pakistan, only 27 percent of women receive antenatal care, 13 percent of deliveries occur in a health facility, and a "mere" 18 percent of births are attended by "skilled" practitioners (Tinker 1996).

To borrow Wan's (1982) definition, access is a multifaceted concept, involving *awareness* that one's condition needs medical attention, *availability* of services in terms of time and distance, *acceptability* in terms of trust and willingness to use such services, and *affordability* in terms of income and time. In South Asia, lack of access to health facilities is 1.5 times worse than in other regions of the Third World. In Pakistan, only 55 percent of the population has access to health services. On the average, one facility is available for 11,000 people and one bed for 1,500 persons (PFBS 1998). But only one-fifth of the beds is available with facilities in rural areas, where about 68 percent of the people live. In general, the availability of beds is unevenly distributed and not based on the size of the population. This does not assume access to quality services. Infinite stories can be heard from the population regarding the poor conditions of health centers/hospitals and the cruel and disrespectful behavior of health professionals. Due to the increased medicalization of childbirth worldwide, physical abuse of women by medical professionals in hospitals is on the rise (Davis-Floyd 2000). Staff absenteeism, lack of supplies, weak management and supervision, insufficient numbers of female workers, and poor training all contribute to poor quality care (Tinker 1998). Health facilities, particularly the primary and preventive services, are underutilized and get little attention. A study of rural basic health facilities found that about 36 percent of physicians posted in these facilities were absent during normal duty hours, only 48 percent of the positions for female medical officers were filled, and about 38 percent of the facilities did not provide any maternal and child health care because no lady health visitors had been appointed to work in the facility (Tinker 1998). Furthermore, only 23 percent of pregnant women residing in the immediate catchment area reported that they had ever visited a government facility for antenatal care (Parvez, Chaudhry, Rheman, and Khan 1993).

It has become clear that one way to reduce maternal mortality in women having an obstetric complication is to require timely access to a well-equipped hospital (Maine et al. 1991; Koblinsky, Timyan, and Gay 1993). Yet studies show that a majority of women and their families in rural and very poor urban areas continue to rely on local midwives for obstetric care, even if equipped facilities are available (Eades, Brace, Osie, and LaGuirdia 1993). This basic fact is reason enough to think twice before any decisions are made to reconsider investment in the training of local midwives for safe motherhood and reproductive health care. In places where the formal health system is dysfunctional, having access to a *dai* becomes a life-and-death issue. In the BSMI project, men from villages outside of the study area requested that the project train one or two women from their villages to assist women during birth. Men and women of these villages requested training for women to become *dais* so that they could avoid going to the hospitals. No one had "naturally" taken up the role and responsibilities of midwifery in these villages. Instead they would seek a midwife from another village, usually located several miles away or on the other side of the valley.

Contrary to the popular belief that midwives are native death angels in Indonesia (Van Burren in Lefeber and Voorhoeve 1998) and that they are directly responsible for a large proportion of both infant and maternal deaths in India (Lal 1962 in Lefeber and Voorhoeve 1998), a study in Gambia showed that training them had the effect of reducing maternal mortality to half of the pre-intervention rate (Greenwood et al. 1990). As the point of first contact with the health care sector for many women with life-threatening complications, the midwife had a crucial role in facilitating timely and appropriate care. As Eades et al. (1993) showed, the combination of availability and acceptability of TBAs in rural areas increases their potential in improving the health status of women and children in their communities. In Mexico, there were achievements that would have been impossible without the local midwives. For example, in one year (1985) midwives referred 50,708 women with problems during pregnancy to rural clinics or hospitals; 2,744 women were referred to rural hospitals and clinics to give birth there because of complications they recognized they could not handle (Parra 1993).

Why do women and their families prefer their local midwives even when services in a hospital or maternity center are available? A study in Ghana found that even when the midwives referred patients to the health center for a complication, many of the women refused to go due to financial limitations, lack of transport, and expectation of disrespectful or painful treatment from hospital personnel. Thaddeus and Maine (1994) and the BSMI project found similar reasons for the women's refusals to seek emergency services (Towghi and Midhet 2000). Fawcus et al.'s (1996) study in Masvingo, Zimbabwe, showed that delay in seeking care in both the rural and urban areas due to family dynamics and transportation problems were preventable factors leading to a woman's death. Interviews of relatives of women who had died suggest that women waited until symptoms such as puerperal sepsis were too severe before calling for help. Others pointed to economic and childcare responsibilities that made leaving home difficult for women. In cases of induced abortion, women had fear of criminal consequences (Fawcus et al. 1996). A study in Sindh, Pakistan, found that access, cost, and women's lack of autonomy were the major deterrents to using hospitals for delivery in rural areas. Poor treatment by hospital staff, cost, and inconvenience were the main reasons for home delivery in urban areas. Opinions about the perceived safety at home and hospital delivery revealed that 64 percent of urban women felt that hospital delivery was safer, but only 30 percent of rural women felt this to be true (Kazmi 1995). In a situation such as this, a local midwife has little choice but to assist in a high-risk case, not only because there is no time or means to send the woman for higher level care, but also because the midwife often feels a moral obligation to utilize whatever skills she has to help the woman survive.

Another reason why women and their families rely more on local community midwives is due to their shared cultural codes of mutual understanding: they speak the same language, both literally and figuratively (Camey et al. 1996). The culturally determined shared concepts of health and illness in the relationship influence the subsequent quality of compliance and outcome (Heggenhougen and Shore 1986). The negative consequences of culturally uninformed training are well documented by anthropologists (Pigg 1995; Jordan 1989). A qualitative study in Niamey, Niger, found that there was a conflict between delivery techniques that the midwives were taught and the cultural requirements surrounding childbirth. In this case, although both women and midwives are obliged to the same social rules (linguistic taboos, respect, and shame), the technical constraints forced midwives to violate those rules, which made it difficult for the midwives to apply their skills (Jaffre and Prual 1994). This example also illustrates that technical training is insufficient without taking into account the cultural and social dynamics and particularities of practices of midwives as well as the families they serve. Stephens (1992) shows that in southern India, whether or not families choose a *dai* (trained or not) may be influenced by the perception of their own caste in relation to the *dai*'s status, as well as by more practical socioeconomic factors and perceptions of the quality of care offered by the *dai*. A study of the impact of training midwives in an "urban slum" in Visakhapatnam showed that community use of a trained *dai* for maternal care increased by raising the *dai*'s status and not only because of technical improvement in her skills (Stephens 1992). It is not unusual to find that in poor communities, people often do not have faith in hospitals and prefer a local midwife who belongs to the same sociocultural milieu (Khanderkar et al. 1993). The perception about local midwives' experience, kindness, skill, and interest in the welfare of the baby attracted women and families to seek the same midwife, suggesting that a community's insistence to seek a local midwife is not solely an affective response, but is also based on the intent to get good care.

What I am suggesting here is basic: that local community midwives work in a "cultural matrix of a social group" in which the midwife and women belong together. Within this cultural matrix, many visible and invisible practices are conducted during pregnancy, delivery, and postpartum by the midwives (who may or many not be allopathically trained) that not only provide a sense of psychological security and emotional support to mothers (Lefeber 1994), but also play a crucial role in preventing the unnecessary deaths of women.

Safe Motherhood and the Fate of *Dais*

Clearly, women should have timely access to emergency obstetric care, access not only geographically, but also financially, culturally, and psychologically. Limitations in any of these domains influenced whether women and families would call upon a local community midwife.

PHC, emphasizing basic and accessible low-level services linked to and supported by the community, still holds the best hope for a large number of rural and urban communities. While local midwives cannot bring down the rate of maternal mortality without well-equipped and effective referral centers and systems, the fact is that it is largely women living in remote and poor areas who rely most upon them (Parra 1993). For example, it became clear in the BSMI project that in situations where women have limited means to pay for transport, or if they live where roads are rough, vehicles are scarce, and they are therefore unlikely to be linked to a formal health system, these drawbacks in addition to the unavailability of a local midwife can become a life-and-death issue. Hence, policy decisions that fail to consciously consider how TBAs are integral to family and community decisions around women's health care have immediate and long-term consequence for women's lives in the Third World. This is particularly true in the context of structural adjustment policies that curb social spending (Sadasivam 1999). Peabody (1996) warned, "From a purely economic viewpoint, structural-adjustment policies and economic reform policies are viewed as short-term austerities that lead to long-term growth and development. These intertemporal trade-offs, however, are not always acceptable in health" (823). The quantitative data available on the impact of structural-adjustment programs provide a restricted view of the situation. In many countries, there are no reliable data (Lundy 1996) and available data do not assess the impact on people's lives or the despair that the programs bring with them. For example, in Pakistan many of the auxiliary health workers don't belong to the community they are assigned to serve, impeding their ability to do the work. They often want to relocate as soon as they are posted in a rural health center.[5] In this unquantifiable situation, the discontinuation of investment in local midwives (who provide their services irrespective of training) would be a failure of moral conscience. Also, while we may locate availability of crucial medical services, user-oriented health services for rural and poor urban women are not always guaranteed, posing further obstacles in obtaining even basic health care (Simmons et al. 1990).

Conclusion

In Pakistan, programmatic decisions to use *dais* have been largely defined by the need to meet targets, be they immunization rates for child survival or contraceptive prevalence rates in family planning programs. *Dais'* success in such programs is largely described in terms of levels of targets met; and failure to meet such targets have led to conclusions that it may not be cost-effective to train them, that it is better to train educated women as midwives, or that it is better to invest in literate PHC providers. Yet, studies indicate that local midwives have a key role in reducing maternal mortality and morbidity, even if overall national rates remain high (Parra 1993).

Capabilities of local community midwives continue to be evaluated based on the notion that they assist with delivery only, without regard to the eclectic nature of their roles and the context in which they carry out their midwifery functions. It is also assumed that the continued existence of midwives is due to the absence of modern health services. But the dynamics of health-seeking behavior among women and their families are more complex, as reflected by medical anthropological research; and understanding these dynamics is relevant to the success of any restructuring strategy in the health system (Uzma, Underwood, Atkinson, and Thackrah 1999). As Piper (1997) suggested, conditions are so varied throughout the world that the decision to initiate, invigorate, or discontinue trainings of local midwives should be made only after the complex array of relevant issues, resources, and sociocultural factors, including the wishes of families and the local community midwives, are reviewed.

Training *dais* cannot be used as a single approach to reducing maternal mortality and morbidity (Piper 1997). *Dais* cannot be expected to reduce overall mortality and morbidity rates when poverty,[6] lack of female literacy, and discrimination—which are only a few of the underlying causes of women's reproductive-related mortality and morbidity—persist. There are limits to improving women's reproductive health without dealing directly or indirectly with the structural inequalities that largely work against poor women. But advocating for the necessary change in social structure—the availability of modern health care infrastructure and greater social and economic power for women and rural families—need not occur at the expense of local midwives. Whether we view inclusion of midwives as a low-cost strategy or not for Third World countries, the fact is that local community midwives provide legitimate and viable services and will continue to do so whether a backup system of training, support, and supervision is available.[7] To ignore midwives in reproductive health programs due to a view that they are "obsolete, impractical, or primitive" (Parra 1993) would be unjust to a majority of women who rely upon them.

Acknowledgments

I would like to thank Anju Gurnani and Malek Towghi for their comments and editorial assistance.

Notes

1. Stabilization and structural adjustment are core programs of the IMF and the World Bank in the Third World. "Stabilization programs are short-term programs intended to remedy . . . the balance of payments deficit and inflation. Structural-adjustment programs aim to reactivate economic growth" (Curtis 1998:1624). For countries, such programs

mean cutbacks in credit availability, currency devaluation, reduced public spending, and repayment of debt (Curtis 1998).

2. Pakistan is divided into two major cultural zones and groups. One may be called Indic, and the other Middle Eastern cum Central Asian. In Pakistan, the Muhajirs and the Punjabis are largely influenced by Indic cultural values, and the Balochs (residing predominantly in Balochistan and Sindh) and the Pushtuns/Pathans (primarily in the Northwest Frontier Province) are influenced by Middle Eastern and Central Asian cultural values. While we can argue that these are enormously generalized divisions and that we will find cultural and social complexities that overlap between the two zones, we must understand that to talk about a *dai* or group of *dais* in Pakistan requires the consideration of the existence of complex and overlapping social factors that are regionally and culturally specific. Thus we cannot necessarily talk about a characteristic Pakistani *dai,* in the same that we cannot talk about a characteristic Indian *dai* based on one regional study in India. Moreover, we must be careful when making generalized international comparisons. For example, while a regional study in north India about *dais* may provide clues about Punjabi *dais* in Pakistan, those studies may be less illuminating and programmatically consequential for *dais* and women in Balochistan.

3. Balochistan Safe Motherhood Initiative (BSMI) project reports are available at the Asia Foundation Office in Islamabad, Pakistan. The four-year (1998–2002) health research project, funded by the NIH, tested intervention to reduce maternal mortality in Khuzdar, Balochistan. The project principal and co-investigators, respectively, were Farid Midhet and Fouzieyha Towghi.

4. U.S. Agency for International Development (USAID), United Nations Fund for Population Activities (UNFPA), the World Bank, the Swedish International Development Authority, the Ford Foundation, and the Population Council.

5. Female providers are scarce in rural areas, where women prefer to be examined by women. One-third of physicians registered during 1993 were females, but they are concentrated in the cities (Pakistan, Federal Bureau of Statistics 1996). Most female health professionals are auxiliary workers.

6. To capture the multiple dimensions of poverty (e.g., poor health, illiteracy, and lack of access to safe water, nutrition, and income), Mahbub ul Haq developed the Poverty of Opportunity Index (POPI). This includes indicators of basic human deprivations such as lack of access to income, education, and health. Based on this definition, poverty of opportunity affects more people in each South Asian country, except for India, than poverty based on income alone. The most striking gap between POPI and income poverty exists in Pakistan. Poverty rates have risen in Pakistan in 1990s, a reversal of the declining poverty trend in the mid-1970s and 1980s.

7. For example, women in poor urban areas of Dhaka went first and frequently to local midwives for the care of postpartum morbidities, prolapsed uterus, and vesico-vaginal fistula (Uzma et al. 1999). In Mexico, midwives living far from formal medical structures cared for women's gynecological problems (Camey et al. 1996). In a health care project in central India, midwives were essential to educating women on sexuality and reproduction, treatment of vaginal discharge, and the identification of gynecological diseases (Bang 1989).

References

Arnold, D. (1993). *Colonizing the Body: State Medicine and Epidemic Disease in Nineteenth-Century India.* Berkeley: University of California Press.

Asian Development Bank (ADB). (1997). The Status and Quality of Women's Health Care in Pakistan—A Situation Analysis." Draft report.

Awan, A. K. (1987). "Mobilizing TBAs for the Control of Maternal and Neonatal Mortality in Pakistan." In *High Risk Mothers and Newborns: Detection, Management and Prevention,* edited by Ar Omran, J. Martin, and D. M. Aviado, 340–46. Thun, Switzerland: Ott.

Bang, R. (1989). "Commentary on a Community-Based Approach to Reproductive Health Care." *International Journal of Obstetrics,* supplement 3: 125–29.

Brouwere, V., R. Tonglet, and W. V. Lerberghe. (1998). "Strategies for Reducing Maternal Mortality in Developing Countries: What Can We Learn from the History of the Industrialized West?" *Tropical Medicine and International Health* 3, no. 10: 771–82.

Camey, X. C., C. G. Barrios, X. R. Guerrero, R. M. Núñez-Urquiza, D. G. Hernández, and A. L. Glas. (1996). "Traditional Birth Attendants in Mexico: Advantages and Inadequacies of Care for Normal Deliveries." *Social Science and Medicine* 43, no. 2: 199–207.

Curtis, E. (1998). "Child Health and the International Monetary Fund: The Nicaraguan Experience." *Lancet* 352: 1622–24.

Davis-Floyd, R. (2000, March). "Anthropological Perspectives on Global Issues in Midwifery: Mutual Accommodation or Biomedical Hegemony?" *Midwifery Today:* 12–16, 68–69.

Eades, C. A., C. Brace, L. Osie, and K. D. LaGuirdia. (1993). "Traditional Birth Attendants and Maternal Mortality in Ghana." *Social Science and Medicine* 36, no. 11: 1503–7.

El Hakim, S. (1981). "Sudan: Replacing TBAs by Village Midwives." In *Traditional Birth Attendant in Seven Countries,* edited by A. Mangay-Maglacas and H. Pizurki, 131–67. Geneva: WHO.

Favin, M., B. Bradford, and D. Cebula. (1984). *Improving Maternal Health in Developing Countries.* Geneva: World Federation of Public Health Association.

Fawcus, S., M. Mbizvo, G. Lindmark, and L. Nystrom. (1996, November–December). "A Community-Based Investigation of Avoidable Factors for Maternal Mortality in Zimbabwe." *Studies in Family Planning* 27, no. 6: 319–27.

Gardezi, H. N., and A. Inayatullah. (1969). *The Dai Study: The Dai Midwife—A Local Functionary and Her Role in Family Planning.* Lahore: Family Planning Association of Pakistan.

Greenwood, A. M., A. K. Bradley, P. Byass, B. M. Greenwood, R. W. Snow, S. Bennett, and A. B. Hatibnjie. (1990). "Evaluation of a Primary Health Care Programme in the Gambia: The Impact of Trained Traditional Birth Attendants on the Outcome of Pregnancy." *Journal of Tropical Medicine and Hygiene* 93: 58–66.

Heggenhougen, K., and L. Shore. (1986). "Cultural Components of Behavioral Epidemiology: Implications for Primary Health Care." *Social Science and Medicine* 22: 1235.

Jaffre, Y., and A. Prual. (1994). "Midwives in Niger. An Uncomfortable Position between Social Behaviors and Health Care Constraints." *Social Science and Medicine* 38, no. 8: 1069–1073.

Jeffery, R. (1988). *The Politics of Health in India.* Berkeley: University of California Press.

Jeffery, R., and P. M. Jeffery. (1993). "Traditional Birth Attendants in Rural North India: The Social Organization of Childbearing." In *Knowledge, Power, and Practice: The Anthropol-*

ogy of Medicine in Everyday Life, edited by S. Lindenbaugh and M. Lock, 7–31. Berkeley: University of California Press.

Jordan, B. (1989). "Cosmopolitical Obstetrics: Some Insights from the Training of Traditional Midwives." *Social Science and Medicine* 28, no. 9: 925–44.

———. (1993 [1978]). *Birth in Four Cultures: A Cross-Cultural Investigation of Childbirth in Yucatan, Holland, Sweden, and the United States,* 4th ed. Prospect Heights, IL: Waveland Press.

Justice, J. (2000). "The Politics of Child Survival." In *Global Health Policy, Local Realities: The Fallacy of the Level Playing Field,* edited by L. M. Whiteford and L. Manderson, 23–38. Boulder, CO: Lynne Rienner.

Kazmi, S. (1995). "Pakistan: Consumer Satisfaction and Dissatisfaction with Maternal and Child Health Services." *World Health Statistics Quarterly* 48, no. 1: 55–59.

Khanderkar, J., S. Dwivedi, M. Bhattacharya, G. Singh, P. L. Joshi, and B. Raj. (1993, September). "Childbirth Practices among Women in Slum Areas." *The Journal of Family Welfare* 39, no. 3: 13–17.

Koblinsky, M., J. Timyan, and J. Gay. (1993). *The Health of Women: A Global Perspective.* Boulder, CO: Westview Press.

Lefeber, Y. (1994). *Midwives without Training: Practices and Beliefs of Traditional Birth Attendants in Africa, Asia, and Latin America.* Assen, the Netherlands: Van Gorcum.

Lefeber, Y., and H. W. A. Voorhoeve, eds. (1998). *Indigenous Customs in Childbirth and Childcare.* Assen, Netherlands: Van Gorcum.

Lundy, P. (1996). "Limitations of Quantitative Research in the Study of Structural Adjustment." *Social Science and Medicine* 42: 313–24.

MacCormack, C. P. (1994 [1982]). *Ethnography of Fertility and Birth.* London: Academic Press.

Maine, D., A. Rosenfield, J. McCarthy, A. Kamara, and A. O. Lucas. (1991). *Safe Motherhood Programs: Options and Issues.* New York: Columbia University.

Mangay-Maglacas, A., and H. Pizurki, eds. (1981). *The TBA in Seven Countries.* Geneva: WHO, 97–131.

Mangay-Maglacas, A., and J. Simons. (1986). *The Potential of the Traditional Birth Attendant.* WHO Offset publication no. 95. Geneva: WHO.

Mani, S. B. (1980, December). "A Review of Midwife Training Programs in Tamil Nadu." *Studies in Family Planning* 11, no. 12: 395–400.

Midhet, F., S. Becker, and B. Heinz. (1998). "Contextual Determinants of Maternal Mortality in Rural Pakistan." *Social Science and Medicine* 46, no. 12: 1587–98.

Midhet, F., and F. Towghi. (1999). *Balochistan Safe Motherhood Initiative: Results of Health Intervention Research Project.* Islamabad, Pakistan: Asia Foundation Office.

Mosley, W. H. (1983, February 28–March 4). *Will Primary Health Care Reduce Infant and Child Mortality? A Critique of Some Current Strategies, with Special Reference to Africa and Asia.* Paper presented at the IUSSP Seminar on Social Policy, Health Policy and Mortality Prospects, Paris.

MotherCare. (1993, August). *Nigeria Maternal Health Care Project Qualitative Research.* Working Paper 17 B.

Nieof, A. (1988). "Traditional Medication at Pregnancy and Childbirth in Madura, Indonesia." In *The Context of Medicine in Developing Countries,* edited by S. Van der Geest and S. R. Whyte, 235–52. Amsterdam: Kluwer Academic.

———. (1992). *Women as Mediators in Indonesia.* Nijhoff: KITLV Verhandelingen, Den Haag.

Pakistan, Federal Bureau of Statistics. (1996). *Pakistan Integrated Household Survey 1995–1996.* Islamabad: Pakistan, Federal Bureau of Statistics.

———. (1998). *Compondium on Gender Statistics Pakistan.* Islamabad: Pakistan, Federal Bureau of Statistics.

Parra, P. A. (1993). "Midwives in the Mexican Health System." *Social Science and Medicine* 37, no. 11: 1321–29.

Parvez, M. A., M. A. Chaudhry, F. Rheman, and M. M. A. Khan. (1993). *Utilization of Rural Basic Health Services in Pakistan.* Study conducted for the Ministry of Health, Government of Pakistan, and WHO-EMRO. Islamabad: Ministry of Health, Government of Pakistan, and WHO-EMRO.

Peabody, J. W. (1996). "Economic Reform and Health Sector Policy: Lessons from Structural Adjustment Programs." *Social Science and Medicine* 43: 823–35.

Peabody J. W., M. O. Rahman, P. J. Gertler, J. Mann, D. O. Farley, and G. M. Carter. (1999). *Policy & Health: Implications for Development in Asia.* Cambridge: Cambridge University Press.

Phillips, J. F., R. Simmons, J. Chkaraborty, and A. L. Chowdhury. (1984). "Integrating Health Services into an MCH-FP Program: Lessons from Matlab, Bangladesh." *Studies in Family Planning* 15, no. 4: 153–61.

Pigg, S. L. (1995). "Acronyms and Effacement: Traditional Medical Practitioners (TMP) in International Health Development." *Social Science and Medicine* 41, no. 1: 47–68.

Piper, C. J. (1997). "Is There a Place for Traditional Midwives in the Provision of Community-Health Services?" *Annals of Tropical Medicine & Parasitology* 91, no. 3, 237–45.

Prevention of Maternal Mortality Network. (1992). "Barriers to Treatment of Obstetric Emergencies in Rural Communities of West Africa." *Studies in Family Planning* 23, no. 5: 279–91.

Robinson, C. R., A. S. Makhdoom, and M. S. Nasra. (1981). "The Family Planning Program in Pakistan: What Went Wrong?" *International Family Planning Perspectives* 7, no. 3: 85–92.

Rogers, M. R., and D. S. Solomon. (1975, May). "Traditional Midwives and Family Planning in Asia." *Studies in Family Planning* 6, no. 5: 126–33.

Rozario, S. (1998). "The *Dai* and the Doctor: Discourses on Women's Reproductive Health in Rural Bangladesh." In *Maternities and Modernities: Colonial and Postcolonial Experiences in Asia and the Pacific,* edited by K. Ram and M. Jolly, 144–76. Cambridge: Cambridge University Press.

Sadasivam, B. (1999). "Cairo Launched Progress on Several Fronts, but Obstacles Remain." *The UNFPA Magazine* 26, no. 2.

Simmons, R., M. A. Koenig, and A. A. Zahidul Huque. (1990, July–August). "Maternal-Child Health and Family Planning: User Perspectives and Service Constraints in Rural Bangladesh." *Studies in Family Planning* 21, no. 4: 187–96.

Stephens, C. (1992). "Training Urban Traditional Birth Attendants: Balancing International Policy and Local Reality." *Social Science and Medicine* 35, no. 6: 811–17.

Thaddeus, S., and D. Maine. (1994). "Too Far to Walk: Maternal Mortality in Context." *Social Science and Medicine* 38, no. 8: 1091–1110.

Tinker, A. (1996). *Improving Reproductive Health in Pakistan and Saving Women's Lives.* World Bank Report.

———. (1998). *Improving Women's Health in Pakistan.* Human Development Network, Health Nutrition, and Population Series. World Bank

Towghi, F. and F. Midhet. (2000). "'Let's See Who Dies This Time—Me or My Child': Perceptions and Actions around Obstetric Bleeding in Khuzdar, Balochistan." Harvard Center for Population and Development Studies Working Paper Series. Cambridge, MA: Harvard Center for Population and Development Studies.

Uzma, A., P. Underwood, D. Atkinson, and R. Thackrah. (1999). "Postpartum Health in Dhaka Slum." *Social Science and Medicine* 48: 313–20.

Van der Most, S. (1982). *Who Cares for Her Health? An Anthropological Study of Women's Health Care in a Village in Upper Egypt.* Leiden: Women and Development Series Egypt.

Viegas, O. A., K. Singh, and S. S. Ratman. (1987). "Antenatal Care: When, Where, How and How Much." In *High Risk Mothers and Newborns: Detection, Management and Prevention,* edited by Ar Omran, J. Martin, and D. M. Aviado, 287–302. Thun, Switzerland: Ott.

Wall, L. L. (1998). "Dead Mothers and Injured Wives: The Social Context of Maternal Morbidity and Mortality among the Hausa of Northern Nigeria." *Studies in Family Planning* 29, no. 4: 341–59.

Wan, T. (1982). "Use of Health Services by the Elderly in Low Income Communities." *Milbank Memorial Fund Quarterly* 60: 82–107.

World Health Organization (WHO). (1978). *The Promotion and Development of Traditional Medicine.* Technical Report Series 622. Geneva: WHO.

———. (1979). *Traditional Birth Attendants.* WHO Offset Publication no. 44. Geneva: WHO.

———. (1997). *Strengthening Midwifery within Safe Motherhood.* Report of a Collaborative ICM/WHO/UNICEF Pre-Congress workshop, Oslo, Norway, May 23–26, 1996. Geneva: WHO, Division of Reproductive Health.

———. (1986). *Prevention of Maternal Mortality: Report of WHO Interregional Meeting.* Geneva: WHO.

Zeichner, C. (1988). "Family Planning in Pakistan." In *Modern and Traditional Health Care in Developing Societies,* edited by C. Zeichner, 75–85. Lanham, MD: University Press of America.

The Contradictions of a Revolving Drug Fund in Post-Soviet Tajikistan: Selling Medicines to Starving Patients

6

SALMAAN KESHAVJEE

If I cannot buy bread when it is being sold, how then will I be able to pay for the treatment or for the medicines? And what does it matter if they are available if I do not have money to buy them?

—RESPONDENT TO HEALTH SURVEY, BADAKHSHAN, TAJIKISTAN, 1996

OVER THE LAST 30 YEARS, many countries have attempted to implement health sector reform, which has often involved shifting the provision of health services from the public to the private sector. Often undertaken to improve the efficiency of health systems in economic crisis, these policies risk limiting access to needed health goods and services, sometimes exposing poor populations to considerable morbidity and mortality.

In this chapter, the implementation of a revolving drug fund in war-ravaged, post-Soviet Tajikistan is discussed as emblematic of the dissonance that may exist between development policies and population needs. Based on a year of qualitative and quantitative research conducted while working as a social researcher with the Aga Khan Foundation (AKF),[1] an international nongovernmental organization (NGO) working in Tajikistan's easternmost province of Badakhshan, the analysis will focus on how this approach to the distribution of medicines was driven less by evidence from the local world than by the global development discourse of privatization and sustainability.

Tajikistan and Badakhshan in the Aftermath of the Soviet Union

Even before the collapse of the Soviet Union, Tajikistan was a poor country. After 1991, with the loss of subsidies from Moscow and the advent of years of civil war, the country was catapulted into significant economic and social crises. By the end of the 1990s, almost 85 percent of the population was living below the poverty line—the GDP in 1998 was US$215—making the country one of the world's poorest nations (Falkingham 2000:10; United Nations Development Programme [UNDP] 1999). By 1996, rapid inflation had led to a situation where purchasing power and food consumption had been highly curtailed, and health, nutrition, and educational services were close to collapsing (World Bank 1998; United Nations Office for the Coordination of Humanitarian Affairs [OCHA] 1998; UNICEF/WHO Mission 1992).[2] Real wages in 1996 were only 5 percent of their 1991 level; wages continued to plummet so that by 1997, they were only 30 percent of their 1995 level (UNDP 1998; International Monetary Fund [IMF] 1998).

In the midst of this crisis, the central and regional governments were not able to afford the cost of providing health services. Not only did access to services decrease, but so did supplies, such as essential medicines, given that pharmaceuticals comprised 13–16 percent of the state health budget (Falkingham 2000). As social sector spending dropped, the effects on the health sector were almost immediate. Life expectancy at birth for both men and women fell during the early 1990s; by 1994, it was 68.5 for women and 63.2 for men (from 72.3 and 67.1 in 1990, respectively; European Observatory on Health Care Systems [EOHCS] 2000:4). By 1995, infant mortality was above 30.7 per 1000 live births (compared to EU average of 5.8 and a former Soviet Union average of 21.7),[3] mostly due to respiratory infections, diarrhea, and developmental disorders causing death in the first few weeks of life (EOHCS 2000). Maternal mortality increased from 41.8 per 100,000 live births to 93.7 in 1995, almost ten times the European Union average. The breakdown in the supply of clean water, proper sewerage, and the public health system led to an upsurge of communicable diseases, including waterborne diseases, tuberculosis, malaria, typhoid fever, measles, and diphtheria (World Health Organization [WHO] 1999, Hampton, Ward, Rowe, and Threfall 1998; UNDP 1998; Keshavjee and Becerra 2000).[4]

In Tajikistan's remote and sparsely populated easternmost semiautonomous province of Badakhshan, the situation was even more tenuous.[5] Known as the "roof-top of the world," Badakhshan is located in the heart of the Pamir Mountains, bordering China to the east, Afghanistan to the southwest, and Kyrgyzstan to the northeast. The region is one of the country's poorest and most inaccessible areas (EOHCS 2000:4). By early 1993, the population of Badakhshan was near starvation (Keshavjee 1998). The situation was exacerbated by the movement of a large number of ethnic Pamiri refugees into the region, which led to a health and nutritional crisis. If not for the provision of humanitarian assistance of the AKF and a consortium of nongovernmental organizations including the United Nations World Food Program (UNWFP), Médecins sans Frontières (MSF), the International Committee of the Red Cross (ICRC), and the International Federation of the Red Cross (IFRC), many Badakhshanis would have surely perished. AKF provided three meals a day to Badakhshan's more than 200,000 inhabitants, and MSF, ICRC, and IFRC provided essential medicines, additional food supplies, heating fuel, and clothing.

Despite phenomenal amounts of food assistance, a nutrition crisis ensued. Not only did levels of rickets go up as vitamin D–fortified milk disappeared, but so did acute and chronic malnutrition (from 3.0 to 5.8 percent and from 40.3 to 44.8 percent, respectively), as well as childhood weight deficit in children 6 to 59 months old (from 19.2 to 27.4 percent; Keshavjee 1998).[6] In addition to the nutritional deficit, there was also a concurrent increase in incidence of communicable diseases between 1991 and 1995: lab-proven diarrheal diseases increased from 10.6 per 100,000 to 91.1 per 100,000, newly reported pneumonia increased from 2,747 per 100,000 to 6,752 per 100,000,[7] and newly reported malaria increased from 8.3 per 100,000 to 350.5 per 100,000 (Keshavjee 1998).

As in other parts of Tajikistan, access to health services in Badakhshan was markedly reduced after the collapse of the former Soviet Union. In the hospital, patients had to provide their own food and medications, and even do their own laundry; many ambulatory facilities faced shortages of essential drugs and medical supplies. Although MSF, ICRC, and IFRC tried to fill these gaps, patients were forced to buy medicines from local private pharmacies or at the local bazaar. At the same time, more than 60 percent of the households contacted in a 1996 health survey reported a monthly income (from both formal and informal sources) of less than 1,800 Tajik rubles (approximately US$6) (Keshavjee 1998).[8] In fact, a survey covering almost a quarter of Badakhshan's population conducted by AKF in 1996 found that despite the massive humanitarian assistance, in the previous year almost 23 percent of Badakhshan's households had had to sell household goods in order to purchase food and clothes (Keshavjee 1998).[9]

The story of Maryam was typical of those who needed health care services. A 40-year-old unemployed factory worker, Maryam was living in Badakhshan's capital of Khorog. I interviewed her shortly after her daughter died from diarrhea in the summer of 1996. Although her husband was still employed, Maryam's home had very few signs of comfort and looked destitute; despite the cold wind blowing through her house on the day I visited, her young daughter was not wearing warm clothes. It had been a bad year for Maryam's family. In the spring, her son was run over by a car and had to undergo surgery because his leg was broken. He was due for a second operation, but had not returned to the hospital yet because they had been unable to purchase the five meters of gauze that the surgeon had asked them to bring. When I asked Maryam about her deceased infant daughter, she recalled how they had asked her to bring medicines.

> My husband and son were looking for Ringer's solution but could not find it, so the doctors said that they would find it themselves. I got the Ampicillin from the commercial drug store located in the hospital—I have a friend there who gave me the drugs for free. My son borrowed Rheopolyglucine from our neighbor who works in the drug store. Each vial cost 2,500 Tajik rubles. We still have not been able to pay back the money because we do not have it. In any case, we got the medicines too late.

Maryam's daughter died soon thereafter from renal failure. Her story was similar to those of the other 15 families that I interviewed whose infants and children died from diarrheal diseases in the summer of 1996: they all recounted that they were trying to find medicines and raise enough money to pay for them. Maryam aptly summed up the pharmaceutical situation in Badakhshan: "We don't have money for medicines; we only take them when we are totally desperate."

Responding to the Crisis: AKF and the Revolving Drug Fund

In an attempt to address the health crisis in Badakhshan, AKF turned to UNICEF's Bamako Initiative. This approach to health sector reform comes from a resolution adopted by the Health Ministers of the WHO African Region at their Regional Committee session held at Bamako, Mali, in September 1987 (UNICEF 1988). The goal of the Bamako Initiative is to accelerate and strengthen the implementation of primary health care with the goal of achieving universal accessibility to these services (Gilson et al. 2001:37–67; Abel-Smith and Dua 1998:95–109). In order to achieve these goals, the initiative utilizes a strategy of decentralized community-based decision making, user financing of health services under community control, and the provision of essential drugs within the framework of a national drugs policy (Gilson et al. 2001:37–67; WHO 1988; UNICEF 1990). AKF wanted to use this approach as both a mechanism to "rationalize" prescription practices and to make essential medicines available where needed (Keshavjee 1998).

AKF turned to the U.S. Agency for International Development (USAID) as a source of funding and hired an expert on pharmaceutical policies in poor countries to head their program in Badakhshan.[10] In their proposal to USAID, the foundation set as its explicit goals the following:

1. Improved availability and accessibility of essential drugs in project areas.
2. Greater efficiency and effectiveness of clinical case-management and prescribing practices directly at the primary level of health care, and indirectly at all levels of care.

3. The establishment of a monetised [sic] system for purchasing and supplying pharmaceuticals which supports national plans for health sector reform and improved self-sufficiency in financing and resource management.
4. Increased involvement of communities in decision making for essential drugs management (AKF, cited in Keshavjee 1998).

While many of these aims were laudable in the post-Soviet context, they were fraught with considerable discursive biases (Kanji and Hardon 1992; Keshavjee 1998).[11] Nevertheless, the following discussion focuses primarily on the revolving drug fund as a cost-sharing mechanism for distributing medications.

From the very start, AKF saw that "policies that propose user charges for social services are politically sensitive and require a supportive context," and therefore proposed that the contents of the new policies be publicly debated to "raise awareness and encourage acceptance." The process would involve a representative from each of Badakhshan's regions in order for local communities to become "encouraged and enabled to participate in the actual management of the pharmaceutical supply." Community participation in the scheme was considered essential since funds from the sales of medicines would have to be collected at the community level and pooled at the central level. Although 100 percent cost recovery was not expected initially, the plan envisioned a system where the proceeds from the sale of medicines would be used to purchase new medicines. The price list for the medicines would be defined by district management committees who would also identify and "handle" patients who were too poor to pay (Keshavjee 1998).

Part and parcel of the revolving drug fund is the training of health care providers and managers in order to ensure that prescription practices are in keeping with the project. With the view that "health professionals often resist change," AKF set out initially to obtain a technical consensus for the implementation of the revolving drug fund by establishing an Oblast[12] Committee on the Rational Use of Essential Drugs. This committee would include senior officials from the Health, Planning, and Finance ministries, NGOs and donors active in the health sector, and one community representative from each district.[13]

In addition to the establishment of the above committee, AKF's aim was to create a list of essential drugs adapted to the needs of Badakhshan and to establish therapeutic protocols based on the WHO-supported MSF treatment manual[14] and the assistance of a therapeutics consultant. According to the AKF proposal, certificates would be issued to the health staff to "motivate them to adopt new prescribing procedures," and "only health units whose staff have successfully completed the course will be included in the project" (AKF, cited in Keshavjee 1998). Thus, participation in the revolving drug fund (RDF), envisioned to be the major if not the only source of medicines for Badakhshanis, would involve compliance with the AKF/MSF/WHO-sponsored prescription guidelines.

The fact that AKF saw the implementation of the revolving drug fund as more than just the provision of pharmaceuticals was evident from the outset. For them, like their USAID donors, the fund was seen as a way of engineering social change. In their application to USAID, AKF wrote:

> The strategic use of essential drugs to catalyse [sic] the start of these reforms is an opportunity that perhaps should not be missed. In many ways, *the timing for such an initiative seems right,* and if the RDF project can serve to change the old ways of thinking at the many levels of this society, then the project will have made a significant contribution. . . . Although it is unlikely that the project will ever recover more than 50–60% of the actual drug costs, it is imperative that both government and communities make the mental switch that the old system is not coming back, and that any new, viable system will require more community involvement in management as well as in contribution (AKF, cited in Keshavjee 1998; emphasis added).

Thus, the solution to the regional health crisis became a much larger project with a broader underlying mandate, namely, to "change the old ways of thinking."

Defying Logic: Creating Unhealthy Health Policies

The inability of states to fund social services—coupled with the absence of private health sector funding sources such as insurance, employers, or local charities—has led NGOs in many poor settings to turn to the idea of "community financing": people would pay for social goods and services. Community financing of health care, usually involving user fees, is meant to "screen out" people seeking care for minor ailments (considered to be inappropriate demand) and target resources for those who require care. Also, in addition to tapping another source of revenue for the health system, user fees are seen as a way of getting people more involved in their health care delivery, increasing their awareness of health care, and encouraging them to use preventive measures more. Coupled with changes in prescription practices and the creation of an essential drugs list, this approach is aimed at creating a "rational" approach to drug use.

So, why charge for medicines? The largest costs in the formal health care system are pharmaceuticals and personnel. Of these, pharmaceuticals are the largest variable cost and are an easy target for reducing recurrent costs. For example, since the collapse of the Soviet Union, they have constituted 13 to 16 percent of the health costs in Tajikistan (Falkingham 2002). When charging for health services, user fees are usually levied on medicines because it is believed that patients prefer to pay for a commodity rather than a service, and because the availability of efficacious drugs is thought to attract people to a given health center (Litvack 1992). Hence the focus of the Bamako initiative on payment for medicines.

The question that needs to be asked is whether requiring sick people to pay for medicines will worsen social inequalities in access to health care. According to Carrin and Vereecke (1992), community financing of medicines can contribute to greater equity by ensuring greater availability of essential drugs, and it can contribute to more prudent and less wasteful use of drugs (45). Through cost recovery, the poorer part of the population may improve the availability of health resources and the provision of services at their local clinics, providing that they can pay for the charges. To some extent, there is truth to these assertions. For example, 91 percent of people surveyed in a household study in Rwanda said they would pay higher fees in order to ensure availability of drugs (which were available only 55 percent of the time) (Shepard, Carrin, and Nyandagazi 1987). Similarly, 93 percent of households interviewed in Honduras expressed a willingness to pay a fee for pharmaceuticals (Cross, Huff, Quick, and Bates 1986). Furthermore, if people know that they will have access to good quality care, they are willing to pay (Igun 1979; Kloos et al. 1987; Stock 1983).

Be that as it may, as Litvack (1992) points out, willingness to pay does not constitute ability to pay (Litvack 1992:203). Indeed, she argues that at times charging for health goods and services can be problematic, since some of the patients "screened" out by this mechanism will actually require medical attention and will delay seeking treatment until their illnesses are serious, thereby increasing the cost of treatment and potentially reducing their chances for survival (Litvack 1992:4). Experience from Western Europe shows that user charges secure little extra revenue, are inequitable, deter sick as well as healthy people, have adverse consequences on health outcomes, and are rarely well accepted by the public (Mossialos and Le Grand 1999:187).

In poor countries, the situation is similar. For example, in an evaluation of a self-financing public pharmacy in Fianga (Chad), Carrin, Autier, Djouater, and Vereecke (1992:92–93) found that while the overall use of drugs had increased, there were strong indications that poor households had difficulties financing drug treatments, especially when they involved the use of antibiotics. This led to limited utilization or the foregoing of treatment altogether. This was often the case for episodes of childhood diarrhea. In Swaziland, a fee increase preferentially led to reduced utilization of health services by patients with diarrheal diseases, sexually transmitted diseases, and acute respiratory infections, rather than affecting patients suffering from less severe conditions (Yoder 1989). Experience from Africa suggests that richer patients are less influenced by user fees than poorer ones (Dahlgren 1990), and that there might be a greater role for fees within hospitals rather than in the provision of primary health care (Gilson 1997). Sadly, a study of three countries with Bamako Initiative projects (Benin, Kenya, and Zambia) found that in all three countries, the programs failed to protect the most poor from the burden of payment (Gilson et al. 2001).

In looking at the revolving drug fund as health policy, it is clear that it did not make sense for Badakhshan at the point that it was implemented. Firstly, selling medications to a population barely surviving on humanitarian assistance—and, by AKF's own data, facing a worsening nutritional crisis—seems incongruous with the phenomenology of post-Soviet Badakhshan. Even with humanitarian assistance that included free medicines and food, malnutrition and the incidence of communicable infectious diseases had increased. In this nutritional, economic, and health context, it seems unlikely that a revolving drug fund itself would contribute to better health. In fact, using a Living Standards Measurement Survey conducted in Tajikistan in 1999, Falkingham (2002) has shown that not only was the cost of treatment cited as the main reason for not using health care by one-third of respondents, but 70 percent of respondents also noted that the main reason they did not obtain required medicines was their inability to pay for them (51–52). Falkingham concludes that this finding

> has implications for any revolving drug schemes to be developed in Tajikistan, and elsewhere in the region, and underscores the importance of establishing careful exemption policies that protect the poor, especially children and women—the most frequent consumers of essential pharmaceuticals (2002:52).

In Badakhshan, the findings are similar, with many respondents to a 1996 Pharmaceutical Use Survey reporting that despite needing to purchase medicines, they did not have the resources with which to make the purchase (Keshavjee 1998). In fact, only 31 percent of respondents reported that they were able to find money to purchase medicines that were prescribed by the doctor but were not provided to them free. This proportion was as low as 14 percent in one of Badakhshan's poorer regions. Thus, while the demand for health care initially appears inelastic, both quantitative and ethnographic research indicates that price does play a role in the demand for health care, and the demand becomes much more elastic as patients' incomes fall. This is also true in other poor-country settings (c.f. Akin, Griffin, Guilkey, and Popkin 1986; Sauerborn, Nougtara, and Diesfeld 1989; Habib and Vaughan 1986; Bitran 1988; Gertler, Locay, and Sanderson 1987; Gertler, Locay, Sanderson, Dor, and van der Gaag 1988; Gertler and van der Gaag 1988). As Falkingham (2002) concluded in her assessment of access to health care in Tajikistan, "Official and informal payments are acting both to deter people from seeking medical assistance and, once advice has been sought, to deter them from receiving the most appropriate treatment" (53).

Secondly, the main purpose of the revolving drug fund as conceived by AKF was not to promote health equity; it was to make medicines available and have communities "contribute" and "participate" more. Even if the medicines are subsidized, as the AKF revolving drug fund proposal advocated, it still meant that individuals and families were using scarce resources for essential medicines at a time of great hardship and uncertainty. As a Dental Clinic Survey conducted in 1996 discovered, many surveyed individuals said that they would forgo immediate treatment if they did not have money (Keshavjee 1998). Hardon and Kanji rightly note that although programs like the Bamako Initiative accept that a proportion of the community will not be able to pay for services and should be exempted, "Mechanisms and criteria for exemption are, however, simplistic and fail to reflect the complex power relationships that exist at the local levels of health care" (1992: 114).

The outcome of reduced health care use in Badakhshan has the potential to be devastating on the poorer segments of the population, half of whom are children (Falkingham 2002:46). Writing about infant mortality in Kyrgyzstan, Uzbekistan, and Tajikistan soon after the collapse of the Soviet Union, Victoria Velkoff (1992) suggested that lower levels of medical care usage could have a larger impact on infant mortality rates than even a substantial decrease in nutritional intake. She notes:

> If we take the average levels for these three republics, a 20% decrease in nutritional intake would result in an increase in infant mortality rates of less than one death per 1000 live births, or a 2% increase . . . [while a] change in the average level of medical care usage of 20% would result in an increase of over 13 and a half deaths, or 30% (152).

From the very beginning, the Bamako Initiative was caught up in a debate about equity (Gilson 1988; McPake 1993; Reddy and Vandermoortele 1996). In their analysis of the initiative in three countries, Gilson et al. (2001) found that the critical factor underlying the equity problem was "the failure to establish the protection of the poorest as a clear goal of the activities" (53). AKF's approach to the health crisis in Badakhshan was rooted in the discourse of developing "sustainable" projects that have the prospect of becoming self-sufficient; in the long run, to paraphrase AKF's proposal, it is to make it clear that the "old days are over." Indeed, having worked closely with AKF in the initial formulation and planning of the revolving drug fund, I know that the program was viewed as the only viable alternative in a situation where the population could potentially be left with no medicines as humanitarian assistance programs ended. The Geneva-based leadership felt that it was incumbent upon them to pursue sustainable options, especially within a context of great civil uncertainty, the threat of continued war, a collapsed economy, and a reduced flow of international donor assistance.[15] As testament to AKF's commitment to serving the best interests of the population, the organization continues to subsidize medicines in those districts of Badakhshan that have a functioning revolving drug fund (Chandani 1998).[16] That being said, the text of AKF's application to USAID indicates that AKF's approach placed an emphasis on community financing and changing mindsets, without explicit and sufficient protection for Badakhshan's poorest inhabitants—those most vulnerable to ill health.

Lessons for International Health Policy

Clearly, the task of reorganizing the health care system in Tajikistan—and specifically in Badakhshan—is a daunting one. There is a need to reform areas of the health sector that lead to detrimental outcomes (e.g., overprescription of antibiotics leading to antibiotic resistance, and risk of nosocomial and iatrogenic infections) or that could lead to the improvement of health delivery to the population (e.g., the creation of a "general practitioner" specialty, better primary-care facilities, and increased out-of-hospital treatment). There is also a need to improve the operational efficiency of the health care system. As Seedhouse (1995) points out, however, any reform "*must aim to reconstruct an existing structure or system in order to enable it to achieve its original end(s) in an improved way*" (Seedhouse 1995:2; emphasis added).

While the impetus for schemes such as the revolving drug fund may lie in the desire to improve access and availability of health care, their discursive roots lie in a different economic and social context. For example, in the United States, medical financing has been on the political agenda since the 1970s (Starr 1982). Questions arose about whether the high costs of Medicaid could be ameliorated by cost sharing, since it would discourage patients from "overusing" the health system and seeking "unnecessary" medical care. In this context, the debate was framed as one between inefficiency or moral hazard (overconsumption) and risk protection (Arrow 1968; Pauly 1968; Zeckhauser 1970; Feldstein 1973). Some cost sharing was suggested because the gains from the reduced risk that free care provided were modest (Newhouse et al. 1993:138). Even in this context, however, the RAND Health Insurance Experiment conducted in the 1970s and 1980s found that cost sharing reduced all types of interactions with the health system—physician visits, dental visits, prescriptions, and hospital admissions—and that health among the sick poor was adversely affected (Newhouse et al. 1993:338–339).

In the case of post-Soviet Badakhshan with its high rates of communicable diseases, issues of moral hazard do not fully apply to that health system. In fact, if Velkoff (1992) is correct about the increases in infant mortality that could result from reduced medical care usage, the risk is so high as to make the implementation of user fees irresponsible.

In the end, policy makers have to ask whether a given health policy addresses the needs of the population, and what kind of health outcomes are likely to result. Free market-based programs like the revolving drug fund face major challenges in ensuring equitable outcomes. Firstly, the mandate of the revolving drug fund is to create a "sustainable" structure that can ultimately survive in the absence of donor support.[17] Since in Tajikistan, as in many poor countries, a large percentage of the population simply does not have the resources with which to purchase health care, "sustainable" means that the population is relegated to inadequate health care services or none at all.

Secondly, programs like the revolving drug fund instill a much more subtle change within both the health care system and the society: namely, the notion that health and well being are commodities that must be purchased. This means that health increasingly takes on an "exchange value," with those who can afford it having the best health care (c.f. Nichter 1989). The corollary is that the most weak in the society, the poorest, will have the least access to medicines, while those who control various forms of capital will have access to more "advanced" medicines and medical care, leading to an inequitable distribution of health care.[18] On a micro level, this will occur in Badakhshan and will be particularly disadvantageous to the more indigent, whose unequal health outcomes will not be accidental.

Thirdly, approaches that rely on market mechanisms of distribution—that is, ability to pay—risk creating other, more dangerous inefficiencies. For example, if people would only receive medicines if they pay, it drives poorer users of health care away from preventive medicine and toward emergency use. Since the health system in any society is part of a social matrix that is inextricably linked to all the other systems, defining the purpose of the health system is not easy. It is not only involved in the goals of a given government, but also to prolong life and minimize suffering. In a fee-for-service system, this becomes viable only insofar as individuals are able to pay for care.

Selling medicines in the post-Soviet context is certainly not a new phenomenon. As we know, medicines were sold during the Soviet period, but they were sold at affordable prices. To develop a system to sell medicines to a population without the means to purchase them—a population receiving more than 80 percent food assistance—is to ignore the political economy of health in the post-Soviet context. Speaking of the transition that took place in Hungary in 1990, Orosz (1990) argued that issues of social and territorial inequalities in health are evaded by health policy makers. "To put it simply," she noted, "health policy has been 'fiscalized' under the pressure of the economic crisis, while the population's critical health status and the ailing health-care system demand a much broader perspective" (856). Instead of social responsibility, Orosz argues, "A commitment to narrowly interpreted economic efficiency is becoming more pervasive at the expense of medical efficiency and the reduction of inequalities" (Ibid).

Implementers of health policies and programs—including NGOs like AKF—need to design programs appropriate to the lived reality of the regions in which they work. In many settings, inequality of access leads to inequality of outcomes, and it is often the poorest members of the population that endure the highest disease morbidity and mortality (Farmer 1999). This means that health programs need to be based on sound quantitative and qualitative data, rather than on approaches rooted in other social, economic, and cultural contexts. Ethnography is an essential tool in this process because it not only provides an experience near reflection and analysis of what is at stake in the local world (Kleinman 1995), but when applied to policy-making bodies themselves, it also allows for an analysis of the cultural systems and socioeconomic interests that shape development discourse and practice (Ferguson 1994; Escobar 1995).

Notes

1. This research involves a pharmaceutical use survey and a dental clinic survey, both conducted in Badakhshan in 1996 (Keshavjee 1998).

2. The rate of inflation reached 635 percent in 1995; in 1996 it was 42 percent (World Bank 1998).

3. According to EOHCS (2000), reported IMR in Tajikistan is likely an underestimate of the actual IMR because prevailing Soviet-era definitions do not count premature and low birth weight newborns who did not survive the first week. It is also in the interest of hospitals not to record neonatal mortality (EOHCS 2000:4).

4. In 1997, 3,540 cases of measles were reported in Tajikistan (WHO 1999). Rates of diphtheria are much higher in Tajikistan than in other republics, with 1,464 cases reported in 1996 (Vitek and Wharton 1998).

5. With a land surface of 64,100 square kilometers (about half of the country), Badakhshan has only approximately 216,000 inhabitants.

6. Material is taken from an AKF internal report, "Health and Nutrition Survey, Autonomous Oblast of Gorno Badakhshan (Tajikistan)," July–August 1996, February 1997 version (Keshavjee 1998).

7. These data are based on data collected from the Khorog Central Polyclinic (Keshavjee 1998).

8. Because the pharmaceutical use survey relied on individual honesty and self-reporting, the values may be an underestimation of the true household income.

9. Material is taken from "Health and Nutrition Survey, Autonomous Oblast of Gorno Badakhshan (Tajikistan)," July–August 1996, February 1997 version (Keshavjee 1998).

10. They hired Mr. Najmi Kanji, who has written extensively on pharmaceuticals in poor countries. (See Kanji 1989, 1992; Kanji and Hardon 1992; and Hardon and Kanji 1992.)

11. As Kanji and Hardon (1992) rightly point out:

> WHO's concept of rational drugs use is mainly defined in medical and financial terms. But people have their own rationales for deciding on therapies. Irrationality, defined from a medical point of view, may be totally rational from the consumer's point of view. . . . People's economic conditions also play an important part in affecting the use of drugs. From the consumer's point of view, the potential adverse effects of irrational use may be irrelevant in the harsh context of his or her daily life. For example, if a drug is said to be good for certain ailments and is easily available through informal distribution channels, many poor people will use it in the hope that they will be able to continue working and thus avoid losing a day's wages and/or production. A small farmer who has a fever cannot afford to follow the "rational" medical advice to go home and rest. He or she is obliged to take antipyretics and to continue working. Similarly, if a drug treatment has been effective before and there are still some tablets left over, then it also makes sense to keep these tablets for the next time round. Both money and time can thus be saved (103).

12. Provincial.

13. According to Kanji and Hardon (1992:94), programs that are implemented in the absence of a national policy or consensus tend to become vertical, resulting in parallel systems of procurement, distribution, and training.

14. This document was used because it was available in Russian.

15. Carrin and Vereecke (1992) point out that the constraint on international aid and on public health budgets forces governments to produce as much health as possible, within predetermined budgets (23).

16. As of the summer of 1998, the revolving drug fund, renamed the Rational Pharmaceutical Policy and Management Project, had been initiated in two of Badakhshan's districts. The preliminary results show that while other aspects of the program are going exceedingly well (e.g., reaching a consensus with physicians and health officials, and teaching local authorities to plan for and order medicines), the populace is only able to pay about 10 percent of the cost of the medicines. AKF subsidizes the remainder of the cost.

17. According to LaFond (1995), most donor ideas about sustainability involve the following:

> They are predicated on the assumption that once initial "start-up" costs are met, donors will "hand over" all project responsibilities to government. Ordinarily these responsibilities consist of operational costs and support activities such as supervision and management. According to

the traditional definition sustainability occurs when government absorbs these responsibilities and is able to maintain project benefits. . . . The majority of donor perceptions of sustainability are reflected in the following definition employed by the United States Agency for International Development: *Sustainability is the ability of a health project or programme to deliver health services or sustain benefits after major technical, managerial and financial support has ceased* (27–28).

18. For there to be equity, Carrin says, "An acceptable long-run goal is the equal utilization of health care among those patients who have a similar need for treatment in the event of a given illness" (Carrin and Vereecke 1992: 68).

References

Abel-Smith, B., and A. Dua. (1998). "Community Financing in Developing Countries: The Potential for the Health Sector." *Health Policy and Planning* 3, no. 2: 95–108.

Akin, J. S., C. C. Griffin, D. K. Guilkey, and B. M. Popkin. (1986). "The Demand for Adult Outpatient Services in the Bicol Region of the Philippines." *Social Science and Medicine* 22, no. 3: 321–28.

Arrow, K. J. (1968). "The Economics of Moral Hazard: Further Comment." *American Economic Review* 58: 537–39.

Bitran, R. (1988). *Health Care Demand Studies in Developing Countries: A Critical Review and Agenda for Research.* Arlington, VA: Resources for Child Health Project, John Snow Inc.

Carrin, G., and M.c Vereecke. (1992). *Strategies for Health Care Finance in Developing Countries—With a Focus on Community Financing in Sub-Saharan Africa.* London: Macmillan.

Carrin, G., P. Autier, B. Djouater, and M. Vereecke. (1992). "Direct Payment for Drugs at the Public Pharmacy in Fianga (Chad)." In *Strategies for Health Care Finance in Developing Countries—With a Focus on Community Financing in Sub-Saharan Africa,* edited by G. Carrin with M. Vereecke, 75–95. London: Macmillan.

Chandani, Y. (1998). "Utilizing Prescribing Patterns to Determine Rational Drug Use in Khorog, GBAO, Tajikistan." Master's thesis, Department of Epidemiology and Public Health, Yale University.

Cross, P. N., M. A. Huff, J. D. Quick, and J. A. Bates. (1986). "Revolving Drug Funds: Conducting Business in the Public Sector." *Social Science and Medicine* 22, no. 3: 335–43.

Dahlgren, G. (1990). "Strategies for Health Financing in Kenya—The Difficult Birth of a New Policy." *Scandinavian Journal of Social Medicine,* supp. no. 46: 67–81.

Escobar, A. (1995). *Encountering Development: The Making and Unmaking of the Third World.* Princeton, NJ: Princeton University Press.

European Observatory on Health Care Systems (EOHCS). (2000). *Health Care Systems in Transition: Tajikistan.* Copenhagen: WHO Regional Office for Europe.

Falkingham, J. (2000). *Women and Gender Relations in Tajikistan.* London: Department of Social Policy, London School of Economics.

———. (2002). Poverty, Affordability, and Access to Health Care. In *Health Care in Central Asia,* edited by Martin McKee, Judith Healy, and Jane Falkingham, 42–56. European Observatory on Health Care Systems Series. Buckingham: Open University Press.

Farmer, P. E. (1999). *Infections and Inequalities: The Modern Plagues.* Berkeley: University of California Press.

Feldstein, M. S. (1973). "The Welfare Loss of Excess Health Insurance." *Journal of Political Economy* 81: 251–58.

Ferguson, J. (1988). "Cultural Exchange: New Development in the Anthropology of Commodities." *Cultural Anthropology* 3: 488–513.

———. (1994). *The Anti-Politics Machine: "Development," Depoliticization, and Bureaucratic Power in Lesotho.* Minneapolis: University of Minnesota Press.

Gertler, P., L. Locay, and W. Sanderson. (1987). "Are User Fees Regressive?" *Journal of Econometrics* 36: 67–88.

Gertler, P., L. Locay, W. Sanderson, A. Dor, and J. van der Gaag. (1988). *Health Care Financing and the Demand for Medical Care.* Working Paper no. 37. Washington, DC: World Bank Living Standards Study (LSMS), World Bank.

Gertler, P., and J. van der Gaag. (1988). *Measuring the Willingness to Pay for Social Services in Developing Countries.* World Bank LSMS Working Paper no. 45. Washington, DC: World Bank.

Gilson, L. (1988). *Charging for Government Health Care: Is Equity Being Abandoned?* London: London School of Hygiene and Tropical Medicine, EPC publication no. 15.

———. (1997). "Review Paper: The Lessons of User Fee Experience in Africa." *Health Policy and Planning,* 12, no. 4: 273.

Gilson, L., D. Kalyalya, F. Kuchler, S. Lake, H. Oranga, and M. Ouendo. (2001). "Strategies for Promoting Equity: Experience with Community Financing in Three African Countries." *Health Policy* 58: 37–67.

Habib, O. S., and J. P. Vaughan. (1986). "The Determinants of Health Services Utilization in Southern Iraq: A Household Interview Survey." *International Journal of Epidemiology* 15, no. 3: 395–403.

Hampton M. D., L. R. Ward, B. Rowe, and E. J. Threfall. (1998, April–June). "Molecular Fingerprinting of Multidrug-Resistant Salmonella Enterica Serotype Typhi." *Emerging Infectious Diseases* 4, no. 2: 317–20.

Hardon, A., and N. Kanji. (1992). "New Horizons in the 1990s." In *Drugs Policy in Developing Countries,* edited by N. Kanji, A. Hardon, J. W. Harnmeijer, M. Mamdani, and G. Walt. London: Zed Books.

Igun, U. A. (1979). "Stages in Health-Seeking: A Descriptive Model." *Social Science and Medicine* 13A, no. 4: 445–56.

International Monetary Fund (IMF). (1998). *Republic of Tajikistan: Recent Economic Developments.* IMF Staff Country report no. 98/16. Washington, DC: International Monetary Fund.

Kanji, N. (1989). "Charging for Drugs in Africa: UNICEF's Bamako Initiative." *Health Policy and Planning,* no. 4: 110–20.

———. (1992). "Action at Country Level: The International and National Influences." In *Drugs Policy in Developing Countries,* edited by N. Kanji, A. Hardon J. W. Harnmeijer, M. Mamdani, and G. Walt. London: Zed Books.

Kanji, N., and A. Hardon. (1992). "What Has Been Achieved and Where are We Now?" In *Drugs Policy in Developing Countries,* edited by N. Kanji, A. Hardon, J. W. Harnmeijer, M. Mamdani, and G. Walt. London: Zed Books.

Keshavjee, S. (1998, September). "Medicines and Transitions: The Political Economy of Health and Social Change in Post-Soviet Badakhshan, Tajikistan." Ph.D. diss., Harvard University.

Keshavjee, S., and M. C. Becerra. (2000, March 1). "Disintegrating Health Services and Resurgent Tuberculosis in Post-Soviet Tajikistan: An Example of Structural Violence." *Journal of the American Medical Association* 283, no. 9: 1201.

Kleinman, A. (1995). *Writing at the Margin: Discourse between Anthropology and Medicine.* Berkeley: University of California Press.

Kloos, H., A. Etea, A. Degefa, H. Aga, B. Solomon, K. Abera, et al. (1987). "Illness and Health Behavior in Addis Ababa and Rural Central Ethiopia." *Social Science and Medicine* 25, no. 9: 1003–1019.

LaFond, A. (1995). *Sustaining Primary Health Care.* London: Earthscan Publications.

Litvack, J. I. (1992). "The Effects of User Fees and Improved Quality on Health Facility Utilization and Household Expenditure: A Field Experiment in the Adamaoua Province of Cameroon." Ph.D. dissertation, Fletcher School of Law and Diplomacy.

McPake, B. (1993). "User Charges for Health Services in Developing Countries: A Review of the Literature." *Social Science and Medicine* 36, no. 11: 1397–1405.

Mossialos, E., and J. Le Grand. (1999). "Cost Containment in the EU: An Overview." In *Health Care and Cost Containment in the European Union,* edited by Elias Mossialos and J. Le Grand, 1–154. Ashgate: Aldershot.

Newhouse, J. P., and the Insurance Experiment Group. (1993). *Free for All? Lessons from the RAND Health Insurance Experiment.* Cambridge, MA: Harvard University Press.

Nichter, M. (1989). "Pharmaceuticals, Health Commodification, and Social Relations: Ramifications for Primary Health Care." In *Anthropology and International Health: South Asian Case Studies,* 223–76. Dordrecht: Kluwer Academic Publishers.

Orosz, E. (1990). "The Hungarian Country Profile: Inequalities in Health and Health Care in Hungary." *Social Science and Medicine* 31, no. 8: 847–57.

Pauly, M. V. (1968). "The Economics of Moral Hazard." *American Economic Review* 58: 231–37.

Reddy, S., and J. Vandermoortele. (1996). *User Financing of Basic Social Services: A Review of Theoretical Arguments and Empirical Evidence.* New York: Office of Evaluation, Policy and Planning, United Nations Children's Fund.

Sauerborn, R., A. Nougtara, and H. J. Diesfeld. (1989). "Low Utilization of Community Health Workers: Results from a Household Interview Survey in Burkina Faso." *Social Science and Medicine* 29, no. 10: 1163–74.

Seedhouse, D. (1995). "The Logic of Health Reform." In *Reforming Health Care: The Philosophy and Practice of International Health Reform,* edited by D. Seedhouse. New York: John Wiley & Sons.

Shepard, D. S., G. Carrin, and P. Nyandagazi. (1987). *Self-Financing of Health Care at Government Health Centers in Rwanda.* Cambridge, MA: Harvard Institute for International Development.

Starr, P. (1982). *The Social Transformation of American Medicine.* New York: Basic Books.

Stock, R. (1983). "Distance and the Utilization of Health Facilities in Rural Nigeria." *Social Science and Medicine* 17, no. 9: 563–70.

UNICEF. (1988). *Recommendations to the Executive Board for Programme Cooperation, 1989–1993, The Bamako Initiative.* E/ICEF/1988/P/L.40. New York: UNICEF.

———. (1990). *The Bamako Initiative Planning Guide.* New York: Bamako Initiative Management Unit, UNICEF.

UNICEF/WHO Mission. (1992, February 17–21). *The Invisible Emergency: A Crisis of Children and Women in Tajikistan.* New York: Report of UNICEF/WHO mission with participation of UNDP, UNFPA, WFP (unpublished).

United Nations Development Programme (UNDP). (1998). *Tajikistan: Human Development Report 1998.* UNDP.

United Nations Development Project (UNDP). (1999). Human Development Report 1999, Oxford University Press, New York.

United Nations Office for the Coordination of Humanitarian Affairs (OCHA). (1998). *Tajikistan Humanitarian Situation Report May 1998.* Accessed at www.reliefweb.int/files, June 12, 1998.

Velkoff, V. A. (1992). *Trends and Differentials in Infant Mortality in the Soviet Union for the Years 1970–1988.* Dissertation thesis, Princeton University.

Vitek, C. R., and M. Wharton. (1998). "Diphtheria in the Former Soviet Union: Reemergence of a Pandemic Disease." *Emerging Infectious Diseases* 4, no. 4: 539–50.

World Bank. (1998). *Tajikistan.* Accessed at www.worldbank.org/gtml/extdr/offrep/eca/tajcb.htm, June 1998.

World Health Organization (WHO). (1988, September 7–14). *Guidelines for Implementing the Bamako Initiative.* Regional Committee for Africa, 38th Session, Brazzaville. AFR/RC38/18 Rev. 1.

———. (1999). *Country Health Report: Republic of Tajikistan.* Copenhagen: WHO Regional Office for Europe.

Yoder, R. A. (1989). "Are People Willing and Able to Pay for Health Services?" *Social Science and Medicine* 29, no. 1: 35–42.

Zeckhauser, R. J. (1970). "Medical Insurance: A Case Study of the Tradeoff between Risk Spreading and Appropriate Incentives." *Journal of Economic Theory* 2, no. 1: 10–26.

Equity in Access to AIDS Treatment in Africa: Pitfalls among Achievements

7

ALICE DESCLAUX

WITH MORE THAN 30 MILLION PEOPLE living with HIV in Africa, or 70 percent of the world's cases, the African continent is facing a major catastrophe. In addition to its associated high human suffering, the HIV/AIDS pandemic represents a critical issue to current public health, especially when considering access to highly active antiretroviral therapy (HAART). In this chapter, I illustrate some of these issues regarding social values underlying health interventions on the basis of ethnographic data from Senegal and comparative analysis with data from neighboring countries.

The International Issue of Access to HAART in Africa

The last five years have witnessed the effects of globalization and inequalities between high- and low-income countries on access to AIDS treatment in Africa. From 1996, when the effects of HAART were first shown, potent drugs commercialized at high prices in developed countries were first offered at the same—or sometimes higher—prices in African countries, where the average income can be 30 times lower. Welfare protection or health insurance in these countries does not cover HAART; furthermore, the majority of the population is without even this limited welfare protection. This situation, a new kind of exploitation of underdeveloped countries, was modified by the efforts of activists and public health specialists, and the prices for some antiretrovirals (ARVs) were reduced significantly (Katzenstein, Laga, and Moatti 2003).

In 2000, Access Initiative, managed by the World Health Organization (WHO) and UNAIDS, allowed price reductions under certain conditions in a range of countries. At the same time, the commercialization of generic medicines created a competitive market permitting further price reductions. The struggle of low-income countries for access to medicines, however, is not over; present negotiations for the World Trade Organization's TRIPS agreements ('T Hoen 2003) may open or close the possibility for these countries to buy, sell, or produce the medicines they need.[1] Although low-cost and efficient drugs have been discovered, their price, which is now 30 times cheaper than the price for triple-combination therapy was four years ago, is still high compared with average incomes in Africa (Moatti et al. 2003). Special regimens needed for some HIV patients, along with medicines used for opportunistic infections or diseases not related to HIV, are not available in these conditions. The availability of low-cost drugs depends partly on political will, which can differ greatly between countries that import generic drugs and those where the government refuses to provide HAART to AIDS patients, and on international measures that shape such issues as external debt and access to multilateral loans. Access to treatment also depends on availability and efficiency of care, from technical skills and means to human resources. The Global Fund to Fight AIDS, Tuberculosis and Malaria is expected to provide the resources to create or enlarge access to comprehensive AIDS care, which includes HAART, and to reduce inequalities in the provision of care in African countries. But much remains to be done; it is presently estimated that in 2003 only 30,000 persons are receiving HAART in sub-Saharan Africa, when the actual need is estimated at about 4 million (Moatti et al. 2003).

Availability and affordability of HAART in Africa depend mainly on political, legal, and economic factors; the control of medicines is the visible part of important present changes in the production of equalities and inequalities regarding access to resources, according to health and trade policies. International health policies implemented in African countries confront not only commercial interests, but also differing conceptions concerning the responsibility for the provision of health services and the role of government in public health. Beyond these discrepancies, there are different perceptions of equity and different social constructions of AIDS that should be analyzed in a sociopolitical history of international access to HAART. These changes are also related to the commercialization of health and the political management of diseases, in both developed and low-income countries.

From International to Local Access to Treatment

If the survival of an African AIDS patient depends on international power relationships and on the legal control of resources, it also depends on the local management of access to care and medicines. Since the publication of international guidelines for HAART implementation in Africa (International AIDS Society 1999), several pilot projects and national programs have begun to provide access to HAART. These programs have been set up by governments through National AIDS Committees under the UNAIDS Initiative (in Uganda and Côte d'Ivoire); with the participation or technical support of UNAIDS (as in Nigeria and Mali); with complementary financial support from international foundations (in Botswana); by local NGOs (as in Burundi and Burkina Faso); by international humanitarian organizations (as in Malawi, South Africa, and Tanzania); or by government services and research institutions (as in Cameroon and Senegal). Most programs are managed and executed by a group composed of various representatives from international and local institutions.

Putting medical strategies into practice obliged program promoters to weigh the question of equity in the provision of treatment with limited resources and in conditions contingent on political will and national financial resources. HAART programs provide various categories of terms and conditions for access to treatment. The first programs that were set up, as in Uganda, asked the patients to pay the total cost of treatment out of pocket (Katabira 1997). Such programs made possible the securing of price reductions, thanks to the provision of medicines through a centrally managed agency, but they were not accessible to the majority of patients. Some programs initiated by humanitarian organizations, such as Médecins sans Frontières (MSF) offered free medicines, for a specified period—from 18 months to five years (MSF 2003). They were inspired by the strategy of "creating a breach" with the aim of demonstrating the feasibility and efficiency of the provision of treatment, thereby inducing governments to take over the programs. National programs tried to combine the goals of accessibility and durability and provided medicines at subsidized rates under various conditions. The diverse modalities of access to programs and the pricing of medicines have resulted in the social and economic selection of patients who can get treatment, and thus of those who cannot.

Publications on pilot projects in sub-Saharan Africa have until now mainly emphasized the feasibility and efficiency of HAART, adherence to treatment, and the risk of creating viral resistance, as these factors were being discussed at the international level (World Health Organization [WHO] 2001; *AIDS* 2003). HAART programs have also provided observations and experiences about failures and pitfalls in the management of equity that can endanger the health of some categories of population. It is important to describe and analyze these limitations because, for an African AIDS patient, access to HAART can signify survival or imminent death. Moreover, studies and practices in West African countries such as Mali (Imane 2002) and Burkina-Faso (Bronsard 1998) have shown that, lacking a well-run and easily accessible HAART program, patients manage to get ARVs directly from their families living in developed countries, from NGOs and the informal market, or through prescriptions by private practitioners who do not always follow international recommendations for the clinical management of HAART. As HAART requires a high level of adherence and strictly defined prescriptions and follow-ups, these irregular uses of medicines may be not only inefficient but can also lead to adverse side effects or increased risk of viral resistance, jeopardizing the patient's later ability to recover. Therefore, the mismanagement of equity in the provision of HAART results in the loss of opportunities to improve health and exposes a number of patients to iatrogenic conditions.

This anthropological analysis provides insights into the categorization of population groups by the health system and the subsequent medical control of the "social body" in Senegal. It also provides insights into concepts underlying equity and its management that are rooted in the culture of international health or in contemporary African culture. The perceptions and practices pertaining to the equity of programs at the local level stem from the dialectics between these two cultural backgrounds and from the power relationships and negotiations or confrontations among the different institutions mentioned above.

This analysis will be centered on the *Initiative Sénégalaise d'Accès aux ARV* (or Senegalese Initiative for Access to ARVs, or ISAARV), launched in 1998 in Dakar by the National AIDS Committee under the authority of the Ministry of Health. This pilot project was the first to be entirely designed and set up by a national team of health professionals, on a budget provided by the government, and at a time when most international institutions were reticent about access to HAART in Africa. The pilot project was organized on an empirical basis, and its effects were evaluated by epidemiologists and social scientists between 1998 and 2001, leading to a redefinition of the scope and means for provision of treatment. Research in medical anthropology was conducted, mainly among patients undergoing treatment, to discern the social effects of the program (Desclaux, Lanièce, Ndoye, and Taverne 2002).[2]

The results of these studies were, until 2002, regularly discussed with the team managing the program. In Dakar, the program was partly revised based on results from epidemiological and anthropological studies, and has evolved according to local changes and reductions in the international prices of drugs. However, the features and results of ISAARV must be carefully considered from a critical point of view, since this program has been considered as a model for the establishment of other national programs in West and Central Africa, in spite of its limitations, which will be described below.

The ISAARV Program

The Establishment of a Pilot Project

ISAARV was the first pilot project of its kind and its promoters had to face strategic choices, confronted as they were by uncertainties as to the feasibility, efficacy, and acceptability of antiretroviral therapies, as well as by the prevailing material and financial constraints. The project was designed to be integrated in three hospital services. The health professionals responsible for the execution of the program (physicians, biologists, virologists, pharmacists, and social workers) were invited to participate in its definition and planning. They set up a management board composed of four committees in charge of program planning, patients' inclusion, and follow-up (Eligibility Committee); therapeutic and medical decisions (Medical Committee); nonmedical aspects and social research (Welfare Committee); and drug management (Pharmaceutical Committee) (Desclaux et al. 2003).

ISAARV was designed to be accessible to all persons requiring treatment with antiretroviral drugs, regardless of their nationality or socioeconomic status, provided they were residents in Senegal. Drugs were financed both by the government and by the patient—the amount to be paid by the patient was calculated according to his or her personal resources. Patients selected by a physician on the basis of immunovirologic and clinical criteria underwent an "inclusion" interview by a social worker, with the aim of assessing the patient's economic resources and social support network, identifying other HIV-infected persons in the household, and ensuring that the patient had correctly understood the constraints of three-drug regimens. The results of the survey were discussed by the Eligibility Committee, which endorsed the decision to provide treatment and determined the cost (including cost of medicine) to be borne by the patient. Personal, household, and family incomes and expenses were considered in the determination of this amount. Children, health professionals, and active members of self-help groups for people living with AIDS (PLWA) were exempted from financial participation.

When the program was launched in 1998, the price for a triple-combination therapy was about 300,000 FCFA (US$457)[3] per month: the establishment of a unique provision system by the Pharmaceutical Committee and the Ministry of Health's National Procurement Pharmacy had decreased by half the price of drugs in Senegal, drugs that had been previously available only through private drug sellers.

Achievements of the Program

The number of patients included in the program slowly increased during the pilot period, from 60 in April 1999 to 300 in November 2001 to 1,051 in March 2003. Clinical outcomes such as viral resistance and adherence were similar to those observed in developed countries (Laurent et al. 2002). The level of viral resistance was not greater than in developed countries, which could be explained by the use of regimens based mainly on triple combination therapy, a well-managed patient follow-up, and an adequately accessible program (Touré-Kane Ndeye et al. 2002). The level of adherence was high, similar to levels obtained in industrialized countries: average adherence among 158 patients during a 24-month study period (November 1999 to October 2001) was 91 percent (Lanièce et al. 2003). Factors that may explain this good adherence include the experimental nature of the program, recent inclusion in a small cohort of patients, and the fact that most of the patients had never previously received ARVs. Patients were highly motivated because they were symptomatic at the time of their inclusion in the program and they considered getting treatment a privilege. Patients' adherence was supported mainly through counseling by the pharmacist. Two main factors were found to reduce adherence: the type of drug combination (as in industrialized countries, simplified treatment regimens, especially with nonnucleoside reverse transcriptase inhibitors (NNRTI), appear to be better managed and better accepted) and the cost of treatment. Overall adherence was best among patients receiving free treatment.

Social Impact of Equity Management in ISAARV

Financial difficulties soon appeared to be the main barrier for patients' inclusion and adherence, both in questionnaire inquiries and qualitative surveys among patients and in the daily management of the program. Difficulties regarding access to treatment had three kinds of consequences: noninclusion of patients in the program, adherence problems, and social hardship of included patients due to payments requested as family support.

Noninclusions

During the first year, there were seven rates for the same triple-combination treatment (Table 7.1), and the minimum monthly cost for patients (subsidized at 93.5 percent) was 21,000 FCFA (US$28), while the legal minimum wage in Senegal at that time was 36,250 FCFA (US$48.3).

Table 7.1. Patients' User Fees for Medicines (in FCFA)

	ISAARV Period				
	From August 1998	*From Nov. 2000*	*From Feb. 2001*	*From July 2001*	*From Jan. 2002*
Cost of a three-drug regimen	320,000	100,000	100,000	60,000	Unknown
Rates paid by patients	198,000	100,000	100,000		
	150,000	60,000	60,00	60,000	
	64,000		40,000	40,000	
	50,000	20,000	20,000	20,000	20,000
	40,000		10,000	10,000	
	21,000	5,000	5,000	5,000	5,000
		0	0	0	0

Note: US$1 = 640 FCFA; 1,000 FCFA = US$1.56.

Although low compared with the cost of drugs paid by the Ministry of Health, this amount was an obstacle for many patients; in 2001, 30 percent of ISAARV patients had no income and two-thirds of them lived below the poverty line. Patients for whom antiretroviral treatment was medically indicated, but who did not meet economic criteria, were excluded from the selection process, either before or after their financial needs were assessed. Moreover, to avoid raising false hopes, medical doctors generally conducted an informal selection prior to the social survey on the basis of the patients' presumed ability to pay.

Nonincluded patients have remained invisible, and their number cannot be estimated. The lack of material and organizational means for the follow-up of patients restricted the capacity of health services to keep information about them, information that could have led to their inclusion when conditions for access changed. Data from qualitative interviews show that noninclusion in the program was felt by some patients as an exclusion, leading them to stop seeking treatment in ISAARV services. Instead, they turned to other health professionals or to traditional practitioners—some of whom are available in the same hospital services—to experiment with folk medicines. Some patients, often with the help of health professionals, found strategies to get access to treatment, most often by joining PLWA self-support groups. For other patients, the attitudes of health professionals based on denial, silence, and the conscious or unconscious restriction of access to preinclusion (for instance, through limiting access to HIV testing) act as a kind of regulation and can be viewed as the "shadowy side" of the program.

Adherence Problems

The analysis of factors influencing adherence in Senegal showed that adherence among patients receiving the same treatment decreased as the amount of their financial participation increased (Lanièce et al. 2003). This trend was noted during the first year of the study and, to a lesser extent, during the second year. Just as treatment interruptions due to financial problems have been reported in other African settings (Delaunay, Vidal, Msellati, and Moatti 2001), financial obstacles led to prolonged discontinuations of treatment in ISAARV until, following a decision of the Eligibility Committee, patient fees were reduced. The effect of such interruptions on patients' health are deleterious, since a very high level of adherence is required by HAART (more than 90 percent of prescribed intakes) to avoid treatment failures or emergence of viral resistance. In some cases, the economic difficulties of the patients were observed soon after enrollment. After a few months, patients could recognize that they had undertaken costs that were too high for their income, especially when they had to face other unexpected expenses or when the family members supporting them had other priorities. Besides poverty, precariousness is another characteristic of the household economy in

African countries, which appears as a structural limitation to paying for the cost of treatment. Moreover, in urban settings, where households are more often composed of nuclear than of extended families, individuals have fewer opportunities to receive family support (Mary 1997).

For patients who have overcome the acceptance stage of treatment and adapted the management of their personal resources to the monthly HAART payments, problems might arise later when they have lost the social status lent by the "sick role." When the physical stigma of the disease disappears under HAART, the patient is expected to return the help received from his family, who often does not understand why the patient must still pay for treatment or why he or she does not face his or her social obligations again, such as sharing family expenses. These economic difficulties lead to the exclusion of some patients during the first year of ISAARV.

Compensations for Family Support

Many patients had to solicit help from their families to meet the monthly cost of their medicines and were often supported by relatives or friends, who made monthly contributions. Asking help from family members obliged patients to reveal their HIV status in a society where HIV/AIDS is still a stigmatizing disease. Disclosure of status had different consequences, leading some patients to leave their families and others to reinforce links with some family members. Disclosure and the request for financial help in many cases reactivated previous family conflicts. Patients dependent on the financial help of the family had to obey family requests; they were often asked to conform to social norms or to respect religious prescriptions, as if obedience were to compensate for economic support.

In other cases, the question of intrahousehold resource allocation led patients to unavoidable dilemmas, such as when the costs for treatment make it impossible for a household to meet other priorities, such as the illness of a family member. In many cases, these situations jeopardized the patients' health; in most cases, they created anxiety and additional social suffering for AIDS patients.

Analyses of a System

Limitations of a System Aiming at Equity

It is difficult to assess whether the sliding fee set up in ISAARV helped to treat more patients than a "low cost for all" scheme. The overall recovery rate was low: it was estimated at 12 percent of the costs for medicines during the first year. The sliding fee appeared to be time consuming and resource consuming, inaccurate, and inefficient. Due to difficulties in assessing the resources available to an individual or a household in a social context in which most active adults have no declared salary and hold irregular or casual jobs, financial assessments were lengthy, difficult to conduct, and imprecise. Patients felt these inquiries were intrusive and presented a risk of breach of confidentiality. Long discussions of cases in the Eligibility Committee often reflected subjective perceptions or expected social values. Many patients, in the meantime, had to apply for a price reduction because they could not come up with the fee requested from them. In 2000, an experiment was begun using "scores" based on simplified criteria in order to shorten the financial assessments, and the number of price categories was reduced. However, this simplification could not meet the increasing number of inclusions. The "scoring" was abandoned, and the multileveled price scale was progressively replaced by a two-rate system.

Meanwhile, other studies were undertaken to discover the magnitude of the patients' economic burden. Besides payment for medicines, patients included in ISAARV had to pay direct medical costs (including costs of medical visits, biological and radiological examinations, hospitalization, travel, and medicines, but excluding the purchase of ARV) of an average of 5,200 FCFA (US$8.10) per month (Canestri et al. 2002). This amount was far beyond the capacities of the Senegalese population: in Dakar, 83 percent of the population have no welfare protection. Moreover, people who do have protection are reluctant to use it because they fear confidentiality will be breached.

After the November 2000 Price Reductions

The patients' contributions to the cost of their treatment evolved according to the prices imposed by pharmaceutical companies. Prices fell after November 2000, and a government subsidy of 100 percent was introduced. Following the reduction of antiretroviral drug prices early in the second year, the average contribution made by patients already on treatment was cut fourfold, and minimum participation was canceled. The sharp decrease in the cost that patients had to pay contributed significantly to the improvement in adherence during the second year (90 percent in year 2 versus 83 percent in year 1). When interviewed, patients reported that financial difficulties were the leading cause of treatment interruption in the first year, but only the fifth cause in the second year.

Low Prices and Free Treatment as the Final Choice

The ISAARV pilot project gave an opportunity to quantify the limits and failures of an ARV access program that required payment by patients. It also provided an estimate of prices that patients can bear and of the amount needed to support patient access to ARV, in addition to the cost of drugs. Following an evaluation of the program and the reduction of international prices for medicines, ISAARV changed its method of pricing to reach more patients. In November 2002, to provide access to patients in need of treatment, to ensure their adherence, and to mitigate onerous inclusion processes, 95 percent of the patients included in ISAARV were provided treatment free of charge, and 5 percent were provided treatment for a payment of 5,000 FCFA (US$7.80).

Discussion

Multilevel pricing for medicines can be viewed as an economic experiment that will survive neither the difficulties met in its application in Senegal nor the evaluation of the process and tools used in ISAARV. Other as yet unevaluated schemes aimed at equity in access to HAART are still in use.

Selection Based on Social Criteria

In most African countries that have implemented comprehensive AIDS programs, pricing includes a "standard" price for usual patients and waivers or exemptions for patients belonging to different categories and groups. In Mali, for instance, a multilevel price scale has been planned, combined with a fee exemption for active members of PLWA self-help groups and for health professionals. However, until the implementation of this system, usual patients are asked to pay 45,000 FCFA (US$70.30) per month—which represents a 50 percent subsidy for triple-combination therapy at local cost. In Côte d'Ivoire, initial pricing considered "priority categories" that included women who had previously participated in clinical trials for the prevention of mother-to-child transmission, members of PLWA organizations, and, more recently, public-sector health professionals—who had to pay 10,000 FCFA (US$15.60) per month for triple-combination therapy in 1999, which represents a 95 percent subsidy in this country. In addition, those considered poor (under unspecified criteria) who could obtain a partial waiver were asked to pay 80,000 FCFA (US$125), which represented a 60 percent subsidy (Delaunay et al. 2001) until April 2001, when this fee was reduced to 25,000 FCFA (US$39.10) for people with several dependants. In Burkina-Faso, the Ambulatory Treatment Center, which provides HAART in Ouagadougou, has established four fees: free access to orphans; 5,000 FCFA (US$7.80) for pregnant women, health professionals, the poor, students, and school children; 10,000 FCFA (US$15.60) for government employees; and 20,000 FCFA (US$31.20) for businessmen and traders (Alzouma 2002). No published information is available as to how patients are categorized in practice.

The variety of criteria in neighboring countries with similar social and economic contexts is surprising. Moreover, the analysis of the use of categorizations and social criteria for ISAARV patients showed that they did not correspond to clear-cut definitions and were applied in a rather arbitrary manner. The choice of exempted categories is based on various logics (social productivity, level of income and inability to pay, merit, deontology) embedded in social values that are expressed differently according to context. In some cases, such as Mali, where the minimum cost for most patients is nearly twice the minimum wage, not being classified in such categories may lead to exclusion from HAART programs.

Recent studies in the context of primary health care or hospital care in different settings have shown that exemptions or waivers for treatment or hospital charges were seldom offered to patients who would have needed them and had the right to obtain them (Meng, Sun, and Hearst 2002; Kivumbi and Kintu 2002; Paphassarang, Philavong, Boupha, and Blas 2002). The Bamako Initiative policy considered exemptions and waivers as a way to achieve equity, but evaluations of its implementation in West Africa show that measures for the poor were foreseen, but still not in effect ten years after its introduction (Ridde 2003). Several economic studies of cost-recovery policy in West Africa conclude that neither governments nor local health professionals are really interested in translating the rhetoric of equity into practice devoted to health access for the poor (Dumoulin and Kaddar 1993; Jaffré and Olivier de Sardan 2003). These observations challenge the capacity of "positive discrimination" based on social criteria to ensure equity in access to HAART.

Low Prices or Free Treatment for All Patients

Since the use of social criteria for achieving equity is limited, the best proposition might be to provide low-cost or fully subsidized treatments. Numerous ethical and social arguments favor the free provision of HAART in countries that are already severely affected by AIDS (Farmer et al. 2001). The experience of ISAARV has shown that there are also medical and technical arguments to defend this proposition (Taverne, Lanièce, and Desclaux 2002). As a crippling chronic disease if untreated, AIDS reduces the ability of patients to maintain their financial autonomy. The economic situation in African countries, the impact of AIDS on household budgets, and the cost of treatment regimens for opportunistic infections mean that most patients, despite returning to paid work while on treatment, still cannot afford their drugs. Therefore, AIDS should be considered a "social disease," which means, in health care systems of many African countries, that its treatment should be provided free as it is for tuberculosis or leprosy.

Multilevel payment systems or exemptions and waivers may appear as alternatives, but they are limited solutions (Vinard 2002), since they leave many patients untreated who will remain unknown and unaccounted for in program evaluations. The risk of increasing inequalities between the rich and the poor, or between people from different, unclearly defined categories, can only be removed by granting subsidies covering the entire cost of treatment to a large proportion of the patients' population. In Dakar, the provision of heavily subsidized treatment had other advantages: it protected patients from getting irrational treatment regimens. It also contributed to lower demand for antiretroviral drugs on the informal market, and therefore reduced the risk of viral resistance.

Implications

Paying for Treatment: Meaningful for Whom?

The issue of economic access to HAART has questioned the necessity and meaning of patients' user fees. In addition to cost-recovery needs to sustain programs, three main reasons for the implementation of user fees are given by public health professionals involved in West African HAART programs. First, many professionals and some of their colleagues from developed countries argue that patients would consider free medicines to be worthless, leading to low adherence (Desclaux 2001). Second, some consider that receiving free treatment might be humiliating for patients (Desclaux 2001). Third, it has been said that "traditional African solidarity" can help individuals to bear the economic burden of treatment (Groupe de Gorée 2001). This discourse is more than an adaptation to necessity; it promotes payment as having its own value, as leading patients to a better adherence and bringing health professionals to show more respect to patients, as well as obliging families to increase their support of members affected by AIDS.

These three dimensions of the meaning of payment are challenged by the experience and analyses of ISAARV. Our experience in Dakar shows that the assertion that paying for drugs out of pocket leads to increased adherence is not supported by evidence. The provision of free ARVs can be felt as an insult to one's dignity only if it is seen as an act of condescending charity, rather than as a right to health and a social imperative. Family solidarity is active in Dakar, but it is limited by poverty and insecurity, and requesting payment from patients creates an additional burden. In African societies, where AIDS is stigmatized, support from families is not to be taken for granted. Moreover, it may seem paradoxical that the fully subsidized provision of ARVs by governments or welfare systems in Europe and other wealthy countries does not give rise to such comments; in those countries, access to ARVs is seen as a social and human right, and patients do not feel humiliated when they get them free of charge.

Since these discourses are refuted by local experience, as seen in Dakar, their origin should be sought in the medical culture of public health in Africa, in the context of World Bank policies, the Bamako Initiative, and their subsequent interpretations. Some scientists consider that the Bamako Initiative, which was supposed to ameliorate health services by setting up cost recovery and financial autonomy (WHO 1988) and which was only partially implemented, has promoted neoliberal measures, pleading for the transfer to the community of financial responsibilities previously met by the health system (Turshen 1999). The local plea for user fees, regardless of the reason given, should be analyzed as the expression of politically constructed values. We may wonder if the inability of public health professionals and patients from low-income countries to request free provision of medicines cannot be considered as a submission to an international order of values in which "the poor" should not request more than what is acceptable to the rich.

Double Payment for HIV Patients?

As AIDS patients are requested to pay for ARVs, they are also requested to disclose their status to raise support from their families or to obtain waivers through PLWA self-help organizations. In Mali, fee waivers are granted to "active" members of self-help groups. "Active" status may be defined differently according to each group, but all patients who have publicly admitted their seropositivity, for example during TV or radio programs, are considered "active," as are persons who participate in preventive and educational activities. The declared logic for such favorable treatment is the contribution, through public disclosure, to the destigmatization of AIDS through the "trivialization" of seropositivity, which is encouraged by international agencies such as UNDP and UNAIDS. Although the role of PLWAs in increasing AIDS awareness has been shown in African countries and elsewhere (UNAIDS 2000), evidence is needed to support that public disclosure of HIV status for all AIDS patients is more efficient for advocacy than protection of confidentiality. People whose autonomy is not protected by their social status may suffer from the adverse reactions of family members or coworkers to the disclosure of their seropositivity. Their dependants may also pay a price for this public disclosure, such as subsequently suffering themselves from stigma. Then, we may wonder if public disclosure is not a "second payment" to access treatment, and a form of confession of having a disease still frowned upon. Such a symbolic logic may not be supported by international agencies, but it does correspond to old and deeply rooted perceptions of disease as a retribution for misconduct that can be cured through penitence and sacrifice. Disclosure as an alternative to financial contribution is not an accepted form of payment for drugs to treat other diseases, and we may wonder if this "double payment" is not an indirect form of ostracism toward AIDS patients.

Social Impact of "Community-Based" Management of Equity?

In countries such as Mali and Côte d'Ivoire, where active membership in PLWA self-help organizations provides waivers or free treatment, many AIDS patients turned to these groups when requesting access to HAART programs. This situation has led to social changes for these associations, strengthening their position vis-à-vis health services, opening opportunities to reinforce internal distribution of power through the choice of criteria for the election of "active" members that will receive access to free or highly subsidized treatment, or creating new power relations between older and newer members. This evolution might reinforce the identity of PLWA among AIDS patients and improve the chances of self-help groups or individuals belonging to these groups to gain better social acceptance in the health system or in their communities. It might also have other consequences such as conflicts between individual and collective strategies, or legitimacy conflicts between PLWA groups.

The social changes resulting from the delegation of the management of equity to community-based organizations are not well-known, are difficult to anticipate, and depend on local situations. Giving more power to the civil sector in health programs has been promoted by international organizations, such as UNAIDS and UNDP, and by private, bilateral, and multilateral donors, and is at the heart of many development policies widely inspired by neoliberalism. The consequences of this strategy regarding equity in access to HAART remain to be analyzed.

Conclusion

The withdrawal from the health system of patients who cannot afford user fees, which are often beyond the reach of the majority of the population in low-income countries, is not specific to AIDS: this is commonplace for diseases such as cancer, renal insufficiency, or even high blood pressure. Even in cases of frequent diseases that require simple treatment regimens, it has been shown that in the last decade increases in out-of-pocket health costs have driven some families into poverty and increased the hardship of those who are already poor (Kim, Millen, Irwin, and Gershman 2000); this has been termed "the medical poverty trap" (Whitehead, Dahlgren, and Evans 2001). Criticism by public health specialists based on extensive field research and experience has concluded that privatization policies in health care are regressive regarding equity, mainly because sharing the financial burden of the disease is reduced and payment falls more directly on the sick than on healthy individuals (Ridde 2003). It has been shown that strategies such as the Bamako Initiative were based more on ideological orientations than on evidence of its efficacy. Data increasingly show that several aspects of this strategy are prejudicial to the poor. Although the World Bank has taken some of the criticism into consideration, it has not yet been translated into practice.

The high number of people living with HIV/AIDS in sub-Saharan Africa and needing access to HAART emphasizes the importance of social responsibility at the international level when addressing issues of equity in access to comprehensive AIDS care. So far, the economic burden of AIDS in Africa has been mainly shifted to governments, households, and nongovernmental organizations, sparing the private sector (Rosen and Simon 2003); this is also the case for the provision of ARVs. Requesting partnerships among governments, the private sector, and NGOs to support national programs, the Global Fund to Fight AIDS, Tuberculosis and Malaria provides an opportunity for a change in resource allocation that might alleviate the burden on households.

Data from pilot projects showing the achievements, limitations, and pitfalls of different systems of access to AIDS care are becoming increasingly available (*AIDS* 2003). To meet the equity objectives, policy makers should move beyond values resulting from a decade of public health emphasis on user fees and from an international order based on double standards according to the ability to pay. They also should be cautious about strategies delegating management of equity to community-based organizations. Medical anthropological research on values underlying health and public policies and on the social consequences of choices in the delivery of AIDS care is more than ever necessary, at the local and at the international level.

Acknowledgments

The research program was conducted by Programme National de Lutte contre le Sida (Sénégal) / Institut de Recherche pour le Développement (France) / Laboratoire d'Ecologie Humaine et d'Anthropologie (Université d'Aix-Marseille, France) / Institut de Médecine et d'Epidémiologie Africaines (France), and was funded by Agence Nationale de Recherches sur le Sida. Analyses reported here are based on the work and results of a team of scientists and health professionals published elsewhere (Desclaux et al. 2002). My acknowledgments go to this team and to Bernard Taverne, Institut de Recherche pour le Développement, Dakar, for his critical reading of a previous version of this chapter.

Notes

1. For an update on these issues, see the Access to Medicines Campaign website: www.accessmed-msf.org.
2. For details on the research program, see the acknowledgments listed above.
3. US$1 = 640 FCFA.

References

AIDS. (2003). "The Evaluation of the HIV/AIDS Drug Access Initiatives in Côte d'Ivoire, Senegal and Uganda: How Access to Antiretroviral Treatment Can Become Feasible in Africa." *AIDS* 17, theme issue, supp. 3.

Alzouma, A. S. (2002). "Etude comparative des politiques de gestion des antirétroviraux dans cinq pays de l'Afrique occidentale: Burkina Faso, Côte-d'Ivoire, Mali, Niger, Sénégal." M.D. (pharm.) diss., Faculté de Médecine, de Pharmacie et d'Odontostomatologie, Université de Bamako.

Bronsard, G. (1998). "Les traitements antirétroviraux au Burkina Faso." DEA diss., Laboratoire d'Ecologie Humaine et d'Anthropologie, Université d'Aix-Marseille.

Canestri, A., B. Taverne, S. Thiam, C. Laurent, A. Ndir, and R. Schiemann. (2002). "Coûts directs du suivi médical à la charge des patients hors antirétroviraux." In *L'initiative sénégalaise d'accès aux médicaments antirétroviraux. Analyses économiques, sociales, comportementales et médicales*, edited by Alice Desclaux, Isabelle Lanièce, Ibra Ndoye, and Bernard Taverne, 55–66. Paris: ANRS.

Delaunay, K., L. Vidal, P. Msellati, and J. P. Moatti. (2001). "La mise sous traitement antirétroviral : l'explicite et l'implicite d'un processus de selection" In *L'accès aux traitements du VIH/sida en Côte d'Ivoire: Aspects économiques, sociaux et comportementaux*, edited by Philippe Msellati, Laurent Vidal and Jean-Pierre Moatti, 87–113. Paris: ANRS.

Desclaux, A. (2001). "L'observance en Afrique: Question de culture ou 'vieux problème de santé publique'?" In *L'observance aux antirétroviraux*, edited by Yves Souteyrand and Michel Morin, 57–66. Paris: ANRS.

Desclaux, A., with I. Lanièce, I. Ndoye, and B. Taverne, eds. (2002). *L'initiative sénégalaise d'accès aux antirétroviraux. Analyses économiques, sociales, comportementales et médicales.* Paris: ANRS. Accessed at www.ird.sn/activites/sida/ISAARV.pdf (French version), September 6, 2003.

Desclaux, A., M. Ciss, B. Taverne, P. S. Sow, M. Egrot, M. A. Faye, et al. (2003). "Access to Antiretroviral Drugs and AIDS Management in Senegal." *AIDS* 17, supp. 3: S95–S102.

Dumoulin, J., and M. Kaddar. (1993). "Le paiement des soins par les usagers dans les pays d'Afrique sub-saharienne: rationalité économique et autres questions subséquentes." *Sciences Sociales et Santé* 11, no. 2: 81–119.

Farmer, P. F. Léandre, J. S. Mukherjee, M. S. Claude, P. Nevil, M. Smith-Fawzi, et al. (2001). "Community-Based Approaches to HIV Treatment in Resource-Poor Settings." *Lancet* 358: 404–409.

Groupe de Gorée. (2001, October). "Place des antirétroviraux dans la prise en charge des personnes infectées par le VIH en Afrique." Initiative internationale. *Aspects sciences de l'homme et de la société.* Paris: IMEA, 74 pp.

Imane, L. (2002). "Modes de circulation, significations et usages du traitement antirétroviral à Bamako." DEA diss., Laboratoire d'Ecologie Humaine et d'Anthropologie, Université d'Aix-Marseille.

International AIDS Society. (1999). "Consensus Report: Place of Antiretroviral Drugs in the Treatment of HIV-Infected People in Africa." *AIDS* 13: IAS1–IAS3.

Jaffré, Y., and J. P. O. de Sardan, eds. (2003). *Une médecine inhospitalière: Les mauvaises relations entre soignants et soignés dans cinq capitales d'Afrique de l'Ouest.* Paris: Karthala.

Katabira, E. (1997). "Les traitement antirétroviraux en Ouganda." In World Health Organization, *Les incidences des traitements antirétroviraux: Consultation informelle*, edited by Eric van Praag, Susan Fernyak, and Alison Martin Katz, 119–24. Geneva: WHO.

Katzenstein, D., M. Laga, and J. P. Moatti. (2003). "The Evaluation of the HIV/AIDS Drug Access Initiatives in Côte d'Ivoire, Senegal and Uganda: How Access to Antiretroviral Treatment Can Become Feasible in Africa." *AIDS* 17, supp. 3: S1–S4.

Kim, J. Y., J. V. Millen, A. Irwin, and J. Gershman, eds. (2000). *Dying for Growth: Global Inequality and the Health of the Poor.* Monroe, ME: Common Courage Press.

Kivumbi, G. W., and F. Kintu. (2002). "Exemptions and Waivers from Cost Sharing: Ineffective Safety Nets in Decentralized Districts in Uganda." *Health Policy and Planning* 17: 64–71.

Lanièce, I., M. Ciss, A. Desclaux, K. Diop, F. Mbodj, B. Ndiaye, et al. (2003). "Adherence to HAART and Its Principal Determinants in a Cohort of Senegalese Adults." *AIDS* 17, supp. 3: S103–S108.

Laurent, C., N. Diakhaté, N. F. N. Gueye, M. A. Touré, P. S. Sow, M. A. Faye, et al. (2002). "The Senegalese Government's Highly Active Antiretroviral Therapy Initiative: An 18-Month Follow-Up Study." *AIDS* 16, no. 10: 1363–70.

Mary, A., ed. (1997). *L'Afrique des individus. Itinéraires citadins dans l'Afrique contemporaine (Abidjan, Bamako, Dakar, Niamey).* Paris: Karthala.

Médecins sans Frontières. (2003). *Programs.* Accessed at www.msf.org/countries.index.cfm, September 6, 2003.

Meng, Q., Q. Sun, and N. Hearst. (2002). "Hospital Charge Exemptions for the Poor in Shandong, China." *Health Policy and Planning* 17: 56–63.

Moatti, J. P., B. Coriat, Y. Souteyrand, T. Barnett, J. Dumoulin, and Y. A. Flori, eds. (2003). *Economics of AIDS and Access to HIV/AIDS Care in Developing Countries: Issues and Challenges.* Paris: ANRS.

Paphassarang, C., K. Philavong, B. Boupha, and E. Blas. (2002). "Equity, Privatization and Cost Recovery in Urban Health Care: The Case of Lao PDR." *Health Policy and Planning* 17: 72–84.

Ridde, V. (2003, January 9–10). "Entre efficacité et équité : qu'en est-il de l'Initiative de Bamako? Une revue des expériences ouest-africaines." Paper presented at the 26th Journées des Economistes Français de la Santé, Santé et Développement, Clermont-Ferrand. Accessed at www.cerdi.org/Colloque/PDFSante2003/ridde.pdf, April 28, 2003.

Rosen, S., and J. L. Simon. (2003). "Shifting the Burden: The Private Sector's Response to the AIDS Epidemic in Africa." *Bulletin of the WHO* 81, no. 2: 131–37.

Taverne, B., I. Lanièce, and A. Desclaux. (2002, July 7–12). "Free Access to Anti-Retroviral (ART) Medication in Africa." Poster presented at the 14th International AIDS Conference, Barcelona. Abstract MoPeG 4193. Accessed at www.ird.sn/activites/sida/MoPeG4193.pdf, September 9, 2003.

'T Hoen, E. F. M. (2003). "TRIPS, Pharmaceutical Patents and Access to Essential Medicines: Seattle, Doha and Beyond." In *Economics of AIDS and Access to HIV/AIDS Care in Developing Countries. Issues and Challenges*, edited by J. P. Moatti, B. Coriat, Y. Souteyrand, T. Barnett, J. Dumoulin, and Y. A. Flori, 39–67. Paris: ANRS.

Touré-Kane Ndeye, C., L. Vergne, C. Laurent, N. Diakhaté, N. F. N. Gueye, P. M. Gueye, L. M. Diouf, P. S. Sow, M. A. Faye, F. Liégeois, A. Ndir, et al. (2002). "Faible taux de survenue de souches VIH-1 résistantes aux ARV chez des patients sous traitement antirétroviral au Sénégal." In *L'initiative sénégalaise d'accès aux médicaments antirétroviraux. Analyses économiques, sociales, comportementales et médicales,* edited by A. Desclaux, I. Lanièce, I. Ndoye, and B. Taverne, 157–67. Paris: ANRS.

Turshen, M. (1999). *Privatizing Health Services in Africa.* New Brunswick, NJ: Rutgers University Press.

UNAIDS. (2000). *Enhancing the Greater Involvement of People Living or Affected by HIV/AIDS (GIPA) in Sub-Saharan Africa: Best Practices.* UNAIDS/00.38 E. Accessed at www.unaids.org/html/pub/publications/IRC-pub01/JC274-GIPA-ii_en_pdf.htm, September 9, 2003.

Vinard, P. (2002). *ISAARV: Rapport de mission sur les aspects économiques.* Report. Montpellier: ALTER.

Whitehead, M., G. Dahlgren, and T. Evans. (2001). "Equity and Health Sector Reforms: Can Low-Income Countries Escape the Medical Poverty Trap? *Lancet* 358: 833–36.

World Health Organization. (1988, September 7–14). "Guidelines for implementing the Bamako Initiative." Regional Committee for Africa, 38th session, Brazzaville, AFR/RC38/18.

———. (2001, May 22–23). "International Consultative meeting on HIV/AIDS antiretroviral therapy: Report of the meeting." Geneva: World Health Organization.

8

Contracepting at Childbirth: The Integration of Reproductive Health and Population Policies in Mexico

ARACHU CASTRO

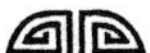

IN 1995, THE MEXICAN MINISTRY OF HEALTH LAUNCHED a new Program on Reproductive Health and Family Planning for the period 1995 to 2000 (Secretaría de Salud 1995) that merged the objectives of Mexico's national program on health reform with ongoing ideas stemming from the international women's health movement. These ideas advocate for reproductive health policies grounded in a broader human development approach that guarantees access to sexual and reproductive health services while committing to human rights (Sen, Germain, and Chen 1994). These ideas were reflected a year earlier at the 1994 International Conference on Population and Development (ICPD) held in Cairo, which set a landmark for the promotion of reproductive choice. This conference acknowledged and emphasized a woman's right to make decisions concerning her reproduction—such as if and when to have children—free of discrimination, coercion, and violence. To better respond to women's needs, ICPD adopted a Program of Action, agreed upon by Mexico and 178 other countries, that focused on women's and men's needs and rights rather than on achieving demographic targets (ICPD 1994). One of its objectives was to promote the integration of reproductive health services, such as counseling and testing for sexually transmitted infections during a woman's visit to a family planning clinic, or providing contraceptives to women after childbirth or an abortion.

The aim of this chapter is to bring a critical perspective on how the integration of reproductive health services, intended to improve women's lives, was implemented in Mexico, and the implications it had for women at the time of giving birth in Mexican public hospitals. Were the new policies leveling the playing field for poor women? Or were their implementation highlighting and reproducing existing social inequalities? A combination of ethnography and epidemiology proved most valuable to address these questions. In 1998, I worked with a team from the Population Council in Mexico to study the high proportion of cesarean sections in public hospitals in Mexico. I conducted fieldwork in four public hospitals in Mexico City, relying on in-depth semistructured and unstructured interviews with OB/GYNs, nurses, and women having just delivered, and on participant observation in maternity wards.[1] The interviews included questions on indications for cesarean sections and the decision-making process involved, use of medical technology at the time of birth, training of residents, prenatal care, and instruction in the use of contraceptive methods during the hospital stay. The results of the major objective of that study, which was to explain the high proportion of cesarean sections in public hospitals in Mexico, have been published elsewhere (Castro 1998, 1999a, 1999b; Castro, Heimburger, and Langer 2002). Throughout that study, we observed a correlation between cesarean sections and tubal ligations, which led to this current exploration.

The Integration of Reproductive Health Services

Mexico adopted official policies in support of family planning activities in the 1960s (Brambila 1998), much before other Latin American countries. These measures included sterilization, which received significant opposition from several sectors of Mexican society, but which became one of the most popular methods of contraception in less than 20 years (MacGregor 1981). The literature on the social conditions under which women are sterilized in Mexico dates back to the 1980s and 1990s (Bronfman, López, and Tuirán 1986; Bronfman 1989; Bronfman and Castro 1989; Figueroa Perea 1994).

In 2000, female sterilization —mostly a tubal ligation performed surgically— was the most frequently used contraceptive method in Mexico: 44 percent of women who use modern contraceptive methods are sterilized (which represents about one-third of the fertile-age female population). The second most used method is the intrauterine device (IUD), with 20 percent of women using it among all those who use a contraceptive method. Other methods are used by less than 10 percent of women (Encuesta Nacional de Salud [ENSA] 2003). These numbers indicate an increase in the proportion of women users of sterilization (41 percent in 1995) and a decrease in those who wear an IUD (22 percent in 1995) (Secretaría de Salud 1996).

In Mexico, health services are channeled through the social security sector (for salaried workers), the private sector, and the public sector (for those, most often poor, who do not qualify for social security and who cannot afford to pay for medical care). The public sector includes different types of hospitals, some administered by the Ministry of Health (SSA) and others by the Mexican Institute of Social Security (IMSS). Both types of public hospitals are open to 59 percent of the population; in Chiapas, 84 percent of the population qualifies, technically, to use these public institutions (ENSA 2003).

The large increase in initiating or continuing contraception right after giving birth is the stated major goal of the Program on Contraception after an Obstetric Event (*Programa de Anticoncepción Posevento Obstétrico*), and is part of the Program on Reproductive Health. Already in 1994, 51 percent of contraceptives provided in SSA public hospitals were "delivered" immediately after giving birth (Secretaría de Salud 1996). In public hospitals administered by IMSS—which are called *IMSS-Oportunidades*, formerly *IMSS-Solidaridad*—85 percent of contraceptives in 2002 were provided immediately after birth, up from 45 percent in 1993 (IMSS 2002). This program promotes the use of contraceptive methods to all women giving birth in public hospitals in Mexico, and OB/GYNs are encouraged to do so. As a third-year female resident explained in an interview:

> I don't like to insert an IUD after birth or after a cesarean section, either way it will come out. We only do it because it's an *indication*, an *order* from the Ministry of Health, but I personally don't like it.

Although this program does not promote the mandatory provision of a contraceptive method, it has been planned to increase the coverage of women contracepting at childbirth and after an abortion, and has clearly defined population goals (Secretaría de Salud 1995).

The integration of reproductive health services, and in particular of labor and contraception, has led some public hospitals to restrict the use of surgical contraception to the immediate postpartum period, during a cesarean section, or after an abortion—thus limiting the opportunities, mostly in poor women, to make reproductive choices. In July 1998, one of the largest public maternity hospitals in Mexico City stopped performing tubal ligations at interval—meaning "in between" pregnancies. This practice has actually been discouraged by the World Health Organization (WHO) on the grounds that the information and informed consent necessary to perform surgical contraception should be given and obtained "preferably during the prenatal period, although it is possible following birth if the client has fully recovered and is lucid. It should *not* be done during birth, or when the woman is under stress" (WHO 1992; emphasis in the original). A qualitative study conducted in Mexico showed that women sterilized at interval have an increased amount of information and a decreased degree of regret with the permanent method than women being sterilized at the time of birth (AVSC 1998).

Still, tubal ligations and IUDs are the methods most frequently proposed by OB/GYNs to women in labor due to their long-acting effect and to the positive perception that these health care professionals have of methods that require a passive or nonexistent role of women in assuring their effectiveness. Their use is often supported on the grounds that a large number of women do not visit hospitals for prenatal or postnatal care. In fact, providing a method during childbirth is often perceived by health care providers as the only time in which it can be done:

> I would prefer to give the patient an appointment one month following birth and insert an IUD then. The problem is that if patients here don't even come for prenatal care, much less will they come to have an IUD inserted.

Therefore, the moment of birth, whether vaginal or cesarean, becomes the golden opportunity for OB/GYNs to offer a contraceptive method. Our interviews and participant observation suggest that health care providers often place more energy in the promotion of contraceptive use immediately after birth than in the promotion of postnatal visits, which could bring several benefits both to the woman and her newborn.

The Fears of Integration

I argue that the integration of reproductive health services in Mexican public hospitals yields two questionable outcomes. First, a proportion of women giving birth in these institutions leave the hospital with a contraceptive method that is provided without sufficient information and with limited contraceptive choices, that is sometimes accepted under pressure and, in fewer instances, is provided without the knowledge of the woman herself. Second, these conditions deter some women from seeking obstetric care in public hospitals, especially where there is an already existing environment of fear and distrust toward public institutions, such as in the southern state of Chiapas—thus increasing the risk of maternal mortality and morbidity in cases of birth that require obstetric care.

July 14, 1998. In a large public maternity hospital in Mexico City, Antonia arrives in a wheelchair at the operating room. She is 23, mother of a young child, and is 37 weeks pregnant with twins, one of which is breached. She is going to have a cesarean section, just like she had the first time she gave birth. Soon after the anesthetist places an epidural, most of her body starts to numb. A male surgeon arrives in the operating room and asks Antonia how many children she has. She responds one. The surgeon bluntly asks her if she's going to "get tied" this time—"*¿y te vas a ligar ya?*" Antonia says no, and the surgeon looks at her in dismay and leaves. Twelve minutes later the cesarean section begins. Two residents are performing the surgery, and there are a total of nine people around Antonia, including myself. The male surgeon comes back. Six minutes later, two healthy girls are born. While the residents are stitching Antonia, the male surgeon asks her: 'Aren't you going to get tied?' Upon Antonia's firm and negative response, he gets mad at her and leaves.

We observed several cases like Antonia's and heard many more stories similar to hers, not only in Mexico City, but also from distant places such as Chiapas (Graciela Freyermuth 1998, personal communication). In the summer of 1998, at meetings with demographers and other social scientists working at different institutions throughout the city, I started to hear the rumor that the most recent demographic and health survey—ENAPLAF, or *Encuesta Nacional de Planificación Familiar 1995*—was having a delayed release due to a certain number of problems with the data set. The rumor also said that about one-third of women having given birth had left the hospital with a contraceptive method that had been forced upon them. The majority of these women had learned, either at the hospital or much later, that health care providers had inserted an IUD into their bodies; a minority, probably less than 5 percent, had been sterilized without their consent.[2]

I was interested in working with the data set and testing my hypothesis, based primarily on ethnographic research, that women undergoing a C-section had an increased probability of having a tubal ligation. In Mexico, the number of C-sections had increased in public and social security hospitals from 12.7 percent in 1990 to 24.8 percent in 1995, and in private hospitals the average for the country was 51.8 percent in 1997 (Comité Promotor por una Maternidad sin Riesgos 1997). During the same period of time, maternal mortality was relatively stable, fluctuating around 50 deaths per 1,000 registered live births (Lezana 1999; Secretaría de Salud 2000). Ironically, obstructed labor, the leading cause of maternal mortality in Mexico, which can be prevented by a timely C-section, accounted for 39 percent of maternal deaths. This indicator rose to 48 percent in the states with highest incidence of maternal deaths: Chiapas, Hidalgo, Oaxaca, Puebla, Querétaro, Quintana Roo, San Luis Potosí, and Veracruz (Reyes, Lezana, García, and Bobadilla 1998). Because the increase in cesarean sections was not leading to a decrease in maternal mortality, we have reasons to believe that some are performed without an absolute medical indication, and that resources for reproductive health services are unequally distributed within the country.

As an OB/GYN explained, when a woman has had three cesarean sections,

> We give her, really quick, the information about the risk of uterine rupture. We propose the definitive method at the third cesarean; we are forced to insist that she get her tubes tied. We insist by saying, "look, your uterus can burst, and you'll make orphans of your babies." It's difficult to make our society believe that you can have just one child. So, at the second cesarean we propose the idea, but we don't insist, and at the third, we have to insist. When, in spite of insisting on the risks and benefits of surgical contraception, they say no, the patients have to sign a paper in which they state that they decided not to be sterilized against the advice of the physician. In general we insist a little bit more with C-section deliveries because of the ease of going ahead and combining the surgical procedures.

The main explanation brought forward by OB/GYNs is that the woman is already cut open and the surgical sterilization does not entail an additional risk. Secondly, OB/GYNs rightly argue that the body of a woman is not capable of supporting various cesareans, due to the risk of uterine rupture; therefore, women who have undergone multiple C-sections should put a permanent end to their fertility. However, the claim that women should not have more than one, two, or three cesarean sections may depend more on the physician's perception of the ideal number of children than on actual clinical recommendations; one physician stated, "Why three? First of all, because physically a woman's body cannot bear more than that, and secondly, three is the ideal number of children."

The practice of combining a C-section with a tubal ligation is also customary in other hospitals: "Right now we see fewer and fewer patients with more than three cesareans, because the majority of health institutions give a definitive contraceptive method at the time of the third cesarean." Another OB/GYN explained:

> Even though a woman already had three cesareans and still does not want a definitive method of sterility, in our field no family planning method can be forced on anyone. If I explain to the patient that it is not in her best interest to have more than three C-sections, and she still insists on having four or more children, then that is completely voluntary. In that type of situation, the patient signs a paper stating that all the risks she could incur were perfectly explained to her, but even so she is consciously agreeing not to have surgical contraception as a permanent means of fertility regulation. We've had a few of these situations—patients who come to us with more than two cesarean sections—but as a general rule, most women with a history of C-sections decide to have a tubal ligation.

Although ethnographic work repeatedly confirmed the hypothesis linking C-sections with tubal ligations, the support of these findings increased after I obtained an electronic copy of ENAPLAF 1995 at the Colegio de México in March 1999. Not only was I interested in testing the hypothesis statistically, but I also wanted to learn more about other items included in the survey—such as the context in which contraceptive methods were offered, including women's informed consent. To my surprise, all the figures related to these latter questions had been erased from the database. Fortunately, there was enough information to build a logistic regression model, for which I collected data on a total of 3,588 women, 829 of whom had been sterilized. The results of the model showed that the probability of female sterilization increases when the last birth is by cesarean section and when it takes place in a public hospital, with an OR = 2.69 (2.68, 2.71) after controlling for parity and type of birth (Castro 1999a). That is, among women delivering by cesarean section, the poorest are sterilized at the time of birth almost three times as much as women delivering at social security or private hospitals. When comparing public versus social security and private hospitals, the predicted probability of sterilization is higher in public hospitals for both types of birth, as shown in Figure 8.1.

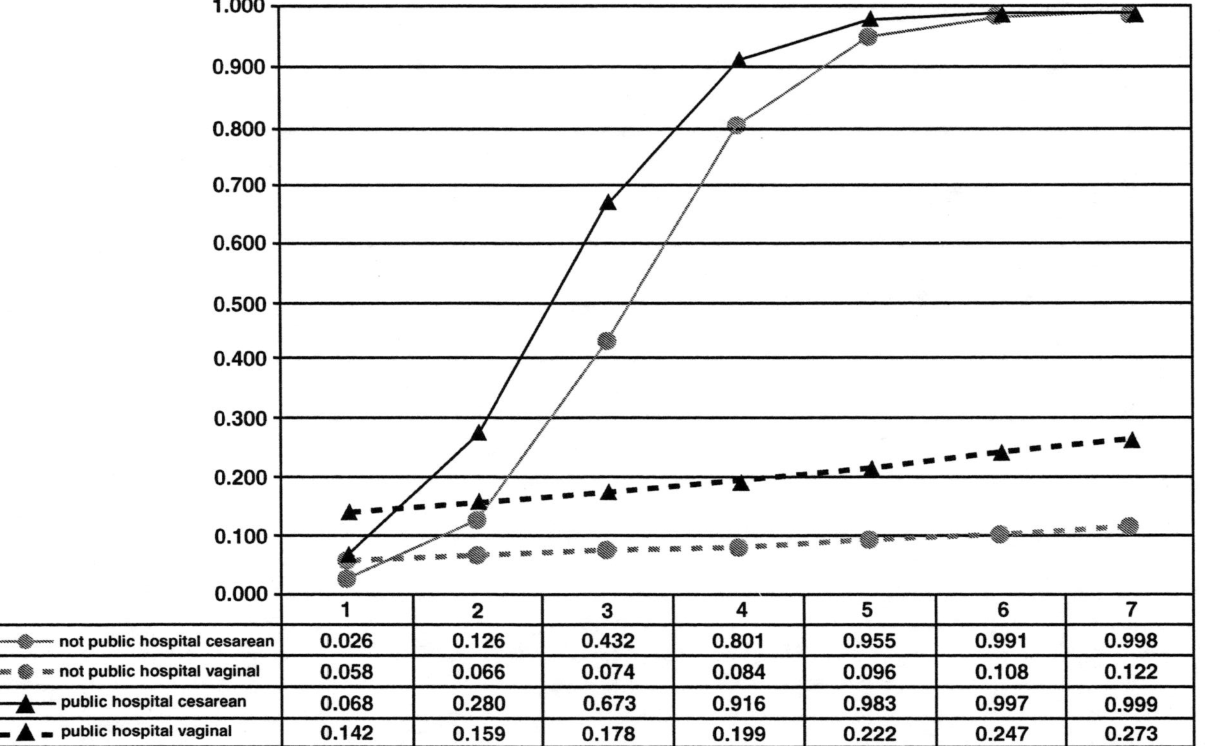

	1	2	3	4	5	6	7
not public hospital cesarean	0.026	0.126	0.432	0.801	0.955	0.991	0.998
not public hospital vaginal	0.058	0.066	0.074	0.084	0.096	0.108	0.122
public hospital cesarean	0.068	0.280	0.673	0.916	0.983	0.997	0.999
public hospital vaginal	0.142	0.159	0.178	0.199	0.222	0.247	0.273

Figure 8.1. Predicted Probability of Sterilization for Women Aged 25 by Type of Birth Delivering in and outside Public Hospitals, Mexico. Source: Based on ENAPLAF (1995).

The statistical analysis therefore confirmed that, in Mexico in 1995, poor women were sterilized more frequently, especially if they were delivering by cesarean section—despite the fact that poor women have proportionately less C-sections than women delivering in social security and private hospitals. Although ethnographic work in Mexico City revealed that most women who had been sterilized had signed a consent form, it is not clear at which moment they had placed their signature. Health care providers explained that some women sign the form after the procedure for the simple reason that they are being asked or induced to "get tied" either during a C-section, like Antonia, or during a vaginal delivery. Moreover, having signed the form, or having been "informed consented" to sign it (George Zeidenstein 1999, personal communication), is not a guarantee that the woman understood the permanent nature of the procedure (Center for Reproductive Law and Policy [CRLP] and Grupo de Información en Reproducción Elegida [GIRE] 1997).

The last Demographic and Health Survey, from 1987, had shown that sterilized women who were younger, living in rural areas, and with less schooling had higher probability of regretting the procedure and of not having consented to it than older, urban, and more educated women (Demographic and Health Survey [DHS] 1987). Although we could not confirm this trend with ENAPLAF 1995 because some of the data had been erased, it is not improbable to think that instances of forced sterilization are still more frequent among poor women.

Increased Fear in Chiapas

In 1998, there was significant international attention brought to the Zapatista movement, originated in San Cristóbal de las Casas in Chiapas on January 1, 1994. Their *Declaración de la Selva Lacandona* with which they launched the uprising said:

> We have been denied the most elemental education so that others can use us as cannon fodder and pillage the wealth of our country. They don't care that we have nothing, absolutely nothing, not even a roof over our heads, no land, no work, no health care, no food, and no education (Comandancia General del EZLN 1993, translated in Farmer 2003).

Chiapas not only has the highest reported maternal mortality in Mexico but also records last in the country in percentage of women receiving some sort of prenatal care (62 percent) or having a cesarean section (14 percent) (ENSA 2003). Complex factors operate in Chiapas in terms of accessing obstetric services.

At a national conference on maternal mortality in Mexico, organized by the Safe Motherhood Committee in the summer of 1998, a physician-anthropologist from Chiapas publicly denounced that indigenous women from Chiapas preferred to die at home from childbirth than be exposed to the abuse exerted upon them in public hospitals throughout the state. She later clarified that these women feared racist denigration, political interrogation, and forced sterilization. These fears have been documented in several publications (Freyermuth 1998; Kirsch and Arana Cedeño 1999; Physicians for Human Rights 1999; Freyermuth 1999; Freyermuth and Manca 2000).

Among the indigenous communities in Chiapas, sterilization is perceived as an intrahospital practice that can place women at risk. Under the rubric of *Misión Chiapas*, an intense birth control campaign initiated in 1995, public hospitals, depleted of essential medicines, are stocked with contraceptive methods. Freyermuth, who has written extensively about these matters, explains that when a woman in Chiapas wants to have a tubal ligation, the hospital arranges for transportation, whereas this arrangement is not provided for laboring women with severe complications who do not want to be sterilized (Freyermuth 1998:78–79). Others have reported that, in Chiapas: "Pressure is placed on physicians to urge poor women to accept birth control and IUDs immediately after they have given birth, irrespective of the patient's wishes or responses" (Kirsch and Arana Cedeño 1999:419). Early in 2003, a Mexican newspaper reported that health care workers employed by *IMSS-Oportunidades*, having to fulfill sterilization quotas, have to entice indigenous women to become sterilized and pay their transportation costs to the hospital from their own pockets, for fear of losing their jobs (Ruíz 2003).

Clearly, the provision of contraceptive methods at the time of birth for poor women is, in Mexico, an instrument of public policy that reproduces all sorts of existing inequalities. The integration of two reproductive health services—birthing and contracepting—uses international "ICPD language" on reproductive choice and convenience for women but is mostly intended to induce fertility decline—a disguised way of exerting population control. The Cairo conference had emphasized the importance of implementing quality care in family planning services instead of focusing on number-driven demographic targets. But as Potter has suggested (1999), target-driven population policies have been so deeply institutionalized in Mexico that it requires time before the focus changes to de facto reproductive choices. Analyzing the structurally violent context in which health and contraception statistics exist resocializes the suffering of those affected by unhealthy policies.

Acknowledgments

I am especially grateful to Ana Langer, as well as other staff from the Population Council Regional Office for Latin America and the Caribbean in Mexico City, for all their support and for facilitating access to health care facilities and documentation. I am indebted to Angela Heimburger for sharing her knowledge of reproductive health policies in Mexico, and to Amy Ratcliffe for her help in building the logistic regression model. I am also thankful to Monique Vledder for her earlier assistance in analyzing the literature on sterilization of poor women throughout Latin America, and to Christina Harding for editing the text. Finally, I wish that Charlotte Ellertson had lived several decades more and continued her extraordinary work on behalf of women's reproductive rights.

Notes

1. Our research procedures were in accordance with the ethical standards of Population Council, the committees on human experimentation of all the participating hospitals, and the Declaration of Helsinki of 1975, as revised in 1983.

2. In 1999, the United Nations Commission on Human Rights (UNCHR; 1999) defined sterilization provided without appropriate consent as a form of violence against women.

References

AVSC. (1998). *Estudio de Caso sobre Consentimiento Informado para la Esterilización en el IMSS.* Report presented to the Instituto Mexicano del Seguro Social, Mexico City.

Brambila, C. (1998). "Mexico's Population Policy and Demographic Dynamics: The Record of Three Decades." In *Do Population Policies Matter? Fertility and Politics in Egypt, India, Kenya, and Mexico,* edited by A. Jain, 157–91. New York: Population Council.

Bronfman, M. N. (1989). "La relación entre población y salud en la crisis." *Cuadernos del CENDES* 12: 87–107.

Bronfman, M. N., and R. Castro. (1989, June). "Discurso y práctica de la planificación familiar: El caso de América Latina." *Saúde Em Debate:* 61–68.

Bronfman, M. N., E. López, and R. Tuirán. (1986). "Práctica anticonceptiva y clases sociales en México: la experiencia reciente." *Estudios Demograficos y Urbanos* 1, no. 2: 165–203.

Castro, A. (1998). *La Operación Cesárea en México: Un Estudio Cualitativo con Mujeres y Profesionales de la Salud.* Mexico City: Population Council Regional Office for Latin America and the Caribbean, 1998.

———. (1999a). "The Impact of the Epidemic of Cesarean Sections in the Fertility Decline in Mexico." Paper presented at the Population Association of America Annual Meeting, New York.

———. (1999b). "Commentary: Increase in Caesarean Sections May Reflect Medical Control, Not Women's Choice." *British Medical Journal* 319: 1401–1402. Accessed at www.bmj.com/cgi/content/full/319/7222/1397#resp2, April 17, 2004.

Castro, A., A. Heimburger, and A. Langer. (2002). *Iatrogenic Epidemic: How Health Care Professionals Contribute to the High Proportion of Cesarean Sections in Mexico.* Working Papers on Latin America, Paper no. 02/03-3. Cambridge, MA: David Rockefeller Center for Latin American Studies at Harvard University, 42 pp.

Center for Reproductive Law and Policy (CRLP) and Grupo de Información en Reproducción Elegida (GIRE). (1997). *Women's Reproductive Rights in Mexico: A Shadow Report.* Report prepared for the 18th session of the Committee on the Elimination of All Forms of Discrimination against Women, New York.

Comandancia General del EZLN. (1993). *Declaración de la Selva Lacandona.* Chiapas, Mexico. Accessed at www.ezln.org/documentos/1994/199312xx.es.htm, April 17, 2004.

Comité Promotor por una Maternidad sin Riesgos (Mexico). (1997). *Cesáreas: Tendencias actuales, y perspectivas.* Mexico City: Secretaría de Salud.

Demographic and Health Survey (DHS). (1987). *Mexico.* Calverton, MD: Macro International.

Encuesta Nacional de Salud (ENSA). (2003). *Encuesta Nacional de Salud 2000.* Cuernavaca, Mexico: Instituto Nacional de Salud Pública and Ministerio de Salud. Accessed at http://xipe.insp.mx/ensa/, April 17, 2004.

Farmer, P. (2003). *Pathologies of Power: Health, Human Rights, and the New War on the Poor.* Berkeley: Univesity of California Press.

Figueroa Perea, J. G. (1994). "Apuntes para un estudio multidisciplinario de la esterilización femenina." *Estudios Demográficos y Urbanos* 9, no. 1: 105–28.

Freyermuth, G. (1998). "Antecedentes de Acteal, muerte materna y control natal ¿genocidio silencioso?" In *La otra palabra: Mujeres y violencia en Chiapas, antes y después de Acteal,* edited by Rosalva Aída Hernández, 63–83. Mexico City: CIESAS, Centro de Investigaciones y Estudios Superiores en Antropología Social.

———. (1999). "Muerte Materna, lo que no dicen las estadísticas de salud." In *Una Nueva Mirada a la Mortalidad Materna en México,* edited by M. C. Elu and E. Santos-Pruneda, 115–50. Mexico City: United Nations Population Fund.

Freyermuth, G., and M. C. Manca, eds. (2000). *Luna golpeada: Morir durante la maternidad: investigaciones, acciones y atención médica en Chiapas, y otras experiencias en torno a la Mortalidad Materna.* Tuxtla Gutiérrez, Mexico: Comité por una Maternidad Voluntaria y Sin Riesgos en Chiapas.

Instituto Mexicano del Seguro Social (IMSS). (2002). *Salud Reproductiva en el Ámbito del Programa IMSS-Oportunidades.* Mexico City: Instituto Mexicano del Seguro Social.

International Conference on Population and Development (ICPD). (1994). *Programme of Action of the United Nations International Conference on Population & Development.* Cairo: ICPD. Accessed at www.iisd.ca/linkages/Cairo/program/p00000.html, April 17, 2004.

Kirsch, J. D., and M. Arana Cedeño. (1999). "Informed Consent for Family Planning for Poor Women in Chiapas, Mexico." *Lancet* 354, no. 9176: 419–20. Accessed at www.thelancet.com/journal/vol354/iss9176/full/llan.354.9176.news.3543.1, April 17, 2004.

Lezana, M. A. (1999). "Evolución de las tasas de mortalidad materna en México." In *Una Nueva Mirada a la Mortalidad Materna en México,* edited by M. C. Elu and E. Santos-Pruneda, 53–70. Mexico City: Comité Promotor por una Maternidad sin Riesgos en México.

MacGregor, C. (1981). "Aspectos de la reproducción relacionados con los derechos humanos. IV. Esterilización por métodos quirúrgicos." *Gaceta Médica de México* 117, no. 7: 272–74.

Physicians for Human Rights. (1999). *Health Care Held Hostage: Human Rights Violations and Violations of Medical Neutrality in Chiapas.* Boston: Physicians for Human Rights.

Potter, J. E. (1999). "The Dark Side of Diffusion: Increasing Returns and the Persistence of Outmoded Contraceptive Regimes." Paper presented at the Harvard Center for Population and Development Studies, Cambridge, MA.

Reyes, S., M. A. Lezana, M. C. García, and J. L. Bobadilla. (1998). "Maternal Mortality Regionalization and Trend in Mexico (1937–1995)." *Archives of Medical Research* 29, no. 2: 165–72.

Ruíz, M. (2003, January 3). "Obliga IMSS a trabajadoras a reclutar mujeres para programa de esterilización permanente." *Cimacnoticias.com, Periodismo con perspectiva de género.* Accessed at www.cimacnoticias.com/noticias/03ene/03010703.html, April 17, 2004.

Secretaría de Salud. (1995). *Programa de Salud Reproductiva y Planificación Familiar 1995-2000.* Mexico City: Programa de Reforma del Sector Salud and Grupo Interinstitucional de Salud Reproductiva.

———. (1996). *Encuesta Nacional sobre Planificación Familiar 1995.* Mexico City: Secretaría de Salud.

———. (2000). *Mortalidad Materna 1988-1997.* Unpublished data. Mexico City: Dirección General de Salud Reproductiva, Comité Nacional par el Estudio de la Mortalidad Materna y Perinatal.

Sen, G., A. Germain, and L. C. Chen, eds. (1994). *Population Policies Reconsidered: Health, Empowerment, and Rights.* Boston: Harvard School of Public Health.

United Nations Commission on Human Rights (UNCHR). (1999, January 21). *Integration of the Human Rights of Women and the Gender Perspective: Violence against Women.* Report of the Special Rapporteur on violence against women, its causes and consequences, Ms. Radhika Coomaraswamy, in accordance with Commission on Human Rights resolution 1997/44. Geneva: United Nations Economic and Social Council.

World Health Organization (WHO). (1992). *Female Sterilization: A Guide to Provision of Services.* Geneva: World Health Organization.

9

How Healthy Are Health and Population Policies? The Indian Experience

IMRANA QADEER AND NALINI VISVANATHAN

Unhealthy Trends

INDIAN POPULATION POLICIES have tried to regulate family size by promoting contraceptives through incentives and penalties, arguing for family planning in the cause of maternal and child health. When these policies adversely affect the welfare and long-term interests of the majority while favoring only a small section of the population, then we *must* consider them to be "unhealthy." This chapter identifies the unhealthy trends in India's health and population policies, assesses the impact on India's people, attempts to understand the underlying politics, and explores the possible lessons. These unhealthy trends began in the mid-1980s and were formalized in the 1990s. The first trend was the drastic cutting of total investments in the welfare sector, especially in health—although the family planning budget remains double that for general health. The second trend was privatizing medical care and introducing user fees and private investment in public hospitals, thereby weakening the referral system and distorting integrated services. The third was emphasizing technological solutions to public health problems, thereby marginalizing the principles of equity and development that underlie comprehensive primary health care (PHC). The fourth was the verticalization of disease and population control interventions, further weakening the integrated approach and promoting imports of drugs and equipment. The fifth comprised transforming reproductive and child health (RCH) services into instruments of population control rather than channels for providing health services to this vulnerable section, and the continuing dependence on female sterilization to limit family size without assessing women's general and gynecological health status.

The Rationale

What are the assumptions behind these policies in the Indian context? The first assumption is that private care is more *efficient* and of *better* quality (World Bank 1993). The *World Development Report 1993* defines "efficiency" purely in terms of cost reduction and not in terms of coverage or self-sufficiency in the long run—a definition that may help the state, but not the majority of the sick. An expert group at the Planning Commission calculated one episode of hospital admission to cost 320 rupees (US$7.30) (excluding food and drugs that may be purchased by patients) for public hospitals and Rs. 735 (US$16.70) for private hospitals (Government of India [GOI] 2001b). Similarly, for "quality," dimensions such as outcome, costs, and patient satisfaction are ignored (Baru, Qadeer, and Priya 2000). Thus, with doubtful quality and increased costs, private care may have value as additional high-tech institutional care, but is not of any epidemiological significance.

The second assumption is that a public-private mix increases *coverage* and is a step toward *equity* (World Bank 1993). However, an area may have both public and private health care institutions, but these are not necessarily accessible to socially and economically deprived people. National statistics definitely show a rise in the overall use of private health care, but they also illustrate that the proportion of the poorest 40 percent (the lowest monthly per capita expenditure [MPCE] groups) opting for admission to public hospitals has gone up from 42.95 to 60 percent between 1989 and 1998, and 16 percent of the sick in this group do not get any treatment (National Sample Survey Organisation [NSSO] 1989, 1998). Thus, restricting the growth of the public sector deprives them even more of health services.

The third assumption is the primacy of *technology* over welfare services and economic and social development. Although the policies state that they "empower" women, they actually propagate the notion that "liberation" comes through the use of contraceptives. Similarly, "targeting" the underprivileged (GOI 1992) is a euphemism for public provision of second-rate (and cost-saving) primary services, now dissociated from the privatized secondary- and tertiary-level care. This goes contrary to the Alma Ata declaration that the choice of technology should be based on the epidemiological needs of population, affordability within the framework of self-sufficiency, and acceptability (WHO and UNICEF 1978). As we shall see later, the current prime movers for technological choice are the interests of the "free market" led by multinational corporations.

The fourth assumption is that the state should change from a *provider* to a *regulator* of health services; however, it is unclear how a state that is unable to perform its current regulatory functions of monitoring, registration, and standardization will become more effective (Baru, Qadeer and Priya) 2000). In fact, the state is now actively promoting the private sector through subsidies for capital investments, imports, products, drugs, contraceptives, services, reimbursements, and social marketing (GOI 2002b). In a situation where "unmet needs" have been officially recognized, opening health services to the "free" market is not justifiable, neither for reducing costs nor for ensuring regulation. Social marketing to promote "socially desirable behavior" is irrelevant for the needy, but it ensures subsidies for the private sector.

Policy Prescriptions

In the above context, the National Population Policy 2000 (NPP) marks a turning point in the history of population planning. On paper it strives for a welfare strategy that is voluntary, target-free, and integrated with the key components of welfare. It promises economic and social development to improve the quality of lives of the people and their welfare through provision of opportunities and choices "to become productive assets in society" (GOI 2000a). However, the NPP leaves many loopholes for political and economic processes to be manipulated by the elite. Thus, while the rhetoric is of integrating communicable diseases and malnutrition, the focus is only on family planning through RCH.

Similarly, the National Health Policy 2002 (NHP) verticalizes disease control programs and, by failing to link health and population planning, lets RCH occupy the entire domain of essential health care. Together, the two policies shift the focus of primary health care from comprehensive care to family welfare (planning). Even while RCH professes to cover maternal and child health, sexually transmitted diseases including HIV, reproductive tract infections, abortion and sterility treatment facilities, gynecological services, treatment for anemia and malnutrition, along with communicable disease control, it is actually restricted to the so-called essential RCH, with contraception becoming the first and the foremost priority (GOI 1997).

Thus, the inherent Malthusian inclination of the policy is reflected in the adoption of a technocentric and demographically oriented objective of achieving a replacement-level fertility rate by 2010 and a stable population by 2045 (GOI 2000a). It is, therefore, not surprising that the demographic obsession that had, in the past, isolated and demonized the Family Welfare Program continues to distort the expressed intent of the NPP. Inevitably, both emergency medical care and childcare services get linked to a small-family norm through incentive schemes rather than to essential services. Instead of ensuring safe abortion, the policy proposes "making abortion attractive" by doing away with the requirement for registering service providers to ensure minimum institutional standards.

In addition, as spacing of births is promoted, a deluge of new technologies has flooded the market. Those technologies that are not accepted by the official program are now promoted through the private market and NGOs. Depo-Provera, Net-En, Norplant, and RU 480 are the controversial hormonal contraceptives in use (Sathyamala 2000; Akhtar 1995). Two U.S. citizens, Stephen Mumford and Elton Kessel (a physician), both with well-known anti-immigrant inclinations and Malthusian views, tested the sterilant action of the malarial drug quinacrine on 25,000 poor women in ten countries (Hieu et al. 1993) without the permission of the national regulatory authorities in at least India. Even after its ban in India, quinacrine sterilization is being pushed through private providers. Thus, while the policy underscores "safety," it offers no regulatory mechanisms to prevent illegal and unethical human experiments.

Regional Policies

The policies at the regional level take their cue from the NPP and make use of loopholes to introduce coercive incentives. The policy of the most populous state of Uttar Pradesh, for instance, proposes to introduce untested and known harmful contraceptives and continues to use camps and campaigns for sterilizations. Even though it has acquired massive World Bank funding, it proposes to introduce user charges for RCH services (Government of Uttar Pradesh 2000). Similarly, Madhya Pradesh makes the two-child family a condition for participating in the local elections to the grassroots democratic institutions—the "Panchayats." It also bans government jobs for those who were married before the age of 18 years (16 in the case of girls) and, in the process, penalizes the very women whom it purports to empower (Government of Madhya Pradesh 2000).

Despite the NPP's emphasis on spacing and a nontargeted approach, demographic compulsions enforce strategies geared to increase sterilizations for the surest results. As the boundaries between goals and targets dissolve, the pressure on doctors to perform increases, especially in states like Uttar Pradesh, Bihar, Rajasthan, and Madhya Pradesh that are considered major blocks in bringing down overall fertility rates. The illiterate poor become the targets in the name of "reaching out to the poor." This is the very purpose of transforming the content of primary health care, which now essentially consists of family planning services and basic curative care. Instead of promoting women's health, it uses both maternal and child health services as instruments of population control with unhealthy consequences.

Impact Assessment

Despite prolonged civil strife, Sri Lanka has impressive health and demographic indicators that should set standards for assessing the impact of India's health and population policies.[1] India's demographic achievements over the 1990s were not impressive: an infant mortality rate (IMR) of 68 per 1,000, a life expectancy of 63.6 for men and 64.9 for women, a birthrate of 25.8 per 1,000, a death rate of 9.0, estimated maternal mortality of 54.0 per 10,000, and an under-six mortality of 94.5 per 1,000 (GOI 2002c). The repeated failure to achieve policy objectives has made demographers question unrealistic goals. They point out that population momentum will slow growth rates (Visaria and Visaria 1996), taking 60-odd years to move from replacement-level fertility to a stable population. This makes the objective of achieving a stable population by 2045 unrealistic (Visaria 2002).

Vulnerable Populations

In a country where the estimates of absolute poverty are around 34.7 percent (United Nations Development Programme [UNDP] 2003), the significance of these two health policies cannot be underestimated, especially when an almost equal proportion of the population is barely above the poverty line. An expanding "free" market can only reach the middle and upper classes (about 300 million), while the rest are either sold dreams through the media or appeased—and, if neither works, the state resorts to control and coercion. Who are the vulnerable sections in India? The poor lie within the Scheduled Castes and Tribes (8.08 and 16.08 percent of the population, respectively; Kulkarni 2002) and a significant proportion of the backward castes and sects among the Hindus and Muslims. The economic differentials are reflected in the MPCE categories, where the lowest 40 percent and the highest 20 percent respectively spend Rs. 3,336 (US$76.10) and Rs. 10,350 (US$236) in rural areas and Rs. 4,728 (US$107.80) and Rs. 21,183 (US$483.20) in urban areas (NSSO 2001).

Absolute and relative poverty generate extremely unhealthy environmental conditions that are conducive to disease.[2] Inadequate access of the poor to education brings the average literacy rates to 65 percent (75.85 percent for males and 54.1 percent for females) in the 2001 census (GOI 2001a). India's socioeconomic realities not only indicate a substantive proportion of underprivileged, but also a subset within them of the most vulnerable—the poorest women, children, and men who constitute over 33 percent of India's population. These averages, therefore, contain inherent inequalities when seen through the lens of economic and social stratification.[3]

Gender Dimensions

Patriarchy pervades these hierarchies to create gender inequality around work, sexuality, entitlement, inheritance, access to opportunities, and freedoms. Patriarchal biases also consolidate social divisions and the inherent aggression and frustration by providing a common outlet through violence against women. Women bear the double burden of working and caring for the family under conditions of daunting poverty where procuring drinking water and food, collecting firewood and fodder, and cleaning are demanding tasks. In addition, socially, women's fertility is seen as their prime function, making them an easy target for the state. The result is declining sex ratios, especially for those under six. The overall female-to-male sex ratio in 2001 was 933 but the 0–6-year child sex ratio was 927. Of 577 districts, 48 had a ratio less than 849 and only in eight was the ratio 1,000 or above (GOI 2001a). The situation has worsened since 1991, and ratios under 880 were reported from rich states like Haryana, Punjab, Gujarat, and Delhi (Nanda 2002).

Pushing the two-child norm in a patriarchal society promotes the killing of female fetuses and infants in order to acquire a balanced family within the prescribed limits, if not one with many sons (Dasgupta 1998). This norm also promotes the misuse of technologies such as ultrasound and amniocentesis. The postabortion minor complications, like uterine and cervical erosion and hemorrhage, and major complications, such as delayed infections, sepsis, embolism, and other life-threatening sequelae, were 3.1 and 1.0 percent respectively in the 1980s (Indian Council of Medical Research [ICMR] 1981). Since then, provision of abortion services remains inadequate, a significant proportion of induced abortions are failures, hospital studies still report deaths following postabortion complications (Vasundhara, Shah, and Misra 2000), and practitioners continue to report bleeding, secondary infertility, and irregular periods (Bandewar 2003). In rural areas, antenatal and natal care by trained personnel, including trained traditional birth attendants, is available to only 43.8 and 33.6 percent of the women (GOI 2002c). Overall couple protection rate is only 55.1 percent, of which 36.2 percent is through sterilizations (International Institute for Population Sciences [IIPS] 2000).

The overuse of sterilization among women is yet another form of gender discrimination. A hospital-based study that followed up sterilized women over several months showed that the procedure had an adverse impact on both physical and mental health status (Purkayastha and Bhattacharyya 1992). A reproductive health survey of women in the state of Karnataka records higher prevalence of morbidity symptoms in sterilized women across all economic strata and demographic characteristics (Bhatia and Cleland 1995). Evaluating sterilization practices and procedures followed by 55 Harayana gynecologists, Tewari and associates found that most of the doctors relied on lay staff to counsel patients and administer informed consent forms, and left it to the general practitioners to assess the patient's eligibility for surgery (Tewari and Rathee 1997). Official guidelines, however, require surgeons to interview the patient prior to surgery (Government of India, Ministry of Health and Family Welfare 1989). These guidelines state the criteria to be used by medical personnel for selecting men and women candidates for sterilization. For women, the lower age limit stipulated is 20 years, reflecting a social milieu where early marriages, if not unions, are common. Nevertheless, it is questionable whether a 20-year-old woman can anticipate a need to reverse the procedure for such reasons as infant and child mortality, or even a second marriage in the event of widowhood or divorce.

In the United States, EngenderHealth, formerly the Association for Voluntary Surgical Contraception, warns against accepting women for the procedure at an early age (EngenderHealth 2002). Women who are less than 30 years old are more likely to consider reversal (Westhoff 2002). Counseling and informed consent are critical steps in the protocol followed before surgery is scheduled in the United States (Baill, Cullins, and Pati 2003). Long-term studies of the effects of tubal ligation have been conducted mainly in the United States. A prospective cohort study followed U.S. women for five years and concluded that sterilized women were no more likely than nonsterilized women to suffer from menstrual abnormalities (Peterson et al. 2000). These findings have challenged the validity of a post–tubal ligation syndrome centered on menstrual changes.[4] Yet, psychological and cultural factors and the issues of procedural safety are not comparable across settings, where there are gross disparities in health care resources.

By making gender the thrust of population policies, the state ignores the importance of poverty and blames certain marginalized groups, whose relatively higher fertility is symptomatic of their condition rather than the cause (Kulkarni 2002). The acceptance of family planning methods is greater among the educated upper-class women due to lower IMR, maternal mortality rate (MMR), child mortality, and son preference. Yet, the Family Planning Program (FPP) targets the poor and the less educated in isolation and irrespective of any welfare inputs. This is in spite of a number of studies that show the lowest family size or fertility among the poor (Patel 1994; Rao 1997), and goes against substantive arguments that favor developmental inputs to promote generating demand for family planning services in situations where levels of productivity as well as literacy among women are low (Kim, Sinha, and Dev Gaur 2002). Not surprisingly, an important recommendation for legislative changes to ensure property rights for women, by an earlier draft of the NPP (GOI 1993), was deleted from the final document. Why does the Indian State follow these regressive policies?

Funding Pressures

In Uttar Pradesh, USAID has invested US$30 million over the 1990s in a special project—State Innovations in Family Planning Service Agency (SIFPSA)—to improve family welfare service in 28 districts (U.S. Agency for International Development [USAID] 1997). The World Bank has been actively funding the same through its India Population Project. Between 1994 and 2002, US$79 million were given to five states—Uttar Pradesh, Madhya Pradesh, Andhra Pradesh, Karnataka, and Delhi (GOI 2000b). Another Rs. 4950 million (US$13.1 million at the current exchange rate) were given to Uttar Pradesh for five and a half years in 2002 (GOI 2002a). Uttar Pradesh, Madhya Pradesh, Rajasthan, and Bihar are the most poorly developed states—both socially and economically. They contain over 40 percent of India's population and have the highest levels of IMR, MMR, and child mortality rates. Owing to strong patriarchal values, acceptance of family planning is linked to two or more surviving sons (Satia and Jejeebhoy 1991).

A study conducted in 1999 in eight states, including Uttar Pradesh, Rajasthan, and Madhya Pradesh, to assess the impact of the paradigm shift after ICPD found some improvements in the provision of services. While there were marked interstate variations among the eight states, the three states under consideration demonstrated that the official mindset remained unchanged, the lowering of targets by auxiliary nurse midwives (ANMs) was not appreciated, and officially fixed targets continued in practice. Coercion of workers was also reported in Uttar Pradesh. Sterilization remained the mainstay of the program, and safety of abortion was negligible (Health Watch Trust 1999).

USAID's own evaluation of its project SIFPSA shows that, of the 28 districts covered, the focus was only on six, and nine were a second priority. This not only left out 13 of the project districts, but also the remaining 42 districts of Uttar Pradesh. Hence, the evaluator's claims of improved performance and personnel capacity have to be judged while keeping in view the concentration of funds in a limited area (USAID 1997).[5]

Yet another study from Uttar Pradesh estimates 31 percent unmet needs in comparison to a national estimate of 18 percent, serious deficiencies of women doctors and PHC equipment, poor ANM functioning, and the use of mini-camps for catching up with goals. Only half the respondents reported a visit of paramedics over the past three months, and 70 percent believed that they are not of much use anyway (Prasad, Khan, Ram and Patel 1993). A recent report of a campaign against oppressive population policies in Uttar Pradesh interviewed 1,689 persons in 31 districts. It dispels illusions of any progress since 1993. A fear of coercion, the nonavailability of all kinds of health and family welfare services including abortions, and the need for strategy change if the no-target approach has to succeed were evident in the study (Health Watch UP-Bihar 2002). The role of the U.S. government and private foundations in introducing an aggressive sterilization campaign in the 1970s provokes a comparison, of women's experience, between these two democracies.[6]

In the United States, sterilization has become the leading method of permanent contraception, and approximately 11 million women (15 to 44 years) are users (Farrington 2003). Its popularity was established in the 1970s when surgical advances made tubal sterilization highly safe and effective. At the same time, its appeal was enhanced by the availability of insurance coverage and concerns over the safety of the oral contraceptive pill, both of which resulted in the large-scale acceptance of the method, particularly by black and Hispanic women (Westhoff 2002). In India, political exigency, not medical rationale, led to the shift from the relatively simple and safe procedure for vasectomy to female-centered surgical procedures that carry greater risk for complications and long-term morbidity. During the same period, the popularity of the method spread worldwide. For women in societies, where reversible methods were scarce, expensive, or too obtrusive, sterilization was both right and reliable.

The median age at sterilization in India (26.6) is not much below that in the United States (28.8) but only 2 percent of the Indian women have education beyond secondary schools in contrast to 33 percent of the women in the United States (EngenderHealth 2002). Discrete demographic data that characterize sterilized women, however, do not portray the clinical protocols followed before surgery in different regional settings, or the medical response to surgical complications and ongoing morbidity related to menstrual dysfunction. After more than three decades and tens of millions of tubal ligations, Indian family planners have gathered little epidemiological evidence on the long-term side effects of the procedure. The predominant users are women with little schooling and low and unstable incomes, who are often residents of urban slums and shantytowns, and who were within reach had the government shown an interest in tracking their health status. Nag (1973), in a review of the early years of the Indian sterilization program, found complications in 20–30 percent of men (pain and discomfort) and 50 percent of women (menstrual disorders). When women were followed up postsurgery, general physical and mental health problems and menstrual disorders were documented as well as improved conjugal relations (Das Gupta, Jain, Prasad, and Vidyabhushan 1970).

Women behind the Numbers

The Health Watch survey cited above collects 38 fully documented reports of complications and deaths due to negligence of reproductive health care providers and of cases of contraceptive failure where, instead of penalizing those responsible, the state had protected them and pressurized the victim's family to withdraw cases. Some of these case briefings are as follows (Health Watch UP-Bihar 2002).

- **Chutki Devi** of Barabanki district went to a health center for an abortion. She was instructed to take pills and was told that the pregnancy was still in an early phase, so the abortion would be safe. After two days of taking the pills, she developed severe abdominal pain and died on her way to the health center. The doctor at the district hospital said she was four months pregnant and should not have undergone abortion.

- **Leelawati**, 29 years, went to her district hospital at Kushinagar for sterilization. She died immediately after surgery, and the family was refused a death certificate.
- **Rajrani** of Dewa was refused hospitalization and brought back home. With the help of a midwife, she delivered twins but fell unconscious and died by the evening. Both her babies also died.
- **Rampyari**, 30 years of age, was asked to pay Rs. 1,000 (US$22.80) at the district hospital and, when she could not do so, she was thrown out. She delivered outside the hospital gate.
- **Dhokhia** had her abortion and then a tubectomy at the Manikpur government hospital. Just after the operation, she was thrown out by the doctor and the nurse and also badly beaten as she was complaining. Her stitches became septic and she had to spend Rs. 1,500 (US$34.30) for treatment.
- **Rani Jaiswal**, 15 years old, was abducted and forcibly taken to an RCH camp where the doctors operated on her without bothering to check. She was neither given a certificate of sterilization nor any postoperative care. Stitches were not removed for 42 days. An FIR was lodged in the police station against the abductor.

Despite an improved policy that recognizes the importance of well-being and equity in fertility declines, what makes the mode of implementation so contrary to its stated purpose?

Politics and Policies

The FPP has a checkered history. Beginning as a voluntary program, with a clinic and then cafeteria approach, it slipped into an extremely coercive population control drive that treated human beings, especially the poor, without respect or dignity. During the National Emergency (1975–1976), the FPP touched the nadir when the poor were caught and sterilized like animals (Banerji 1997). The political fallout of this was a national election that threw out the oppressive regime of the Congress Party and brought in a new regime. In time, the new regime and its successors became increasingly dependent on international loans and accumulated huge debts. Funding thus became an instrument of domination by agencies such as the World Bank and International Monetary Fund (IMF), and the multinational drug and equipment companies linked with them. The agencies proposed restructuring the Indian economy, with its large consumer market, through structural adjustment policies (SAP), with the agreement of an elite establishment fully vested in this arrangement.

This alliance used an aggressive strategy of population control, blaming the victim and diverting attention from economic issues to justify expanding the contraceptive market. Despite accumulating evidence pointing out the structural roots of the problem and contradicting the alliance's myths, the return to Malthusianism became widespread.[7] Divisive forces used the demographic profile itself to divide people on religious grounds. Ignoring the fact that the largest minority was also the poor and the least literate, who had a fast-declining fertility rate (Kulkarni 2002), the higher fertility of the poor became a source of political propaganda against them (Jeffery and Jeffery 1997). The concept of a "social safety net"—propagated along with SAP—was dropped as soon as South Asia accepted the SAP. However, vigilant activists foiled a move to include a two-child norm in the NPP (Rao 2002). The Uttar Pradesh Population Control Bill 2002 subsequently attempted to codify a number of anti-human rights features of the State Population Policy.

Assessing these issues, actions to counter unhealthy policies must include a series of strategies. The first is mobilizing politically to ensure that the entire set of policies that promote disintegration, commercialization, and technological fixes are reviewed. The second is instituting welfare measures and mechanisms to regulate health markets, with the state assuming responsibility for provision of services. These actions must take priority over subsidizing and supporting the private sector. Significantly, in most First World countries undergoing structural reforms, the state continues to invest 60 to 100 percent in public sector health services (WHO 2002). Third is strengthening primary health care infrastructure to enable an integrated approach to health and family welfare that is critical for success. Fourth comprises channeling contraceptive drugs and services to those with high unmet needs rather than to those not creating the demand. For the latter, there should be an effort to improve economic and social circumstances to bring about shifts in behavior. Finally, basing medical and surgical practices on health outcomes (evidence) is needed, by reevaluating India's dependence on female sterilization through epidemiological studies of short- and long-term health effects. This approach should also be followed in other countries with high rates of female sterilization. Contraceptive donors should be required to fund such research.

Theoretical Lessons

For example, the newfound wealth of "social capital" is currently being projected as a panacea for communities (Organization for Economic Cooperation and Development [OECD] 2001) that do not have economic capital. In India, the metropolises are first breaking and uprooting vulnerable communities, then resettling them afresh, and in the process destroying even their precarious wealth of social capital. An emphasis on a political economy approach that contextualizes the value of social capital, underlining class distinctions, would be much more crucial to policy formulation.

Anthropologists must move beyond understanding the "native" and the "local community" and illuminate the cultures and mindsets of all classes—particularly those that make policies. Little is known about those who do not necessarily understand or care about the underprivileged and yet constantly use them and determine objective reality for them. Such an exposition will clarify the real nature of conflicts and reveal the connecting thread of vested interests. By incorporating the lessons learned from India, the health movement will be strengthened and its struggles consolidated.

Notes

1. In Sri Lanka, while there was an aggressive family planning campaign increasingly using both pills and condoms, traditional contraceptives remained an important source of fertility control (Nichter and Nichter 1996), in marked contrast to the Indian campaign. While Sri Lanka succeeded in creating and maintaining an effective primary health care infrastructure with full support of secondary- and tertiary-level institutions (Dulitha 2001), India has reduced the same to "primary-level care" by neglecting its public sector referral system. In Sri Lanka, the public sector focuses on inpatient care with the private sector dealing mainly with outpatients; but in India the private sector has captured institutional care, to the detriment of a more vulnerable population.

2. For example, in rural India, 70.8 percent use wells, tube wells, and hand pumps, while only 23.2 percent have tap water to drink. In fact, 5.4 percent people drink from tanks, ponds, rivers, and canals directly. There is no provision for latrines or for drainage for 84.4 percent and 62.0 percent of rural households respectively (NSSO 1998).

3. Thus, among the 20 percent of households with the lowest MPCE, only 15.0 percent can access tap water, latrines are not accessible to 94.3 percent, and the Scheduled Castes and Tribes bear the brunt of this deprivation (NSSO 1998). The infant mortality among Scheduled Castes and Scheduled Tribes is 83 and 84 per 1000 live births in comparison to the national average of 72 per 1000 (Kulkarni 2002). Of the lowest 20 percent MPCE groups, only 48.3 percent and 33.3 percent in urban and rural areas respectively reported registration of pregnant women, in comparison to 74.8 percent and 55.9 percent in the highest MPCE groups (NSSO 1998). Also, just 40 percent of poor women received advice from lady health visitors (LHVs) and ANMs; they were far behind the better off in their knowledge and information about immunization and oral hydration. The literate had higher couple protection rates (57.0) in comparison to the illiterate (42.0), but sterilizations were much higher among the illiterate (IIPS 2000).

4. Such changes have been documented by women's groups and health activists in India (Sabla, Swatija, and Meena 2002; Sathyamala 1989), and statistically supported with survey data from college-educated women in the United States (Visvanathan and Wyshak 2000). The late Dr. Malini Karkal, feminist demographer and health activist, observed a trend in earlier menopause for sterilized women in national health surveys.

5. A previous study conducted in 1995 by the same agency had pointed out that 22.2 percent of the public facilities lacked essential sterilization equipment, 45 percent districts were short of workers, and only 38.5 percent of the providers themselves had correct knowledge of contraception. Just 15.4 percent of the sterilized couples received follow-up for needs and only 7 percent of the eligible women reported contact with providers of family planning services in the past six months. Of those who discontinued contraceptive use, 20.7 percent had health problems (side effects), 16.2 percent reported contraceptive failure, and 50.4 percent desired pregnancy (USAID 1995).

6. Deepa Dhanraj's 1991 film, *Something like a War,* documents the role of USAID and the Ford and Rockefeller foundations in the Indian sterilization program as well as live footage.

7. This is reflected in the emergence of a new set of political agents who are today busy "cleaning" the metropolis of the "slum dweller," closing so-called polluting industries, and denying the poor the constitutional right to shelter and work (Roy 2000). Among the well-off who, in the 1960s and 1970s, had accepted Nehru's idea of socialist democracy and the challenge of progress of all, a new value has surfaced. It is respectable today to blame the poor for the ills of the society, be it filth, pollution, or population. It is widely propagated (and believed) that the rich were all through with "subsidizing" the poor, and it is now time to stop "spoiling" them. It is also considered a universal truth that the poor are so because they reproduce more and that their excessive illness is due to their ignorance.

References

Akhtar, F. (1995). *Resisting Norplant: Women's Struggle against Coercion and Violence.* Dhaka: Narigrantha Prabartana.

Baill, I. C., V. E. Cullins, and S. Pati. (2003). "Counseling Issues in Tubal Sterilization." *American Family Physician.* 67: 1287–94.

Bandewar, S. (2003, May 24). "Abortion Services and Providers' Perceptions—Gender Dimensions." *Economic and Political Weekly* 38, no. 21: 2075–2097.

Banerji, D. (1997). "Community Response to the Intensified Family Planning Programme." *Economic and Political Weekly* 12, nos. 6–8: 261–66.

Baru, R. V., I. Qadeer, and R. Priya. (2000, July 15–21). "Medical Industry: Illusion of Quality at What Cost?" *Economic and Political Weekly,* 35, nos. 28–29: 2509–11.

Bhatia, J. C., and J. Cleland. (1995, Jul–August). "Self-Reported Symptoms of Gynecological Morbidity and Their Treatment in South India." *Stud Fam Plann* 26, no. 4: 203–16.

Dasgupta, M. (1998). "Social Development and Fertility Reduction in Kerela." In *Reproductive Change in India and Brazil,* edited by George Martin et al., 37–64. Delhi: Oxford University Press.

Das Gupta, S. K., P. C. Jain, B. G. Prasad, and Vidyabhushan. (1970, August). "Female Sterilization." *J Obstet Gynaecol India* 20, no. 4: 509–16.

Dulitha, F. (2001). "Structural Adjustment Programs and Health Care Services in Sri Lanka—An Overview." In *Public Health and the Poverty of Reforms: The South Asian predicament,* edited by Imrana Qadeer, Sen Kasturi, and K. R. Nayar, 311–26. Delhi: Sage.

EngenderHealth. (2002, May). "Contraceptive Sterilization: Global Issues and Trends. Accessed at www.engenderhealth.org, August 28, 2003.

Farrington, A. (2003). "Permanent Contraception for Women in the United States." *Health and Sexuality* 8, no. 1: 2–12.

Government of India. (1992). *Eighth Five Year Plan, 1992-97*. New Delhi, Planning Commission, 322.

———. (1993). *Draft National Population Policy*. Chairman, M. S. Swaminathan. New Delhi: Ministry of Health and Family Welfare.

———. (1997). *Ninth Five Year Plan 1997-2002*, vol. II. New Delhi: Planning Commission, 138–204.

———. (2000a). *National Population Policy*. New Delhi: Population Commission.

———. (2000b). *Parliamentary Proceedings: Annexure Referred to in Reply to Lok Sabha Unstarred Question*. No. 2690 for 6.12.2000. New Delhi: Lok Sabha Secretariat.

———. (2001a). *Census of India 2001, India Series—I, Provisional Population Total, Paper 1 of 2001 supplement, District Totals*. New Delhi: Office of the Registrar General.

———. (2001b). Working Group on Health Care Services for Tenth Plan. New Delhi: Planning Commission, 40.

———. (2002a). *Annual Report 2001-2002*. New Delhi: Ministry of Health and Family Welfare.

———. (2002b). *National Health Policy*. New Delhi: Ministry of Health and Family Welfare.

———. (2002c). *Tenth Five Year Plan 2002-2007*. New Delhi: Planning Commission, 213.

Government of India, Ministry of Health and Family Welfare. (1989). "Guidelines for Voluntary Sterilization" (No.N.11011/1/84-Ply), March 18, 1986; cited in *Annu Rev Popul Law*. 16: 21, 300.

Government of Madhya Pradesh. (2000). *Population Policy of Madhya Pradesh*. Bhopal: Department of Health and Family Welfare.

Government of Uttar Pradesh. (2000). *Population Policy of Uttar Pradesh*. Lucknow: Department of Health and Family Welfare.

Health Watch Trust. (1999). *Community Needs–Based Reproductive and Child Health in India: Progress and Constraints*. Jaipur: Health Watch Trust.

Health Watch UP-Bihar. (2002). *People, Population Policy, and Women's Health Uttar Pradesh*. Lucknow: Health Watch UP-Bihar, 47–51.

Hieu, D. T., T. T. Tan, P. T. Nguyet, P. Than, and D. Q. Vinh. (1993). "31781 Cases of Non-Surgical Female Sterilization with Quinacrine Pellets in Vietnam." *Lancet* 342, no. 8865: 213–17.

Indian Council of Medical Research (ICMR). (1981). *Short-Term Sequelae of Induced Abortion: A Collaborative Study*. New Delhi: ICMR.

International Institute for Population Sciences (IIPS). (2000). *India—National Family Health Survey*. NFHS—2, 1998-99. Mumbai: IIPS, 136, 187, 195.

Jeffery, R., and P. Jeffery. (1997). *Population, Gender and Politics*. London: Cambridge University Press, 216–54.

Kim, S. U., R. Sinha, and K. D. Gaur. (2002). *Population and Development*. New Delhi: Sunrise Publications, 489–507.

Kulkarni, P. M. (2002, March). "Special Population Groups." *Seminar*, no. 511: 58–66.

Nag, M. (1973, June 18–19). "Sterilization in India, 1965-72: An Overview of Experience, Research Results and Research Needs." Paper presented at the workshop on Behavioral-Social and Public Health Aspects of Surgical Contraception: Research Approaches, Bethesda, MD.

Nanda, A. R. (2002, March). " Not Just a Number Game." *Seminar*, no. 511: 29–32.

National Sample Survey Organisation (NSSO). (1989). *2nd Round, 1986–1987, Report No. 364: "Morbidity and Utilisation of Services."* Table 2, A7. New Delhi: Government of India.

———. (1998). *52nd Round 1995-96, "Maternal and Child Health Care in India," Report no. 445.* Tables 1.1–1.3, A1–A7. New Delhi: Department of Statistics, Government of India.

———. (2001). *55th Round, 1999-2000: Consumption of Some Important Commodities, Report no. 461.* A1–A435. New Delhi: Department of Statistics, Government of India.

Nichter, M., and M. Nichter. (1996). *Anthropology and International Health: Asian Case Studies.* Amsterdam: Overseas Publishers Association.

Organization for Economic Cooperation and Development (OECD). (2001). *Well-Being of Nations: The Role of Human and Social Capital—Education and Skills.* Paris: OECD.

Patel, T. (1994). *Fertility Behavior: Population and Society in a Rajasthan Village.* Delhi: Oxford University Press.

Peterson, H. B., G. Jeng, S. G. Folger, S. A. Hillis, P. A. Marchbanks, and L. S. Wilcox; U.S. Collaborative Review of Sterilization Working Group. (2000, December 7). "The Risk of Menstrual Abnormalities after Tubal Sterilization: U.S. Collaborative Review of Sterilization Working Group." *N Engl J Med.* 343, no. 23: 1681–87.

Prasad, R., M. E. Khan, R. B. Ram, and B. C. Patel. (1993). *Promotion of Family Planning and MCH Care through Dairy Cooperatives in Rural Bihar: Baseline Survey.* Patna: Population Research Center and the Population Council, India.

Purkayastha, S., and P. K. Bhattacharyya. (1992, February). "Aftermaths of Surgical Sterilization with Special Reference to Menstrual Disturbances." *J Indian Med Assoc.* 90, no. 2: 29–30.

Rao, M. (1997, June 21). "Myths of Reproductive Profligacy of Poor: Evidence from Mandya District." *Economic and Political Weekly:* 1447–49.

———. (2002). "Population Policy: From Bad to Worse." *Economic and Political Weekly* 37, no. 22: 2120–22.

Roy, A. K. (2000). "Organising for Safe Livelihoods: Feasible Options." *Economic and Political Weekly* 35, no. 52–53: 4603–4608.

Sabla, S., and M. Sabla. (2002). *Sterilization: A Closer Look.* Mumbai: Initiatives: Women in Development.

Sathyamala, C. (1989, March). *Family Planning Programme and People's Right to Health: A Report on the Socio-Medical Impact of 'Sterilisation' on the Lives of Women in Four Resettlement Colonies in Delhi. A Survey.* New Delhi: Sabla Sangh.

———. (2000). *An Epidemiological Review of the Injectable Contraceptive, Depo-Provera.* Pune: Medico Friend Circle.

Satia, J. K., and S. Jejeebhoy, eds. (1991). *Demographic Challenge: A Study of Four Large Indian States.* Bombay: Oxford University Press.

Tewari, S., and S. Rathee. (1997, March). "Practice of Standards in Female Sterilisation." *J Indian Med Assoc.* 95, no. 5: 136–37, 141.

United Nations Development Programme (UNDP). (2003). *Human Development Report 2003, Millennium Development Goal: A Compact among Nations to End Human Poverty*. New Delhi: Oxford University Press, 246.

U.S. Agency for International Development (USAID). (1995). *Performance Indicators for the Innovations in Family Planning Services Project: 1995 Perform Survey*. U.P. State Seminar Report, Lucknow, Uttar Pradesh, September 1996. New Delhi: USAID.

———. (1997). *Innovations in Family Planning Services Project: Midterm Assessment Report.* Washington, DC: USAID.

Vasundhara, D., R. Shah, and G. Misra. (2000). *Gender and Reproductive Health Research Initiative Mapping a Decade of Reproductive Health Research in India, Abortion in India: An Annotated Bibliography of Selected Studies (1990-2000)*. New Delhi: Creating Resources for Empowerment in Action.

Visaria, L., and P. Visaria. (1996). *Prospective Population Growth and Policy Options for India (1991-2101)*. Ahmedabad: Gujarat Institute of Development Research (Mimeo).

Visaria, P. (2002, March). "Population Policy." *Seminar*, no. 511: 14–28.

Visvanathan, N., and G. Wyshak. (2000, June). "Tubal Ligation, Menstrual Changes, and Menopausal Symptoms." *J Womens Health Gend Based Med.* 9, no. 5: 521–27.

Westhoff, C. (2002, May). Slide Presentation. Cited in "History and Epidemiology of Tubal Sterilization in the United States." *ARHP Clinical Proceedings*: 4–6.

World Bank. (1993). *World Development Report, 1993: Investing in Health.* Washington, DC: World Bank.

World Health Organization (WHO). (2002). *World Health Report 2002: Reducing Risks and Promoting Healthy Life*. Geneva: WHO, 202–17.

WHO and UNICEF. (1978, September 6–12). *Report of the International Conference on Primary Health Care.* Alma-Ata, USSR. Geneva: WHO.

II

NATIONAL HEALTH POLICIES AND SOCIAL EXCLUSION

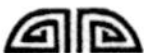

10

Happy Children with AIDS: The Paradox of a Healthy National Program in an Unequal and Exclusionary Brazil

CÉSAR E. ABADÍA-BARRERO

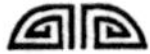

BRAZILIAN CHILDREN AND ADOLESCENTS living with and affected by HIV and AIDS (CALAHA) live in a justice-injustice paradox that is directly related to their illness. Children are infected with HIV and/or become orphans because their families come from underprivileged social classes. Once infected, however, these children benefit from a series of social responses that assure that the care for their infection follows the same protocols that are applied to the uppermost classes not only in Brazil but in any nation. The lives of this group of Brazilian children and adolescents represent a paradox that I have termed "diseases of poverty-privileged responses." While HIV/AIDS enters children's lives due to its association with poverty, HIV/AIDS-infected children receive vanguard medical treatment, food, and shelter as a result of the successful social responses developed by the Brazilian AIDS social movement (Abadía-Barrero 2003).

This chapter deals with the experience of an exemplary program that, instead of perpetuating social inequalities, successfully looks at health as a human right both in discourse and in practice. I studied the Brazilian National Program of Sexually Transmitted Diseases (STDs) and AIDS during a 20-month fieldwork research in which I paid particular attention to the relationship between the social responses around the AIDS epidemic in Brazil and the subjectivities of CALAHA in São Paulo. This chapter's main questions are (1) How can a health policy be truthful to the implementation of health as a human right considering the unequal structure of Brazil? and (2) What happens to people's experiences of illness when their rights are recovered, citizenship is respected, and inequalities are diminished?

The Brazilian National Program of STDs and AIDS

The general principles of the Brazilian National Program of STDs and AIDS are clear examples of the program's commitment to respecting all citizenship and human rights for people living with HIV and AIDS and to providing them with high-quality, public, and free-of-charge health care (Ministry of Health of Brazil 2002:7). Under this ideology, health care means providing adequate diagnosis, prevention, and treatment in tandem, contesting the idea that prevention and treatment are two separate issues when facing AIDS.

Dealing with AIDS care as a human right has been an almost steady process of accomplishments. However, it has been no easy task (for several reviews, see Altman 1995; Barbosa and Parker 1999; Galvão 2000; Parker 1997; Parker, Galvão, and Bessa 1999). In 1991, the first available medicine for the control of the progression of HIV/AIDS, zidovudine (AZT), was distributed to thousands of infected people in Brazil. In 1996, the recently discovered protease inhibitors followed AZT's path and were also included into the antiretroviral (ARV) treatment for all people living with AIDS within the country's public health infrastructure. There are currently more than 135,000 Brazilians receiving the most advanced antiretroviral medications for the treatment of AIDS at no cost. If they had to pay, the large majority—who are poor—would not be able to afford the necessary treatment and, consequently, would be sentenced to an early death.

ARVs are funded by the Ministry of Health. In 2001, the ministry spent US$232 million treating 105,000 people, which represented 1.6 percent of the ministry's budget—less than 0.05 percent of the country's GDP (Ministry of Health of Brazil 2002). At the end of 2003, there were approximately 135,000 people receiving ARVs, yet the ministry will actually be saving millions of dollars. On one hand, when people improve their health (and hence their quality of life), they need less expensive medical care. Since 1996, the need for hospital admissions by patients with AIDS in the public health network has dropped by 80 percent, the need for treatment of opportunistic infections has decreased by 60–80 percent, and the more expensive hospital-based care has to a great extent been replaced by a less expensive ambulatory-based care. The Brazilian Ministry of Health estimates that roughly US$1 billion was saved in the period 1997–2001, when approximately 358,000 AIDS-related hospital admissions were prevented (Ministry of Health of Brazil 2002).

On the other hand, while in developed nations the average cost of ARVs per patient is over US$10,000 per year, as of 2002 the cost in Brazil had been reduced to around US$2,273, and it continues to drop (Reardon 2002). In Brazil, the program's strategy has been to reduce the price of the medications by investing in local manufacturing of generic ARVs, and by negotiating significant price reductions from multinational pharmaceutical companies, holders of the patents of the newest ARVs (Ministry of Health of Brazil 2001, 2002; Reardon 2002). Thus, depending on the exact ARV regime that a patient receives, the price had already dropped from anywhere between 48 and 84 percent during the 1996–2001 period (Ministry of Health of Brazil 2001).

Furthermore, there are other social impacts that reduce costs to the country's social security system. For example, due to the availability of adequate treatment, AIDS-related mortality has been reduced by 50 percent since 1996 (Ministry of Health of Brazil 2002). By receiving adequate health care, healthier citizens living with HIV/AIDS can remain economically productive, there are less social costs when families are not disintegrated because of sickness or death, less money needs to be spent in subsidizing disabled citizens, and fewer orphans are left behind.

In addition to these therapeutic successes, Brazil has also reduced the number of new HIV infections via effective prevention campaigns. While in 1995 the World Bank estimated that "1.2 million Brazilians would enter the new millennium with HIV/AIDS" (Reardon 2002), UNAIDS estimated that only half that number were infected at the end of 2001 (UNAIDS 2002). Thus, Brazil is effectively preventing new infections and has stabilized the rate of infection at a 0.7 percent level, contrary to all predictions.

In short, the Brazilian National Program has received international recognition for several reasons. It is the country where most people living with HIV/AIDS are being treated with optimal health care standards, where more people have had the quality of their lives improved, where fewer people are dying because of AIDS, where fewer people than predicted are becoming infected every year, and where millions of dollars in health care costs are being saved.

What Are the Implications of These Successful Health Care Policies for Brazilian Children Afflicted with AIDS

UNICEF and the World Health Organization (WHO) recognized—as early as 1994—that children suffer as a result of AIDS not only when they are infected themselves, but also when they fall into one or more of the following categories:

> Children whose parents are sick or have died of AIDS; children whose siblings, relatives, or friends have the disease or have died; children whose households are stressed by children from another family who have been orphaned by AIDS; and children such as those on the street, who are at high risk of infection (WHO/UNICEF 1994).

Even though the establishment of categories is an instructive exercise to classify people's experiences, there is a conceptual link that explains the fragile division between the experiences of CALAHA and those considered at risk (i.e., children living on the streets). This link can be seen as a two-way path: CALAHA may end up on the streets, and street children are at high risk to acquire AIDS. In the case of parents' illness or death due to AIDS, if the network of relatives is unable to care for the orphaned child, CALAHA may find the streets to be the only available space in which to "circulate" and survive.[1] Conversely, street children—orphans, abandoned children, or fugitives from their own household—are highly vulnerable to becoming infected or reinfected with the virus and contracting other sexually transmissible diseases, not only from sexual abuse or infantile prostitution, but also because street children are prone to use drugs and exchange sex for protection and satisfaction of emotional needs (Scheper-Hughes and Hoffman 1998; UNAIDS 1999). In addition, Brazilian street children have suffered from other diseases and hazards such as malnutrition; drug use and/or trafficking; peer, institutional, or everyday physical violence; and early death (Gregori and Silva 2000; Inciardi and Surratt 1998; Larvie 1992; Raffaelli et al. 1993), including the infamous murdering of street children by death squads during the 1980s and 1990s (Dimenstein 1991; Martins 1991; MNMMR, IBASE, and NEV-USP 1992).

In order to understand the effects of the program and of these health care policies in the children's subjectivities, I studied children and adolescents at four institutions: two AIDS NGO support houses that shelter CALAHA, one AIDS NGO kindergarten that offers preschool education to children infected with HIV/AIDS and their siblings, and one state-run shelter for street children. In addition, I studied the adults at these institutions and at the medical institutions, as well as the AIDS national program and its policies.

Children, AIDS, and the Paradox: Diseases of Poverty-Privileged Responses

If a child is found on the streets or reported to the authorities—and if the child's HIV status is unknown—they will be directed to the state sheltering system for street children: *SOS criança* (SOS child). If the child is known to be HIV-positive or feared to be infected because his or her mother has died of AIDS, the AIDS NGOs support houses will be contacted to care for the child. However, the driving force behind both living on the streets and living with HIV/AIDS can be traced to the same unequal social and economic factors that have informed the children's present situation—as both situations can be seen as manifestations of the same social ills. Indeed, parents' or children's deaths, sickness, abandonment, or running away from home (the latter usually the result of household violence or neglect) are directly linked to the same structural economic factors that perpetuate widespread poverty, and to political and ideological forces that oppress and marginalize social groups due to age, race, region, culture, gender, and social class.[2]

By working at both the shelter for street children and the AIDS NGO support houses, I was able to analyze the differences between being a poor homeless child and a poor homeless child living with HIV/AIDS, and hence the differences in responses that Brazilian society has constructed around these two groups of children. What happens when the success of the AIDS case is compared with less successful social responses, such as those in the case of street children?

Rogério[3] has lived at the *Siloé,* one of the support houses researched, since he was eight years old. After his mother died when he was five, he lived with his father in one of the city slums—*favela*—yet he mostly remembers his father for his neglectful care and for having given away his two sisters. "I hate him," he told me. By the time we met, he had lived at the Siloé for two years, and through our many exchanges I learned that he is hopeful about his future. I also learned that even though growing up with HIV/AIDS has been difficult, the most difficult aspect of his life is not experiencing AIDS as a sickness, but rather experiencing the stigma and discrimination associated with it, and the many changes in "home" environments, including living at an institution. However, Rogério considers himself happy, and having AIDS has not been an obstacle to achieving successes in school, sports, or socialization. He stands out as an outspoken and confident preadolescent. Rogério was interested in visiting the other places where I was conducting my research. Particularly, he wondered what the lives of the street children were like at the state-run shelter. I told him that if he wanted to, I could take him there one day. This is how our conversation continued.

> Rogério: Are they poor?
>
> César: Yes, they are.
>
> Rogério: Uf, thank God that I am not there. . . . Do they eat? Do they have food?
>
> César: At the shelter they do, but in general when they are on the streets or at home, they don't have much.
>
> Rogério: It can't be Mondays or Wednesdays because I am very busy those days.
>
> César: I am not planning to take you on weekdays. It would have to be on the weekends; you have school.
>
> Rogério: Not only school; on Mondays and Wednesdays I have sports after class, and then in the afternoons I have English lessons. Then, I come back, have a bath, have dinner, and I have to rest, otherwise I can't wake up the next day to go to school.

Rogério's comments illustrate the paradox of AIDS having brought to the lives of many of the infected children upward socioeconomic mobility and life opportunities as a result of adequate and effective social responses. In terms of children's development and hopes for the future, the life options of the child trump the disease. For Rogério, it was better to have AIDS than to be poor; otherwise, he would have most likely ended up at the shelter. Rogério's remarks suggest that to understand the paradox and assess differences in outcome, one has to pay close attention to the satisfaction of economic needs. For him, poverty (symbolized by not having enough food to eat) contrasted with his English and sports classes, the homework for his private school, and his freedom to choose when to rest. Considering that past family histories of both groups of children were overburdened by the same issues—*favela* neighborhoods, dire poverty, unemployment, illegality and imprisonment, drug and alcohol use, physical and emotional violence, and death and murder—Rogério's relief could mean only that in escaping a poor life, one can have access to new options and a different future. Thus, the main determinant of the different outcomes of *happiness* (in the case of AIDS) as opposed to *despair* (in the case of street children) is not simply an issue of having AIDS or not having AIDS, but rather having adequate responses to address the needs of those living with AIDS versus having inadequate responses to address the needs of those living on the streets.

In one of the other institutions, the kindergarten, the paradox diseases of poverty-privileged responses also seemed to explain some troubling situations occurring with mothers every year. Newborn babies of HIV-positive women are cared for following a constructivist pedagogical model that seeks independence, autonomy, and respect for the children's learning and developmental processes. After the first year of being at the kindergarten, some mothers express anger and frustration if their children are found to be HIV-negative. The contradictory response of the mothers, who are angered and frustrated because after a year of kindergarten their children are *now* considered healthy, is explicable when understood through the same paradox: after being diagnosed healthy, the child will have to leave the AIDS NGO kindergarten and the mother will have to search for a spot in one of the municipal or state-run kindergartens. Not only is it extremely difficult to find a place in the public preschool systems, but mothers and families who do so also lose the advantages of being at the AIDS NGO kindergarten, including high-quality education; social work services that provide family counseling, community participation, and empowering projects; privileged health care; excellent nutrition and nurse care during the week; a safe environment; transportation; and much-needed economic aid.

Similarly, within the larger network of AIDS NGO activism for both children and adults, I heard of cases in which people forged a positive HIV test to be able to have access to extra resources or would *try* to become infected—to have access to adequate health care, economic protection, and even disability allowance to afford food (these people would celebrate rather than feel distressed if the HIV test came back positive). In addition, I also knew of cases of HIV-infected people claiming that they would kill themselves if an AIDS cure was ever found, because their lives had gained meaning only after they joined AIDS support networks. People living with AIDS were thankful to AIDS because they had acquired benefits from it, or their lives had acquired a new dimension after receiving help and counseling. Many Brazilians living with AIDS have been empowered; thus, AIDS has transformed many lives in a positive way (Brito and Franco 2000).

Children's Perceptions of the Paradox

I was driving the boys of the Siloé to another of our monthly *gama* visits—that included physical checkups and IV immunoglobuline treatment. As we passed a corner, Bruno (age 13) commented as he looked out the window: "My uncle and I come here and sell fireworks when I am on vacation. Once, when the police started to mess with us, my uncle told them that they bother those who work honestly and not those who steal from people. You see, the police are not fair."

I asked him incredulously: "Do you really come here?"

"Yes, I am poor," he said.

I teased him about the poverty of the Siloé, pointing out that, in reality, their lives were more like "rich" kids than anything else.[4]

"That is true," Bruno said. "The Father [director of the Catholic AIDS NGO] says that there is nothing we don't have at the [house]; that we are rich."

I challenged him: "How is that: you are rich and poor at the same time? How can that be?"

He challenged me: "That is easy, my family is poor."

I explained to Bruno my hypothesis that AIDS could in fact be beneficial because it gives kids "rich-life options," and that AIDS, in the end, could become a positive factor for any kid's life.

"That is right . . . but not always," Bruno wisely answered, and then continued: "That only happens if you live at a support house. If you have AIDS, but you live with your family, then you will have AIDS and be poor."

Bruno's insights show how the AIDS network of help and support follows a sort of "calamitous" path in which the more losses a person has, the better support they receive. For children, the situation proceeds as follows: when a parent dies, the family loses the economic support that the AIDS program was giving to the deceased parent, unless he or she had a pension that can remain with the widowed. However, in either case, as Bruno suggested, *you will have AIDS and be poor* because the economic aid is far from sufficient. If the remaining parent dies and the children are HIV-negative, they will be taken to the state-run shelter—where Rogério felt relieved not to be, and where, for Bruno, it would mean "to be poor without AIDS." In contrast, the most favorable set of responses comes when children are

HIV-positive—*and* both parents die or cannot take care of the children. In this case, the children are sent to a support house to live "rich" lives with AIDS, as Bruno suggested. Thus, children at support houses will exit the confined sphere of poverty, from which a great number of Brazilian children cannot escape.

Working at the shelter for street children, I found conditions that supported Rogério's relief for not being at the shelter and Bruno's insights about the importance of social responses. Children at the state-run shelter for street children "circulate" among the street, home, the shelter, and, in some cases, the youth jail. The future outcomes at any place are bleak. At home, dire poverty, intrahousehold violence, alcoholism, and drug trafficking or consumption are common. On the streets, the risks are multiple, including child prostitution networks, drug abuse, illegal and criminalizing activities, and lack of food and sheltering. At the shelter, the situation is not much different. The child protection system is structured around a criminalizing legal system that links the children's lives to the suspicion of delinquency. A child found on the streets performing serious criminal acts—murdering, or sexual or violent physical assaults—is sent to the youth jail (generally known as FEBEM), and a child found "merely" vagabonding, begging, or performing petty crimes—stealing in general—is sent to the shelter (generally known as SOS child). In addition, both FEBEM and SOS child, which belong to the same division, have been accused of being corrupt bureaucratic organizations that function as political platforms for both electoral purposes and budget cuts (Gregori and Silva 2000). Thus, the shelter option is far from adequate, and children usually take off to the streets or return home.

The shelter's social worker could only remember three children (out of more than 100 with whom she had worked) who made it out of the harsh circles of extreme poverty, illegality, violence, or early death: "One [child] ended up working in a store, another as a security man, and the other got married and had children. Just three." Thus, the majority of street children could not envision anything positive in their future and filled my ethnographic notes with despair, which confirmed the paradox revealed in conversations with Rogério and Bruno. Street children feel, and rightly so, that their future is constrained by a total lack of options, and, given that they are aware of the dreadful experiences of many of their peers, they expect to find themselves negotiating the boundaries of legality and illegality and trying to avoid early death.

Although street children are considered healthy, it is children living with AIDS who can envision hopeful outcomes to their lives. This larger implication of the aforementioned paradox is evidence of the effective reduction in social inequalities accomplished by the social movement behind the AIDS health policies and social support networks in Brazil.

AIDS Care and Biomedicine

As biomedicine has increasingly interconnected with market-based approaches to health—which follow the current globalization/neoliberal economic and political paradigms—private pharmaceutical and technological companies through "scientific" biomedical research determine the current parameters for medical competency (Good 1995) and restrict the physician's freedom to engage in nonbiological aspects of the patient's treatment (Schraiber 1993). Most importantly, under the market-based model, health care has become another commodity (Pellegrino 1999), and consequently its access is an asset of privilege that only a few can afford. Not surprisingly, the links between biomedicine and the market are discussed as exclusionary practices of the Western project regarding health via unequal power relationships and in which the inequalities that exclude the poor are perpetuated (Huertas 1998; Kim et al. 2000).

The influence of private investors in health care, however, has also produced incredible advances in AIDS diagnosis and therapeutics, and has made a very complex infectious disease treatable and controllable after 20 years of the epidemic. Thus, for those who have access to comprehensive AIDS care, suffering due to AIDS is reduced by the therapeutic regime introduced in the late 1990s with the inclusion of protease inhibitors and by the further simplification of the complex regime via improved presentation and form of the ARVs and increases in their length of action. In the children's accounts, such as Rogério's, access to these biomedical achievements has meant proper control of their infection and the possibility for a longer, healthier, and, as Rogério put it, "happy" life. Yet, even though Brazil is one of the world's most unequal countries[5] and the price of the adequate ARV treatment makes it prohibitive to most of the world, Brazil stands out as an exceptional example by treating all people living with HIV/AIDS with such medications. Thus, a closer look at this exception—which has effectively reduced inequalities by incorporating the advancements produced by the wealthy aspect of biomedicine into the universal principles of AIDS care—may show us what is beneficial about AIDS and biomedicine, and how to alter its exclusionary practice.

Latin American social movements theory can help to explain what is at stake in the biomedical practice of AIDS care in Brazil. Latin American social movements neither want to overthrow the democratic state nor integrate with its bureaucratic structures (Escobar and Alvarez 1992; Escobar, Alvarez, and Dagnino 2001; Foweraker 1995). Consequently, these social movements need to be understood as constant revolutions aiming to democratize society—power negotiation occurs while acknowledging the state as the ruling institution. A parallel analysis of the role of the Brazilian AIDS social movement and its national program of STDs and AIDS shows that this social movement is neither *integrationist* nor *separatist*—borrowing Yúdice's (2001) argument for Latin American social movements in general—with the practice of biomedicine, but rather that the movement aims to democratize biomedicine. The Brazilian AIDS social movement acknowledges that biomedical advances are positive for reducing the suffering brought to individuals, families, and communities due to AIDS. Thus, it supports and favors the use of pharmacological measures for the treatment of infected people, while strongly disagreeing with the private orientation of the health care markets and the social exclusion that results from medicines being overpriced or conceived as private goods.

A thorough analysis of biomedicine should stand close to the experience of the ill by understanding not only why biomedicine has many failures and may enhance suffering, but also why it has, or can have, many successes and may reduce suffering. Such moves allow medical anthropology to provide important contributions to program design and evaluation and to dialogue more closely with policies.

Further Implications for Social Science Research: Successes and Failures within the Context of Inequalities

The *democratization* of biomedical practices occurs when therapeutic advancements are made available to all. Thus, while the Brazilian AIDS social movement agrees with the use of biomedical advancements, it *does not identify* with the current commodification of health care. It proposes, instead, to assume health as a human right to be provided within the country's public health infrastructure. Its *strategies* are to entrust local experts with the creation, implementation, and monitoring of responses; to rely on the democratizing tradition of its social movement, which is in charge of organizing effective social responses including the national AIDS program; to invest in local capacity (public health care infrastructure and production of generic versions of the expensive ARVs) to be able to negotiate with the markets; and to enroll in large solidarity networks that can push their cause forward. Thus, it keeps the basic aspects of the Latin American social movement tradition: democracy, identity, and strategy (Escobar and Alvarez 1992). In order to be successful, the movement has needed to recognize the biomedical successes (technological advancements) and its failures (exclusionary and market-based practices).

This democratization of AIDS care in Brazil, however, illuminates problems and posits challenges to the country's health care infrastructure, in particular, and its social security system in general. In the present case, for instance, the right to life of street children received notable recognition during the 1980s and 1990s through national and international mobilizations. Yet, once the official murdering of street children via death squads stopped, the momentum of the right-to-life mobilizations waned and the programs for street children faltered due to budgetary cuts and bureaucratic corruption for power was endorsed to the state (Gregori and Silva 2000). Consequently, street children filled my field notes with saddened accounts of their existence. The AIDS case is the counterexample because it is grounded in a larger social movement, which targets the factors that drive social exclusion, perpetuate inequalities, and deny human rights. Unfortunately, the factors associated with such recovery of rights, exiting of poverty, and fighting off exclusion become desirable. Having AIDS becomes advantageous because it brings adequate responses.

This paradox talks to the many unsolved issues in Brazil and unveils the many antidemocratic social practices still present in the country. If AIDS care is more comprehensive than the care for other diseases, then these effective social responses to AIDS need to be expanded to other health care programs. If health care is more comprehensive than other basic human rights, such revolutionary responses in health care need to be expanded to other social security networks. In the example of the Brazilian AIDS social movement, we see how AIDS has brought adequate responses that in the context of rampant poverty and lack of life options becomes a "privilege." In order for adequacy not to be a privilege, other social services should follow the same pillars of the AIDS care program, universal and free-of-charge access to services. Street children also strive for adequate services, yet they cannot benefit from the effective AIDS responses because they are considered uninfected. Thus, there is a critical challenge to such a successful program that sees the links between health and society at a deeper level, but excludes those who are only at risk. Brazil's most important contribution is, however, demonstrating that breaking pervasive poverty and inequality is possible through promoting a national social movement and making its ideology a general policy.

Acknowledgments

I would like to thank the children and adolescents who participated in this research. I would also like to thank Arachu Castro for her editorial comments and for reviewing several drafts of the chapter. A longer version of this chapter received the Rudolf Virchow Graduate Student Award of the Critical Anthropology of Health Caucus from the Society for Medical Anthropology.

Notes

1. "Child circulation" is a theoretical concept that explains the shared responsibility that poor families in Brazil use to justify childrearing (Fonseca 1986, 1995). The use of institutions can also be seen as another strategy used by families to protect children (Gregori and Silva 2000). These state-run shelters and the AIDS NGO support houses can also be analyzed as strategies within child circulation networks to assure child survival.

2. For the discussion of structural violence and AIDS, see Farmer (1992) and Farmer, Connors, and Simmons (1996); for infectious diseases in general, see Farmer (1999); for

health and inequalities, see Kim, Millen, Irwin, and Gershman (2000). For discussions about street children and marginalization, see MNMMR et al. (1992), Gregori and Silva (2000), and Dimenstein (1991). The theoretical framework of "oppression" follows Paolo Freire's argument regarding the historical reasons that explain the social reproduction of inequalities based on differences in power between rich owners and poor, "oppressed" workers (Freire 1996).

3. All children's names are fictitious to protect their identities. Many of these nicknames, however, were selected by the children themselves. Rogério sent me the phrase, "I have AIDS but I am happy," one year after I finished my fieldwork.

4. I need to make clear, however, that not all the support houses provided adequate responses or a "wealthy" environment. There was much diversity in responses because of the few parameters considered for the establishment of support houses. Some houses have been formally accused of mistreatment and abuses, and some have been closed down. In the other support house researched, children signaled out some internal episodes occurring at the house that were consistent with child abuse. One year after I finished my fieldwork, this other house was required to change its location and administration after several anonymous child-abuse reports. I should also make clear that the "wealth" expressed by my informants referred to middle-class living conditions. I use the extreme wealth-poverty dichotomy because the scarcities at the shelter for street children are all-encompassing.

5. Poverty and inequalities are rampant in Brazil, and are clearly connected to the demographic distribution of the country's AIDS epidemics (Bastos and Szwarcwald 2000; Parker and Rochel de Carmego 2000). Brazil's Gini index continues to be one of the highest in the world (it was 59.1 for the year 2001), which signifies that while the richest 20 percent of the population retains 63 percent of the total income, the poorest 20 percent retain only 2.6 percent (United Nations Development Programme [UNDP] 2001). However, when inequities in race, gender, and region are considered, the Human Development Index, which classifies Brazil as a middle-income country, in fact reveals the country's marked social disparities, with Afro-Brazilian women exhibiting the poorest indexes in life expectancy and literacy level (Paixão 2000). It is not surprising that the face of the epidemic presented a dramatic shift from a homosexual epidemic in the mid-1980s (with a male to female ratio of 17:1 in 1986) to a heterosexual epidemic since the 1990s (with the same ratio being 2:1 in 1997–1999, and dropping even further since then) (Ministério da Saúde 2001). It is thus clear that Brazilian women living in poverty are particularly vulnerable to the epidemic and that, consequently, many children are being born not only infected with HIV, but also poor.

References

Abadía-Barrero, C. E. (2003). "The Cultural Politics of the Brazilian AIDS Social Movement: A Local and Global Revolution." Paper presented at Latin American Students Association (LASA), Dallas, Texas.

Altman, D. (1995). *Poder e Comunidade: Respostas Organizacionais e culturais à AIDS.* Rio de Janeiro: ABIA, IMS/URRJ, Relume-Dumará Editores.

Barbosa, R. M., and R. Parker, eds. (1999). "Sexualidades pelo Avesso." *Direitos, Identidades e Poder.* São Paulo: Editora 34, IMS/URRJ.

Bastos, F. I., and C. L. Szwarcwald. (2000). "AIDS and Pauperization: Principal Concepts and Empirical Evidence." *Reports in Public Health* 16, supp. 1: 65–76.

Brito, N., and E. Franco. (2000). *Fios da Vida: Tecendo o feminino em tempos de aids*. Brasilia: Ministério de Saúde.

Dimenstein, G. (1991). *Brazil, War on Children*. Translated by C. Whitehouse. London: Latin America Bureau.

Escobar, A., and S. Álvarez. (1992). "Introduction: Theory and Protest in Latin America Today." In *The Making of Social Movements in Latin America*, edited by A. Escobar and S. Álvarez, 1–15. Series in Political Economy and Economic Development in Latin America. Boulder, CO: Westview Press.

Escobar, A., S. Álvarez, and E. Dagnino. (2001). "Introducción: Lo cultural y lo político en los movimientos sociales latinoamericanos." In *Política Cultural & Cultura Política: Una nueva mirada sobre los movimientos sociales latinoamericanos*, edited by A. Escobar, S. Álvarez, and E. Dagnino, 17–48. Bogotá: Taurus, Instituto Colombiano de Antropología e Historia.

Farmer, P. (1992). *AIDS and Accusation: Haiti and the Geography of Blame*. Berkeley: University of California Press.

———. (1999). *Infections and Inequalities: The Modern Plagues*. Berkeley: University of California Press.

Farmer, P., M. Connors, and J. Simmons, eds. (1996). *Women, Poverty, and AIDS: Sex, Drugs and Structural Violence*. Monroe, ME: Common Courage Press.

Fonseca, C. (1986). "Orphanages, Foundlings, and Foster Mothers: The System of Child Circulation in a Brazilian Squatter Settlement." *Anthropological Quarterly* 59, no. 1: 15–27.

———. (1995). *Caminhos da Adoção*. São Paulo: Cortez Editora.

Foweraker, J. (1995). *Theorizing Social Movements*. London: Pluto Press.

Freire, P. (1996). *Pedagogy of the Oppressed*. Translated by M. B. Ramos. London: Penguin.

Galvão, J. (2000). *AIDS no Brasil: Agenda de construção de uma epidemia*. São Paulo: Editora 34, ABIA.

Good, M. J. D. (1995). *American Medicine: The Quest for Competence*. Berkeley: University of California Press.

Gregori, M. F., and C. A. Silva. (2000). *Meninos de Rua e Instituições: Tramas, Disputas e Desmanche*. São Paulo: Contexto.

Huertas, R. (1998). *Neoliberalismo y Políticas de Salud*. Barcelona: El viejo Topo.

Inciardi, J. A., and H. L. Surratt. (1998). "Children in the Streets of Brazil: Drug Use, Crime, Violence, and HIV Risks." *Substance Use & Misuse* 33, no. 7: 1461–80.

Kim, J. Y., J. V. Millen, A. Irwin, and J. Gershman, eds. (2000). *Dying for Growth: Global Inequality and the Health of the Poor*. Monroe, ME: Common Courage Press.

Larvie, P. (1992). *A Construção Cultural dos "Meninos de Rua" no Rio de Janeiro: Implicações para a Prevenção de HIV/AIDS*. Rio de Janeiro: AIDSCOM/University of Chicago.

Martins, J. de Souza, ed. (1991). *O Massacre dos Inocentes: A criança sem infância no Brasil*. São Paulo: Hucitec.

Ministério da Saúde. (2001). *Boletim Epidemiológico AIDS*. Brasilia: Ministerio da Saúde.

Ministry of Health of Brazil. (2001). *National AIDS Drug Policy*. Brasilia: Ministry of Health, 1–24.

———. (2002). *Response: The Experience of the Brazilian AIDS Programme*. Brasilia: Ministry of Health, 65.

MNMMR, IBASE, and NEV-USP. (1992). *Vidas em Risco: Assassinatos de Crianças e Adolescentes no Brasil*. Rio de Janeiro: MNMMR, IBASE, NEV-USP.

Paixão, M. (2000). *Os Indicadores de Desenvolvimento Humano (IDH) Como Instrumento de Mensuração de Desigualdades Étnicas: o caso Brasil*. Accessed at www.fase.org.br/acervo_view.asp?id=1283, January 18, 2003.

Parker, R., ed. (1997). *Políticas, Instituições e AIDS: enfrentando a epidemia no Brasil*. Rio de Janeiro: ABIA.

Parker, R., J. Galvão, and M. Secron Bessa, eds. (1999). "Saúde Desenvolvimento e Política." *Respostas frente a AIDS no Brasil*. Rio de Janeiro: Editora 34, ABIA.

Parker, R., and K. R. de Camargo, Jr. (2000). "Poverty and HIV/AIDS: Anthropological and Sociological Aspects." *Reports in Public Health* 16, supp. 1: 89–102.

Pellegrino, E. D. (1999). "The Commodification of Medical and Health Care: The Moral Consequences of a Paradigm Shift from a Professional to a Market Ethic." *Journal of Medicine and Philosophy* 24, no. 3: 243–66.

Raffaelli, M., R. Campos, A. Merrit, E. Siqueira, C. Antunes, R. Parker, et al. (1993). "Sexual Practices and Attitudes of Street Youth in Belo Horizonte, Brazil." *Social Science and Medicine* 37, no. 5: 661–70.

Reardon, C. (2002). "AIDS: How Brazil Turned the Tide: Can Others Emulate Its Success?" *Ford Foundation Report* 33, no. 3: 8–13.

Scheper-Hughes, N., and D. Hoffman. (1998). "Brazilian Apartheid: Street Kids and the Struggle for Urban Space." In *Small Wars: The Cultural Politics of Childhood*, edited by N. Scheper-Hughes and C. Sargent, 352–88. Berkeley: University of California Press.

Schraiber, L. B. (1993). *O Médico e seu Trabalho: Límites da Liberdade*. São Paulo: Hucitec.

UNAIDS. (1999). *Children and HIV/AIDS*. Geneva: UNAIDS, 21.

———. (2002). *Report on the Global HIV/AIDS*. Geneva: UNAIDS, 226.

United Nations Development Programme (UNDP). (2001). *Inequality in Income or Consumption*. Accessed at www.undp.org/hdr2001/indicator/cty_f_BRA.html, February 28, 2003.

WHO/UNICEF. (1994). *Action for Children Affected by AIDS: Programme Profiles and Lessons Learned*. New York: WHO/UNICEF.

Yúdice, G. (2001). "La globalización de la cultura y la nueva sociedad civil." In *Política Cultural & Cultura Política: Una nueva mirada sobre los movimientos sociales latinoamericanos*, edited by A. Escobar, S. Alvarez, and E. Dagnino, 381–410. Bogotá: Taurus, Instituto Colombiano de Antropología e Historia.

11

Between Risk and Confession: The Popularization of Syphilis Prophylaxis in Revolutionary Mexico

KATHERINE ELAINE BLISS

IN 1909 DR. EDUARDO LAVALLE CARVAJAL PUBLISHED an article in the *Gaceta Médica de México* describing current venereal disease prevention programs in Mexico City. A syphilis specialist and a member of the capital's Sanitary Inspection Service, the corps of physicians who were charged with preventing the spread of disease among the city's residents, Lavalle Carvajal argued that sexual hygiene in Mexico was in a sorry state, indeed. Not only did the incidence of syphilis infection seem to be on the rise, but those people at the greatest risk for contracting and spreading the disease, sexually promiscuous men and women, also went to great lengths to avoid all medical examinations. The mere mention of the city's public *sifilicomio* for women, the Hospital Morelos, filled the capital's prostitutes in particular with a sense of terror and dread. Lavalle Carvajal went on to describe a recent episode in which one patient he diagnosed with a sexually transmitted infection was so enraged at having to be confined for medical attention that she mailed him threatening letters filled with pubic lice when she left the hospital. Was there not some way, Dr. Lavalle Carvajal pondered, to convince the Mexican population of the benefits of state-supervised disease prevention (Lavalle Carvajal 1909)?

Thirty-one years after Dr. Lavalle Carvajal shared his concerns about syphilis prophylaxis with the nation's medical elite, Román Barrón sent Mexico's President Lázaro Cárdenas a letter complaining about what was apparently still a deplorable state of sexual hygiene in Mexico City. In 1940 Barrón, a Mexican citizen who had lived in the United States, wrote Cárdenas that he had recently taken several American friends on a tour of his homeland. While enjoying the pleasures of metropolitan life in the revolutionary nation's capital, he said, the men had visited several downtown nightspots. It was in these venues that the men had contracted syphilis from the prostitutes they met there. Rather than chastise his friends for visiting prostitutes or blame the women for the spread of a devastating and potentially life-threatening disease, Barrón wrote to Cárdenas to protest what he considered to be the government's negligence with respect to venereal disease prophylaxis, saying, "In the good name of my country and in your good name, I beg you to turn your attention to this matter."

Barrón's frank description of his young friends' activities and physical ailments stands in sharp contrast to Lavalle Carvajal's dire portrayal of popular reaction to syphilis diagnosis three decades earlier. In 1909, according to the syphilis specialist, men and women ignored their disease status and people of all ages consistently sought to avoid medical examination, diagnosis, and treatment. But by 1940 Barrón felt comfortable writing to no less an official figure than the president of Mexico, complaining openly about his friends' sexually acquired infections. Had something changed to make Mexican citizens see the government as their ally in the struggle to conquer bodily affliction?

Popular perspectives on privacy, sexual activity, and medical treatment represented the greatest challenge to what at least one specialist had called the number-one health problem confronting Mexico's revolutionary government: preventing the spread of the often deadly and intractable venereal disease, syphilis, to Mexico's future generations. As early as 1926, Mexico's Department of Public Health chief, Dr. Bernardo Gastélum, had told audience members at an international sanitary conference that some 60 percent of the nation's population suffered the complications of *treponema pallidum* infection, which included fevers, hair loss, skin lesions, neurological disorders, gastrointestinal problems and premature death (Gastélum 1926). With at least half of the nation's syphilitics living in the capital city, Dr. Gastélum emphasized, it was as important to prevent disease as it was to promote a cure. Since the bacterium spread through sexual/genital contact and through birth from mother to child, he recommended that the government work to protect young women from becoming sexually active before marriage, dissuade men from seeking transitory sexual encounters, and encourage all infected members of the population to seek medical treatment. Doctors believed that even if the weekly injections of the arsenic-derived treatment neo-Salvarsan did not completely eliminate syphilis from the patient's body, it could reduce infectiousness and could prevent victims from developing symptoms of the more advanced stages of the illness. Thus, over the next decade and a half, public health officials worked to reduce the impact of "social disease" in Mexico through a series of steps that included the following measures: establishing public reformatories to dissuade young women from being sexually promiscuous; presenting public lectures on venereal disease transmission and treatment; organizing anonymous, free medical clinics for those who suffered from sexually transmitted disease; deregulating prostitution; and ultimately criminalizing the spread of sexually contagious maladies, a category that included syphilis and such other infectious agents as chancroid and gonorrhea, by 1939 (Bliss 2001).

Dr. Gastélum and his colleagues labored to eradicate syphilis in the capital city in the years after 1926, but Barrón's letter to Cárdenas suggests that by 1940 public policies had had little success in altering popular attitudes toward transient sexual encounters, poor women's occupations, men's leisurely pastimes, or the risk of contracting a deadly disease. Indeed, Barrón's letter to Cárdenas raises questions about the potential for public policy to alter popular private behaviors, on one hand, and about the assumptions people make about the state's relationship to their bodies and to social hygiene, on the other. Unlike such other common diseases as tuberculosis or influenza, syphilis was a disease that was often assumed to "confess" the patient's otherwise private sexual involvement with someone who had had at least one other sexual partner. A print advertisement placed by the department of public health, in fact, urged men and women to get disease treatment, stating that "if you don't confess it, your children will show it." At best, this "confession," whether spoken or expressed through "telling" physical symptoms like chancres, skin rashes, subdermal lumps, or oral lesions, could reveal a daughter's loss of virginity or a boyfriend's prior sexual experience; worse, it could reveal a husband's infidelity or a woman's participation in an undesirable trade such as prostitution, scenarios that often made disease victims reluctant to acknowledge their infections. Syphilitic men and women who were asymptomatic or who were convinced that their health problems were not serious infected sexual partners as well as their children, who at birth entered the world with medical complications and often led a painful trip through adolescence to an early death. Health campaigns thus urged Mexicans to shed their notions of privacy, confess their disease status, and seek medical treatment for the benefit of the nation and its future.

But to what extent did Mexicans actually internalize the new ideas about gender equality, disease prophylaxis, and social reform? Conversely, to what extent did popular ideas about sexuality and syphilis shape or limit the reform agenda that emerged by 1940? To understand these issues, this chapter examines the historical, social, and popular dimension of attitudes toward syphilis and sexuality in early-twentieth-century Mexico. To understand why people like Barrón and his friends were still willing to risk disease "confession" and also how they came to see the government as their ally when they did, it explores the formation of attitudes regarding disease risk, contagion, health, and bodily well-being.

Problematic Prophylaxis: The *Reglamento para el ejercicio de la prostitución* (1867–1926)

Since 1867 the key to the Mexican government's effort to fight syphilis had been the *Reglamento para el ejercicio de la prostitución* (Regulation for the Exercise of Prostitution). Syphilis had long afflicted members of all social classes in Mexico, but it was not until the last decades of the nineteenth century that public officials elaborated a plan to halt the spread of disease and treat those people considered to be at the greatest risk for spreading infection to the general population: female prostitutes. Under the terms of the *Reglamento,* young women over the age of 18 who were sexually experienced and who wished to speculate in sexual commerce were required to register their activities with sanitary authorities, report for weekly physical examinations, and undergo compulsory medical treatment if found to harbor venereal disease. The regulations were inspired by the sanitary measures that French imperial administrators had imposed to protect European soldiers during the Mexico occupation between 1863 and 1867. However, Liberal Party officials had adopted the measures in the years of the Restored Republic under the idea that maintaining regular medical surveillance over women who had multiple sex partners might similarly protect the health of sexually promiscuous Mexican men and their families (Franco Guzmán 1972). The *Reglamento* rested on medical and legal assumptions that the normal Mexican male would be sexually adventuresome, but that a woman who had more than one sexual partner was morally if not criminally deviant and therefore subject to state surveillance. For nearly three-quarters of a century, sexually promiscuous women served as the nation's idealized repository of contagious, sexually transmitted disease.

Over the years that the *Reglamento* was in effect, however, it became clear to medical practitioners that it was of dubious success in curbing the spread of infectious disease through sexual channels. First, the *Reglamento*'s assumption of heterosexuality meant that sanitary legislation completely overlooked and failed to regulate the apparently large number of male prostitutes willing to exchange sex with other men for money in downtown areas of Mexico City (Roumagnac 1906). More vexing to health officials, however, was the apparently cavalier attitude that female prostitutes espoused with respect to disease prevention itself. Most brothel managers, older women known as *matronas,* sought to avoid excessive police attention by registering their new *pupilas,* as women who worked in brothels were known; however, women who worked outside the brothel system were rarely eager to register and enter the rigid regime of licensing, fees, weekly inspections, forced hospitalization, and, by many accounts, police harassment and doctors' abuse. The fact that sanitary legislation effectively acknowledged the sharp differences in social class and decorum that characterized prostitutes and their clienteles also effectively undermined the *Reglamento* (Lavalle Carvajal 1909). In a 1909 article, one inspector complained that first-class prostitutes' habits of wearing several layers of underclothes in imitation of Mexico City's most dignified *señoras* severely limited physicians' potential to inspect them for signs of syphilis or gonorrhea (Lavalle Carvajal 1909). More serious problems for inspectors, however, included the fact that some diseased women sought to cosmetically disguise the lesions that characterized venereal disease, tricking clients and doctors alike.

Others apparently placed their faith in divine intervention, taking matches and burning them in the shape of the cross to ward off disease before heading out for their weekly physical exam (Lara y Pardo 1908). When miracles or disguise failed, prostitutes apparently preferred to bribe officials rather than risk hospitalization (Lara y Pardo 1908). For those who did find themselves placed in the hospital for treatment, escape offered the only relief from the interminable rhythms of medication, confinement, and abuse. Back on the streets, prostitutes convinced male clients that they were disease-free and initiated the cycle of infection all over again (Rivera-Garza 1997).

If prostitutes' ideas about class, work, and the medical establishment limited the *Reglamento*'s potential to halt the spread of syphilis in the Porfirian era, popular male perspectives on sexuality and disease similarly created tension between the state and the sexually promiscuous population. Fathers, brothers, and cousins, for example, took their younger male relatives to visit prostitutes as a rite of passage from childhood to adolescence, exposing their younger male relatives to contagion at an early age. Some doctors blamed early sexual activity on the easy availability of erotic literature and "lubricious spectacles" in the capital; others, like eminent hygienist Dr. Luis Lara y Pardo, blamed Mexico's lower-class male culture. The conviction that sleeping with a virgin was a sure way to avoid syphilis infection also led many men into risky sexual liaisons, according to the *higienista,* who asserted cynically that some men "pay for virginity as if it were a precious jewel! And how often that virginity is long gone!" (Lara y Pardo 1908).

On the eve of revolution in Mexico, thus, it was clear to public health experts—if not to the population at large—that the age-old effort to control the spread of syphilis through the regulation of prostitution was of dubious merit, for men and women routinely engaged in extramarital sexual encounters that fell outside the state's moral and sanitary purview. Was there not, many pondered, a better way to stop the spread of sexually transmitted disease?

Sanitation and Reform: A Revolutionary Approach to Syphilis Eradication, 1926–1937

That the Porfirian regime of preventing the spread of syphilis was showing signs of strain by the outbreak of armed conflict was clear to Mexican health officials, who had relied on the *Reglamento* to contain all promiscuous sexual activity inside brothels and the licensed *accesorias,* or rooms, where independent prostitutes plied their trade. But nearly a decade of fighting, the flow of refugees toward the capital, and the constant passage of armies through Mexico City between 1910 and 1917 strained official surveillance of the syphilis population in Mexico. With thousands of young women visibly practicing unregulated prostitution on the city's streets, public health officials studied and then formulated a revolutionary plan to stall the spread of syphilis in the nation.

Rural warfare was especially devastating to young women, who faced rape by invading armies if they remained at home or abandonment and starvation when parents or siblings died in the conflict. Between 1910 and 1917, thousands of young women traveled to the city on their own, with family members, or to join older female relatives who had already established residence in the capital; others who left their villages to join traveling military units as *soldaderas*, women who provided food and other services for the armies, similarly found themselves alone in the capital after the men with whom they traveled died or left them as they moved on to engage in fighting elsewhere in the republic (Friedlander 1994). As social workers' reports make clear, a startlingly high number of these young women turned to prostitution in the difficult economy that characterized Mexico City in the late 1910s and early 1920s. Young, inexperienced, and completely outside the regulation system, these adolescents, doctors feared, would be the first to succumb to infection and then pass disease along to their sexual partners and offspring (Rodríguez Cabo 1940).

Revolution also transformed the spatial organization of metropolitan sexual commerce, further challenging the state's ability to control syphilis's spread. The *Reglamento* had long enshrined the *matrona* and the brothel as the keys to maintaining control over prostitutes and disease transmission, but between 1915 and 1918 newly established dance halls and cabarets began to compete with long-established bordellos as sites of sexual permissiveness (*Boletín Municipal* 1915). Some cabarets offered special rooms for couples who wished to engage in intimate activity on the premises, while other nightclubs were conveniently located next to hotels that rented rooms at an inexpensive, hourly rate. *Matronas* complained bitterly to city councilors that competition from the new cabarets and young *clandestinas* severely undermined their own beleaguered businesses, which, they claimed, doubly suffered in the postrevolutionary era thanks to municipally mandated shorter hours and steeper licensing fees. As *matronas* shut their brothel doors, increasing numbers of women working outside the confines of the *Reglamento*'s surveillance scheme thwarted official oversight of sexual activity and further challenged the antiquated regime of syphilis prevention.

As proof that the old plan of sequestration and surveillance was failing miserably, public health officials in the early 1920s pointed to the fact that the rates of syphilis among the population were rising at an alarming rate. In 1925 Dr. Adrian de Garay, director of the city's anti–venereal disease dispensaries, estimated that the majority of male and female patients examined in the municipal syphilis clinics were in the first and second stages of the disease. Estimated mortality from syphilis had doubled between 1916 and 1925, and obstetricians at the city's maternity hospitals concluded that a mother's venereal infection was the leading cause of miscarriage. In addition, some 80 percent of children at a local elementary school had tested positive for the infection (de Garay 1925).

Careful study of Mexico City's burgeoning syphilis epidemic led public health officials to posit a new approach to disease prevention and eradication. Mexico's adolescents, considered the population most at risk for developing syphilis and other sexually transmitted infections, were the first targets of the new syphilis eradication campaign. Curing and reforming teenagers who were already infected with venereal disease represented the first line of attack. Health offices infused the old prohibition against registering underage girls as prostitutes with new purpose, sending sanitary police out across the city to arrest those underage *clandestinas* who solicited clients in cabarets and on street corners outside of theaters and public dances. Preventing Mexico's youngest children from engaging in risky behavior represented a second front of the campaign. Elementary school teachers not only inspected schoolchildren, but also awarded ribbons for cleanliness and anatomical knowledge in what was known as the Game of Health. Girls, moreover, were warned of the perils of premature sexual activity by teachers and parents alike.

But since adult men and women still represented the majority of new syphilis cases reported each quarter, sexual education for adults complemented the Department of Public Health's approach to preventing children and adolescents from being exposed to the deadly infections. Public health and education officials used factories, parks, markets, and community centers as venues in which to impress sexually active men and women with information not just about disease prophylaxis, but also about sexual health in general. In conjunction with the Secretariat of Public Education, the public health department published a series of pamphlets for popular distribution. Public officials also promoted radio dramas and films intended to inspire listeners and viewers with sympathy for those characters whose vices had led them to an old age marked by mental degeneration and physical agony (Brandt 1987).

Despite their ambition to change adult sexual behavior overnight, policy makers acknowledged that the Mexican population's sexual habits were well established, and they worked to undermine the population's sexual privacy, noted some 20 years before by Dr. Lavalle Carvajal, by encouraging frank and open discussion of sexuality and sexually transmitted disease among all members of the community. Dr. Gastélum blamed the Mexican popular classes' ideas about sexual secrecy on the Catholic Church, which many revolutionary reformers believed had kept the population in ignorance and superstition. Others posited that outdated social hierarchies were to blame for men's and women's "false modesty" with respect to physical examination and disease treatment. To encourage anyone with a sexually transmitted disease to seek treatment, the clinics were open late into the evening and were scattered around the city so that men and women of all social backgrounds could access the latest in syphilis-combating techniques (Villalobos 1925).

Finally, public officials advocated deregulating prostitution altogether. By educating the public, suppressing laws that endangered women to protect men, and eliminating brothels and thus making prostitutes more difficult to find, experts posited, revolutionary Mexico might ultimately witness new and more equitable relations between classes and between the sexes. Suppressing the *Reglamento* and implementing a new, gender-blind regime of syphilis prophylaxis struck many reformers and *higienistas* as the most appropriate means of promoting community health and social equality. By 1937 the Department proposed suppressing syphilis by abolishing the *Reglamento*, criminalizing disease transmission, and ultimately dismantling the *zona de tolerancia*.

Embodying Reform: Popular Perspectives on Abolitionism, Health, and the Body

Despite the Department of Public Health's vision that new antivenereal legislation represented the ideal fusion of revolutionary ideology and public health practice, deregulating prostitution and criminalizing disease transmission generated considerable controversy among *capitalino* men and women in the late 1930s and early 1940s. Officials posited that abolishing regulations would protect the Revolution's promises to redeem the Mexican people through eliminating "antisocial subclasses" and protecting the right of all citizens to good health. However, the very people supposed to benefit from abolitionism, the prostitutes for whom the *Reglamento*'s antisyphilis provisions had been most onerous, opposed what they perceived to be an attack on their right to work and a threat to their ability to generate a subsistence for themselves and for their children. Clients, likewise, rejected abolitionism as a threat to their own pursuit of good health as defined by engaging in regular sexual activity. Both parties opposed the new health proposals because they believed the measures clashed with their own ideas of welfare and bodily well-being.

Prostitutes actively opposed deregulation for several reasons. First, they seriously questioned the *Departmento de Salubridad Pública*'s position that the measure would guarantee their rights as Mexican citizens to good health. At a 1935 meeting to discuss whether or not they approved of the Department's plan to abolish *Reglamento*, for example, Maria Millán, a veteran prostitute and cabaret dancer, questioned the officials' concern for poor women's health. Referring to her body, ravaged by repeated abuse and exposure to disease, Millán stated: "This life is tragic, the cabaret chews out our guts. And afterwards? When we are no longer attractive, it spits us out!" (*El Gráfico* 1937). And in a 1939 letter to President Cárdenas, Gloria Mendoza echoed Millán's concerns about body and health, noting that the abolition of regulated sexual commerce had complicated prostitutes' already miserable lives by making them vulnerable to greater police corruption, physical abuse, and harassment. Mendoza criticized the Department's equation of good health with being syphilis-free, pointing out that the beatings and mistreatment she and her colleagues regularly suffered at the hands of disreputable policemen posed a greater threat to the women and their families than the risk of disease transmission. Were the women's bodies and their children's lives less important that the national syphilis threat, she wondered?

Men who were accustomed to visiting prostitutes in established vice centers found fault with the new antisyphilis regime as well. While they did not specifically oppose government efforts to criminalize disease transmission, clients' statements reflect that even into the 1930s many *capitalino* men were still convinced that indulging in regular sexual activity was a healthy pursuit that provided physical benefits that offset any risk of acquiring syphilis. Unmarried men argued that it was medically necessary for them to engage in regular sexual activity, and they were among the most vocal opponents of the ban on officially regulated prostitution. As a group of individuals who identified themselves to Cárdenas as "various bachelors" stated, "Those of use who don't have girlfriends—because we have nowhere to take them—must now go visit the prostitutes in their homes." Not only did the "bachelors" object to the inconvenience of searching for prostitutes outside of centrally located brothels, but they stated that they also worried about the impression such visits made on the young children who lived in the city's least expensive tenements, where many prostitutes now resided.

Men and women elaborated alternative notions of health and well-being, in part thanks to the growing visibility and influence of advertising campaigns regarding bodily care, good health, and attractiveness in Mexico over the late 1930s and 1940s. Magazines that targeted male and female readers generated images and information about the benefits of physical exercise, plastic surgery, and disease prophylaxis, suggesting that true happiness—if not national progress—was linked to an image of physical fortitude. Women's magazines such as *Mujer* and *Nosotras* encouraged women to take their health into their own hands and to assume responsibility for the physical well-being of themselves and their children. *Mujer*, a late 1920s publication that advocated the "moral and intellectual elevation of the Mexican woman," recommended that teenaged girls practice swimming and attend dances, "which are necessary for the health of the body as well as the soul." Numerous merchants and international companies also encouraged women to employ the latest cosmetic and technological advances to radiate a personal image of bodily perfection and good health.

Like women, male readers and consumers learned to assume personal responsibility for their own health and hygiene. In fact, male brothel clients began to demand an assurance of hygienic excellence from bordellos during the 1930s. A 1933 pocket guide to metropolitan nightlife, *México de noche: guía para el hombre que quiera divertirse*, for example, provided readers with a dazzling choice of cabarets, bordellos, and "discreet rooms" that, the editors boldly asserted, guaranteed "an absolute principle of moral ethics." Bordello proprietresses promoted their establishments with advertisements that proclaimed their hygienic status as well. Carmen Uribe, for example, assured potential clients that her bordello on calle Mérida was "the safest house in the colony," while another spot on calle Colima promoted itself as "the most discreet and hygienic house in the city" (*México de Noche* 1933).

When Román Barrón wrote Lázaro Cárdenas to complain about his friends' venereal disease infection, Mexican men's and women's perspectives on syphilis, secrecy, and the state's relationship to the population's bodies had changed significantly since Dr. Eduardo Lavalle Carvajal had first lamented the *capitalino* population's resolute ignorance of disease symptoms, prevention, and treatment. Men and women were more likely to recognize venereal disease symptoms in 1940 than they were in 1909, thanks to health information and education programs. They demanded hygienic work and leisure conditions, and could also count on a well-established system of free, anonymous clinics in which they might seek treatment at a low cost to their pocketbooks or to their respectability.

The history of syphilis prophylaxis popularization in Mexico demonstrates that the idea of risk assumed different meanings that changed over time. Understanding the meaning of disease risk is important to historians and social scientists of health for several reasons. On one hand—at least in Mexico—the idea of risk encompassed an individual's calculation regarding the likelihood of acquiring syphilis, gonorrhea, or any other venereal disease from a sexual encounter. On the other hand, popular conceptualizations of risk included the chance that a body would manifest or confess its owner's involvement in deviant or promiscuous sexual behavior by developing disease symptoms. In the Mexican context, even as public health officials worked to reconcile revolutionary ideology and public health practice, peoples' concerns about acquiring disease remained low, but their concerns over having their infection status made public decreased. In an even broader sense, the study of "infection" and "confession" in revolutionary Mexico demonstrates the variety of interpretations regarding "disease risk" among such diverse groups as physicians, public officials, and patients. The history of health policy development also sheds light on the particular ways in which the human body can become politicized in utopian, reformist settings.

By 1940, when legislators criminalized infection through sexual contact and dismantled the *Reglamento*, men and women were less fearful of "confessing" their disease infection or involvement in sexual commerce either as practitioners or clients. However, they did resent the government's efforts to change their sexual behavior or use of sexual services to earn money for their children and families. In protesting the Department of Public Health's new policies, men and women presented their own visions of health and well-being to public officials. For women, this vision included freedom from physical abuse and harassment. For men, this included the ability to have sexual intercourse with a variety of women on a regular basis. Both groups coincided in demonstrating their concerns over protecting Mexico's youngest citizens from exposure to vice and deadly disease. But men and women alike expected the state to provide them with the ability to both pursue good health and risk disease acquisition in the process.

References

Boletín Municipal. (1915). *Boletín Municipal: Órgano del Ayuntamiento de la Ciudad de Mexíco* 1, no. 1 (February 26): 20.

Brandt, A. (1987). *No Magic Bullet: A Social History of Venereal Disease in the United States since 1880.* New York: Oxford University Press.

Corbin, A. (1990). *Women of the Night: Prostitution and Sexuality in France from 1850.* Cambridge, MA: Harvard University Press.

De Garay, A. (1925). "Los dispensarios del departamento: los dispensarios venéreo-sifilíticos." *Boletín del Departametno de Salubridad Pública,* no 4: 91.

El Gráfico. (1937). "La Vida Miserable y Trágica de las Cabareteras Revelada Ante Varios Funcionarios Oficiales." October 19, 12.

Franco Guzmán, R. (1972). "El régimen jurídico de la prostitución en México." *Revista de la Facultad de Derecho en México,* 85–86.

Friedlander, J. (1994). "Doña Zeferina Barreto: Biographical Sketch of an Indian Woman from the State of Morelos." In *Women of the Mexican Countryside,* edited by Mary Kay Vaughan and Heather Fowler Salamini. Tucson: University of Arizona Press.

Gastélum, B. (1926). "La persecución de la sífilis desde el punto de vista de la garantía social." *Boletín del Departamento de Salubridad,* no. 4: 8.

González Rodríguez, S. (1994). "Cuerpo, control y mercancía: fotografía prostibularia." *Luna Córnea,* no. 4: 73.

Lara y Pardo, L. (1908). *La prostitución en México.* Mexico City: Librería de la Vda. de Ch. Bouret.

Lavalle Carvajal, E. (1909). "Profilaxis venérea: medios prácticfos de fácil a plicación y de prontos resultados." *Gaceta Médica de México* 4, no. 5: 308–58.

Madrigal, C. (1938). *Los menores delincuentes: estudio sobre la situación de los Tribunales para Menores, doctrina y realidad.* Mexico City: Ediciones Botas.

México de Noche. (1933). *México de Noche: Guía para el Hombre que Quiera Divertirse.* N.p., 2, 99, 101.

Rivera-Garza, C. (1997, April). "Prostitutes, Sexual Crimes and Society: Mexico, 1867–1930." Paper presented at the Conference on the Contested Terrains of Law, Justice and Repression, Yale University.

Rodríguez Cabo, M. (1940). "El Problema Sexual de las Menores Mujeres y Su Repercusión en la Delincuencia Juvenil Femenina." *Criminalia* 6, no. 10.

Roumagnac, C. (1906). *Los criminales en México: estudio de psicología morbosa*. Mexico City: Librería de Ch. Bouret.

Villalobos, S. (1925). "Tratamiento de las enfermeras sifilíticas en la Sala Armijo del Hospital Morelos." *Boletín del Departamento de Salubridad* no. 2: 85–87.

12

Saving Lives, Destroying Livelihoods: Emergency Evacuation and Resettlement Policies in Ecuador

LINDA M. WHITEFORD AND GRAHAM A. TOBIN

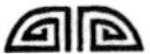

THE TWENTIETH CENTURY HAS BEEN REFERRED TO as the age of displaced persons and refugees. According to the United Nations High Commission on Refugees, the number of people who are forced out of their homes through life-altering events such as geophysical disasters (volcanic eruptions, floods, and earthquakes), political conflicts, ethnic warfare, or economic crises has increased annually. In 2003, one estimate placed the number of refugees at 15 million (*New York Times* June 2, 2003). While people have been forcibly removed from their homes throughout history, only recently has the study of the process and its results been carefully analyzed. In the following chapter, we argue that emergency evacuation and resettlement policies unfairly hurt the most vulnerable populations, the poor and the disenfranchised. Such policies are unhealthy because they make it more difficult for families to recover economic losses, separate them from their kin and support networks, and cause their children to suffer more illnesses than children who are not resettled. The chapter is based on our four years of research following the eruption of Mt. Tungurahua in Ecuador and the subsequent evacuation of 26,000 people living in the shadow of the volcano (Tobin and Whiteford 2002a).

In 1999, Mt. Tungurahua showed every sign of an imminent, potentially catastrophic explosion. In response to professional assessments of the increasing seismic activity, the order to evacuate was given, and in 36 hours the community of Baños and the surrounding villages were emptied. People were forced to flee with a minimum of their belongings, cattle and livestock were sold for a fraction of their worth, homes were boarded up, and chickens, goats, sheep, and other animals were turned loose to fend for themselves. Families desperately tried to stay together and find shelter for what might be a week, a month, or six months.

Military-enforced evacuations usually occur when governments attempt to move populations away from land in dispute or from potential disasters. While there is no uniformly accepted definition of disaster (Shaluf, Fakharu'l-razi, and Said 2003), a major volcanic explosion in a populated area would certainly constitute a disaster. According to Chan (1995:22), there are four common policies used to protect populations from disasters: (1) protection by preventing or modifying the disaster, (2) accommodation through changing human use to avoid the disaster, (3) redirection through population resettlement, and (4) no action. Even though the literature on natural hazards and disasters provides ample evidence to suggest that there are significant political, economic, social, and physical consequences to resettlement policies (Chan 1995; Hansen and Oliver-Smith 1982; Harrell-Bond 1986; Tobin and Whiteford 2001a, 2001b, 2002a, 2002b; Whiteford, Tobin, Laspina, and Yepes 2002a, 2002b), resettlement remains a "popular solution to hazard and disaster management" (Chan 1995:22).

Given the known and often untoward consequences of resettlement policies, the question is why such a policy continues to remain a "popular solution." Our research with some of those evacuated and resettled from around the slopes of the Tungurahua volcano will be used to illustrate the policy and its effects, as we attempt to understand why a policy known to destroy peoples' livelihoods, damage their health, and separate families continues to be employed.

Methodology

An extensive research project was undertaken in several communities around Mt. Tungurahua in Ecuador. This site was selected because of its historical record of disasters and because of the researchers' previous experience in the area (Tobin and Whiteford 2001a; Whiteford et al. 2002a). For this study, two structured questionnaires, one undertaken in June 2000 (131 respondents) and the other in January 2001 (171 respondents), were administered to collect information from evacuees who had resettled in the small community of Quimiag (Tobin and Whiteford 2002a). The survey was also given to permanent residents of Quimiag for comparison purposes. In addition to the structured questionnaires, community leaders, politicians, government officials, and members of the civil defense were consulted, and in-depth interviews with two focus groups were also undertaken to collect further information. Additional research was undertaken in 2002 and 2003 (Whiteford et al. 2002b). Table 12.1 shows the number of children under five years old in both the resettled and local Quimiag samples.

Table 12.1. Population and Number of Children under Five Years of Age

	Number of People	*Mean Number per Household*	*Number of Children*	*Mean Number per Household*
Quimiag Resettlement	108	4.91	18	0.82
Quimiag Locals	137	4.15	16	0.45

Mt. Tungurahua is an active volcano located 120 km south of Quito. The volcano has had four periods of intense activity prior to the current eruptive phase: 1641–1646, 1773–1781, 1886–1888, and 1916–1918 (Hall, Robin, Beate, Mothes, and Monzier 1999). The 1773 eruption produced a large debris flow that descended the Vazcún valley, and the town of Baños narrowly escaped destruction on that occasion. During the 1916–1918 eruptive period, pyroclastic flows moved down both the northwest and north flanks of the volcano. Similarly, in 1886 and 1916, lahars moved through the Vazcún and Ulba valleys (Hall et al. 1999). The volcano then remained relatively dormant until 1993, when seismic activity gradually increased with more violent venting of gas and ash in September 1999. Since then, the volcano has continued to be active, periodically showering ash on the surrounding landscape, initiating lahars, and generating mudslides, while pyroclastic flows remain an ever-present threat.

Quimiag is a small community of approximately 1,700 residents, located in the canton of Riobamba in Chimborazo Province, about 3,000 meters above sea level. Although Quimiag is laid out on fairly level ground, the terrain rises relatively steeply toward the east. There is communal land on these higher slopes, which is used primarily for cattle grazing and growing potato crops. The population is mostly mestizo with some indigenous groups who speak a dialect of Quechua. It was in this community that at least 35 families had resettled after evacuating the agricultural settlements around the town of Baños.

As Singer (1995:81) and others have pointed out, a critical medical anthropology perspective focuses on ways in which international and global forces shape national economies and policies, which in turn shape and are shaped by regional and local history, class structure, and institutions. While evacuation and resettlement policies may appear to be similar, whether they are written for the United States, Canada, or Ecuador, in practice they become very different. Differences in socioeconomic class, access to resources, ethnic identity, and levels of support all shape the local context in which evacuation and resettlement occur. Furthermore, structural forms of power and its distribution are embedded in local as well as international history and perceptions (Farmer 1992, 2003; Kim, Millen, Irwin, and Gershman 2000). Levels of professionalism, decentralization from the central government, and financial support, and even the organization and coordination of bodies responsible for enforcing the evacuation and resettlement policies, reflect distinctive politically defined national priorities (Oliver-Smith 1986b).

In Ecuador, disaster preparedness and management are planned primarily by the country's civil defense system, which at the national level is staffed by paid professionals, while local and regional levels are composed of volunteers who are often retired military personnel. Ecuador is a relatively small country with limited economic resources but seemingly unlimited natural hazards. A country straddling two mountain ranges with numerous active volcanoes, endless lahars, mudflows and landslides, earthquakes, and floods, Ecuador faces significant geophysical threats to its population. Even with the assistance of the U.S. Geological Survey, the European Union, and the U.S. Southern Command, the Ecuadorian government must triage its resources, delegating much of its work to unpaid volunteers.

Recently, researchers have begun to study large-scale population evacuations, particularly of urban areas, in greater detail (Zelinsky and Kosinski 1991). Statistical accounts appeared in the middle of the twentieth century with reports from World War II of the evacuation of cities in Europe and Japan (Zelinsky and Kosinski 1991). In addition to these early descriptions of forced and voluntary evacuations, population movements engendered by disasters have also been documented.[1]

While some social and natural scientists have studied disasters and their social and economic consequences,[2] few have paid specific attention to the history, policies, or processes of evacuations. According to Zelinsky and Kosinski (1991:13), "There has been a deafening silence in the demographic community on the subject of emergency evacuations." Recent concern with disaster preparedness and disaster mitigation, however, has focused attention on these procedures and the consequences of evacuations. As Cernea (2000), Lindell and Perry (1992), Tobin and Montz (1997), Tobin and Whiteford (2001a, 2002a), and Whiteford et al. (2002a, 2002b) have demonstrated, evacuations may produce a series of untoward effects, such as social disruption, increased domestic violence, prolonged economic losses, and increased rates in communicable and stress-related illnesses.

Of the four options identified by Chan (1995:22) to protect populations from hazards, resettling populations is one of the most common even though it is often not successful. If the danger cannot be removed or its potential effect mitigated, then the common option is to move the population away from the hazard zone. However, this can often be accomplished only through the application or threat of military force. Thus, several characteristics combine to make resettlement following forced evacuation due to natural hazards worth our discussion.

Military Involvement and the Threat of Force

Evacuations frequently follow military models, with military personnel brought into a community to force people to leave. This can divide a community into different political camps, frighten some people, and precipitate a level of resentfulness. Furthermore, those with the fewest resources, the poor, and the disabled can be unfairly targeted by the military forces brought in to move them. This situation transpired in Ecuador.

In October 1999, government authorities in Ecuador, in consultation with the director of the Geophysical Institute in Quito (H. Yepes, personal communication 2000), decided that the danger of an eruption and the possible consequential loss of life necessitated an immediate evacuation of the communities surrounding Baños. Some residents who were being affected by ash or threatened by mudflows had already voluntarily evacuated (UN Office for the Coordination of Humanitarian Affairs [OCHA] 1999). The evacuation became mandatory on October 15, 1999. People residing in the hazard risk zone were given approximately 36 hours to leave the area, after which the military enforced the evacuation (CNN 1999) because the civilian civil defense force was unable to force their friends and neighbors to leave. In the 36 hours from when the evacuation was announced to when the community was closed, people left, resisted, hid, were found, and were forced out. Those least able, as well as those least willing, to leave felt the greatest effect of the military force. An estimated 26,000 people were moved to over 60 locations, including private homes, hostels, and government shelters in the provinces of Tungurahua and Chimborazo, where some remained for more than a year. According to the Ecuadorian Red Cross, the Civil Defense set up 125 sites as temporary shelters, and the official count of evacuees in shelters rose to 2,443 early in November (Cruz Roja Ecuatoriana 1999a, 1999b).

Class and Evacuation Strategy

The presence of a potential disaster does not necessarily imply that either the political authorities or local populations will take the threat seriously, particularly in terms of planning to leave their homes and belongings. Therefore, when an evacuation is enforced, people are often in a state of shock, frightened, disbelieving, and ultimately unprepared to leave. During the 1999 evacuation, people first sought to find their family members so that they could evacuate together, then they tried to find family or friends living outside of the evacuated areas to whom they could go for shelter. They piled into cars, stuffed their belongings onto trucks, locked up their houses, and moved in with family members in Ambato, Riobamba, or even as far away as Quito—that is, if they had cars, trucks, and families who would let them live with them. Many of the middle- and upper-class Bañenos left in the first twenty-four hours of the evacuation because they could locate their family members by telephone, they could contact friends and families in other cities to ask them to take them in, and they could move their family and belongings in their own private cars and trucks.

Others were not so fortunate; their family members may have been day laborers working away from home and not accessible by telephone. Thus, in order to evacuate together, families had to wait until they each heard about the evacuation and came home. If they could find others to take them in and public transportation to get there, then they went to stay with friends in other cities. More often than not, by the time the family was reunited, the evacuation was well underway and public transportation was not available. Private trucks rented for the trip went back and forth along the single narrow road between Baños and Ambato (an hour journey each way) ferrying people and their few belongings. Within hours, the road was clogged with people and transportation with few means of travel still available. In the last hours before the military closed the road, military trucks picked up those who were still in and around Baños. Many could not find family or friends to take them, and some were evacuated to government shelters; others were resettled. Official records of the number of people relocated, in shelters, and resettled are unclear regarding how many people went to each place, but in the most rural areas it appears that the poorest just went further into the countryside. They were not found in either the government shelters or the resettled areas.

Structural Violence against the Resettled

While the government made an attempt to resettle people where their children could continue their schooling, the resettled individuals were away from the temperate and lush ecological zone of Baños. Quimiag is in the high sierra, where it is cold, damp, and moist for most of the year. Local Quimiag families contributed housing to the evacuees, but the resettled families had little furniture, no heat, and few blankets. Also, the resettled families had lost their household gardens and chickens, as well as their neighbors and extended families—traditional means of support in times of crisis. Their children got sick more often than those of local families who were not resettled, and local resentment gradually grew. Local Quimiag residents came to believe that the resettled families were receiving "unfair" amounts of support from international and national aid societies, while the resettled families became suspicious of their nonresettled neighbors.

Resettled families had no recourse to settle disputes, a situation epitomized by the apparent generosity of an absentee landlord who offered the resettlement group his land on a steep hillside to plant in potatoes. The resettled families called for a community workgroup (*minga*), and men, women, children, pregnant women, and women with babies on their backs or at their breasts all worked the hillside. After several weeks of cultivating the mountain slope and terracing the fields, they planted the potato crop. They were successful. They crop came in, and the families anticipated food for the winter and potatoes to sell. However, before they could harvest the crop, the landlord took back his land and the crop. The community had nothing to harvest, nothing to eat, and no seed potatoes for the following year. They were on borrowed land with no rights and no official paper to support their claims. Sadly enough, the story is neither apocryphal nor unique to this resettled group.

Agricultural practices in the area were also seriously compromised by hazardous events including volcanic ash. For example, the water supply for agriculture is usually taken from a local canal. However, in January 2000, flow of water in the canal was interrupted due to a landslide. The evacuees were told by agronomists that there would be no water from this source for at least six months, so they collected rainfall and were determined to find water from another source, by whatever means: "*Tenemos que encontrar agua de cualquier manera.*"

Health Outcomes and Resettlement

Resettled families from Baños suffered greater health problems than families from the local community. In virtually every category of illness for which we investigated, incidence levels were much higher for the evacuees (Table 12.2). Two other features stand out. Females invariably experienced higher illness levels than males, and resettled children under the age of five recorded more than twice the percentage of

Table 12.2. Health Statistics: Percentage of Cases per Total Population

	Quimiag Resettlement (N = 108)	*Quimiag Locals (N = 137)*
Males	16.7	20.4
Females	30.6	32.1
Total	47.2	52.6
Males:		
Resp/Cold/Flu	13.9	10.2
Eye/Skin/Throat	13.9	11.7
Stomach/Diarrhea	9.4	2.2
Other Problems	8.3	10.2
Females:		
Resp/Cold/Flu	20.4	21.2
Eye/Skin/Throat	22.2	17.5
Stomach/Diarrhea	13.9	1.5
Other Problems	14.8	13.1
All:		
Resp/Cold/Flu	34.3	31.4
Eye/Skin/Throat	36.1	29.2
Stomach/Diarrhea	23.2	3.7
Other Problems	23.2	23.4

illnesses than local children of the same age group. In particular, resettled children experienced twice as many cold, flu, and upper respiratory infections, and almost three times as many episodes of stomach problems and diarrhea compared to the children from the local community (Table 12.3). These children often suffered from nightmares and other sleep disturbances while their parents struggled to generate income and provide food for the families. While the government resettled the families, they did not provide jobs for them in the community. Families without access to their home gardens, their little group of chickens, and their cow or two found it very difficult to keep their children healthy. Isolated, marginalized, and vulnerable, the children and women's health suffered.

Increased Vulnerability and Marginalization

People in resettled areas are often in limbo; they belong neither there nor somewhere else. Even those communities whose resettlement experience is more successful than what we found in Quimiag find themselves with divided loyalties—belonging to two communities at once, the old and the new. Their marginalization is furthered by not being members of the communities to which they have been resettled, and the resentment from both the resettled group and the local group often further exacerbates the sense of isolation. They are excluded from local and regional politics, marginalized from the quotidian politics of daily life, and fail to share history or families with the local community, and most of the resettled community wants to return home. They are vulnerable because they have no official standing in the community and no external support for being there.

Quimiag evacuees expressed concern about their precarious economic situation especially since they were not generating any income at their new location. Another major problem for some respondents was that they had been forced to sell their land and houses around Tungurahua and hence could not return. Parts of the volcano slopes had been declared too dangerous because of ash and further potential eruptions, so property was sold at often very low prices. Since many of

Table 12.3. Health of Children under Five Years of Age—June 2000

	Quimiag Resettlement		*Quimiag Locals*	
	N	%	N	%
Respiratory, Colds, Flu	5	27.8	2	12.5
Eye, Skin, Throat	3	16.7	—	—
Stomach, Diarrhea	3	16.7	1	6.3
Other Symptoms	4	22.2	2	12.5
Sick Children	7	38.9	3	18.8
Total Children	18	100	16	100

these people rely on agriculture for their livelihoods, this action effectively eliminated any immediate chance of economic recovery.

While 50 percent of the people in the resettlement group had evacuated voluntarily, over 50 percent of the Quimiag resettlement group (52.6) thought that the government had done little or nothing to help in the evacuation. In contrast, 47.4 percent reported receiving shelter, food, clothing, money, or seeds for planting, demonstrating a commitment on behalf of the government to some degree. Most of this group had not returned home because of the volcano (63.6 percent) and because of health risks (4.5 percent). In addition, 27.3 percent reported that they remained in Quimiag because there were either limited resources available at home or better resources currently available at the resettlement area.

The economic status of the resettled group is problematic. If members of the resettled community appear to be doing too well, the local community resents it. Our data suggest that the resettled families in the community suffer significantly more economically than do others—both others who were evacuated elsewhere as well as local residents who were never evacuated (Table 12.4). However, it is apparent that both resettlers and locals experienced severe economic crises during this period due to ongoing problems throughout the country. For instance, median monthly income among the resettled group fell to only 48 percent of pre-evacuation rates, whereas Quimiag locals were still at 78 percent. In addition, 68 percent of the resettlement group recorded agricultural losses, 84 percent economic losses, and 72 percent environmental losses. This compared with 53, 59, and 59 percent respectively for locals. Thus, the ability of resettlers to recover was compromised by diminished economic opportunities.

What emerges is a picture of the poor bearing the greatest burden for a social policy that unfairly targets them because of their relative inability to resist. The resettlement policy so favored by emergency planners is not equally distributed among various groups of the affected population, but rather is concentrated among the working poor. It is the poor who, because they were dependent upon

Table 12.4. Context of Crises: Problems Faced by Households (%)

Crisis	*Quimiag Resettlement*	*Quimiag Locals*
Loss of Home	40.9	N/A
Loss of Crops or Livestock/Inability to Plant	86.4	16.2
Loss of Money/Economic Crises	77.3	63.6
Political Turmoil	68.2	42.4
Disasters—Volcano, Floods, Landslides	68.2	39.4
Family Problems—Illness, Death	59.1	42.4
Theft of Possessions	13.6	3.0

public transportation, had to rely on the military moving them from their homes to a government-sponsored alternative shelter. It is they who find themselves being resettled rather than staying with friends or even in shelters. And it is they whose children suffered the most negative health consequences. Even compared with children in shelters, children whose families were relocated were sick more often.

Furthermore, children in the resettled communities did not have the same access to health care as did children in shelters. The Provincial Health Directorship in the two states to which families were evacuated in 1999 took active responsibility for health in the government-sponsored shelters, particularly that of children. In contrast, those families resettled in small communities scattered throughout the two states did not receive the same level of attention. They were left to visit local clinics, health posts, or other places if they were sick enough and someone could be found to take them.

Resettling families following an emergency evacuation are removed from their extended kin, from schoolmates, and from their routines. They are put into situations where their families are experiencing extreme stress as they struggle to settle into somewhere new, find economically productive ways to support their families, and adjust to new surroundings, people, and expectations. Our data strongly suggest that resettlement is an unhealthy policy for children in many aspects. They fall between the various systems established to protect the youngest and most vulnerable. With scarce resources available, the public health system focuses its attention on the concentration of people evacuated into shelters, leaving those scattered families resettled to fend for themselves.

In this chapter, we have suggested that emergency evacuation and resettlement policies have unhealthy consequences and, furthermore, that they exacerbate already existing social cleavages. Not all people are resettled; usually only those without other resources are identified for resettlement. The identification of the poor and working poor for resettlement is consistent with the cultural values, rooted in history, of using the poor for social experimentation.

Conclusion

Singer (1995:90) has called for "system-challenging praxis" concerned with "unmasking the origins of social inequity" that we find particularly appropriate for this discussion. It is clear that disasters will continue; some argue that they are increasing with the increased human occupation of previously unoccupied hazardous areas (Murphy, Baker, Hill, Perez, and Norris 2001). If we accept as a given that the world has become a more hazardous place in this regard, then the question is "How do we protect those who are most vulnerable?" The unmasking of social policies that reify class-based discriminations while masquerading as aid is one way. Emergency evacuations will continue; resettlement policies will continue to be enforced. But by making public the experiences and stories of those resettled and by demonstrating the unequal and untoward effects of those policies, the basis for their failure is made clear and not obfuscated.

Our research also suggests that there are ways to improve the resettlement experience that are generalizable to the larger hazard preparedness and social science communities. They are aimed at improving the health of those resettled by reducing the stress associated with the experience, and rather than having resettlement be a punishment for those without access to other resources, resettlement could be a positive option. To make it such an option, the following steps could be taken. First, town meetings and discussions should be held to inform community members of hazard risks and the remedial options available, including the resettlement of families in the event of disaster. Second, resettlement strategies should be made available to all members of the community at risk, especially when they are confronted with the potential of catastrophic disasters. Third, resettlement sites should be found that are similar to the site being vacated so that lifestyle, agricultural practices, and so on are transferable. Fourth, resettlement policies should include specific attention to the ongoing health care of the families after they have been relocated. Fifth, resettled families should be provided legitimate ways to own the land on which they are resettled. Finally, government protection should be provided to those families after they have moved.

In short, the process must be anticipated, legitimated, and equally available. Community-based practices and relationships must be transferable. In the case described in this chapter, most families eventually left the resettlement community. Some returned to the volcanic hazard site; others were lost to follow-up and we do not know where they went. Many families tried to make it work; they had already disrupted their families, lost most of the possessions, and committed to the resettlement. However, they could not stick it out. Their children were sick; they had no sense of community, history, or future; and they left. There are many needless losses in this story: those who moved back are still at great risk, they still worry about their children being harmed by the volcano, they have lost faith in their government to help them, and they are worse off than before they were resettled. Not surprisingly, they will fight any new attempts by the government to evacuate them.

The lessons learned from this analysis are applicable to medical anthropologists and other social scientists, as well as to disaster mitigation planners, civil defense authorities, and others in the field of emergency preparedness. The lessons are to situate our research in the larger political and economic context as well as in the lived realities of daily life, to understand the social and cultural cleavages in the fabric of the society being studied, and to document the distribution of power in the society. Failure to recognize and be cognizant of the constraints and possibilities imposed by these contexts limits the efficaciousness and applicability of any recommendation. Unhealthy policies can be transposed into healthy policies, but not until they are identified, documented, and communicated. In the case described in this chapter, the authors have worked with and shared the results of the research with local, regional, and national politicians and policy makers in Ecuador and in the international field of disaster management; with the authorities in Ecuadorian Civil Defense, Geophysical Institute, and the Ministry of Health; as well as with our colleagues in our professional disciplines. We continue to hope and work for the transformation of evacuation and resettlement policies, in the words of one resettled woman, "*Por los niños.*"

Notes

1. For instance, evacuations caused by tropical storms and floods (Belize City, 1961; Darwin, 1974; or the U.S. Gulf Coast areas, 1953–2002), earthquakes (Managua, 1972; India, 2002; Turkey, 2003; or Algeria, 2003), volcanic explosions (Mt. Etna, 2003; Popocatepetl, 2002; Nevado del Ruiz, 1985; Montserrat, 2000–2003), and industrial accidents (such as Three Mile Island, Bhopal, and Chernobyl) evoke memories for many still alive today.

2. See geographers Gilbert F. White (1974), Heinrich Muller-Miny (1959; cited in Zelinsky and Kosinski 1991), and Kenneth Hewitt (1983, 1997); anthropologists Anthony Oliver-Smith and Suzanne Hoffman (1999, 2001), Oliver-Smith (1986a, 1986b, 1996), and Perry and Mushkatel (1984); and sociologists Drabek (1986), Mileti, Bolton, Fernandez, and Updike (1991), and Quarantelli (1998).

References

Cernea, M. M. (2000). "Risks, Safeguards, and Reconstruction: A Model for Population Displacement and Resettlement." In *Risks and Reconstruction: Experiences of Resettlers and Refugees*, edited by M. M. Cernea and C. McDowell, 11–55. Washington, DC: World Bank.

Chan, N. W. (1995). "Flood Disaster Management in Malaysia: An Evaluation of the Effectiveness of Government Resettlement Schemes." *Disaster Prevention and Management* 4, no. 4: 22–29.

CNN. (1999, October 17). "Evacuations Ordered as Ecuadorian Volcano Threatens." Accessed at www.cnn.com/WORLD/americas/9910/17/ecuador.volcano/index.html, October 17, 1999.

Cruz Roja Ecuatoriana. (1999a, October 16). *Ecuador: Informe especial: Un nevo volcán aenaza Ecuador.* Report. Ecuador: Cruz Roja Ecuatoriana.

———. (1999b, November 13). *Erupciones de los volcanes Guagua Pichincha y Tungurahua.* Informe Especial no. 5. Ecuador: Cruz Roja Ecuatoriana.

Drabek, T. E. (1986). *Human System Responses to Disaster: An Inventory of Sociological Findings.* New York: Springer-Verlag.

Farmer, P. (1992). *AIDS and Accusation: Haiti and the Geography of Blame.* Berkeley: University of California Press.

———. (2003). *Pathologies of Power: Health, Human Rights, and the New War on the Poor.* Berkeley: University of California Press.

Hall, M. L., C. Robin, B. Beate, P. Mothes, and M. Monzier. (1999). "Tungurahua Volcano, Ecuador: Structure, Eruptive History and Hazards." *Journal of Volcanology and Geothermal Research* 91: 1–21.

Hansen, A., and A. Oliver-Smith, ed. (1982). *Involuntary Migration and Resettlement: The Problems and Responses of Dislocated People.* Boulder, CO: Westview Press.

Harrell-Bond, B. (1986). *Imposing Aid: Emergency Assistance to Refugees.* Oxford: Oxford University Press.

Hewitt, K. (1983). *Interpretations of Calamity: From the Viewpoint of Human Ecology.* Boston: Allen and Unwin.

———. (1997). *Regions at Risk: A Geographical Introduction to Disasters.* Harlow, UK: Addison Wesley Longman.

Kim, J. Y., J. Millen, A. Irwin, and J. Gershman. (2000). *Dying for Growth: Global Inequality and the Health of the Poor.* Monroe, ME: Common Courage Press.

Lindell, M. K., and R. W. Perry. (1992). *Behavioral Foundations of Community Emergency Planning.* Washington, DC: Hemisphere Publishing.

Mileti, D. S., D. S. Mileti, P. A. Bolton, G. Fernandez, and R. G. Updike. (1991). *The Eruption of Nevado del Ruiz Volcano, South America, November 13, 1985.* Washington, DC: National Academy Press.

Muller-Miny, H. (1959). "Katastrophe und landschaft: Ein beitrag zur kulturlandschaftschumg am beispiel griechischer and deutscher landschaft." *Berichte zur Deutschen landeskunde* 23: 95–124.

Murphy, A. D., C. Baker, J. Hill, I. Perez, and F. H. Norris. (2001). "The Effects of the 1999 Mexican Floods on the Mental and Physical Health of Two Communities." Paper presented at the annual meeting of Society for Applied Anthropology, Merida, Mexico.

UN Office for the Coordination of Humanitarian Affairs (OCHA). (1999, 18 October). *Situation Report no. 3.* Geneva: OCHA. Accessed at http://stone.cidi/org/disaster/99b/0137.html, October 18, 1999.

Oliver-Smith, A. (1986a). *The Martyred City: Death and Rebirth in the Peruvian Andes.* Albuquerque: University of New Mexico Press.

———. (1986b). "Introduction: Disaster Context and Causation: An Overview of Changing Perspectives on Disaster Research." *Studies in Third World Societies* 36: 1–34.

———. (1996). "Anthropological Research on Hazards and Disasters." *Annual Reviews in Anthropology* 25: 303–28.

Oliver-Smith, A., and S. M. Hoffman, eds. (1999). *The Angry Earth: Disaster in Anthropological Perspective.* New York: Routledge.

———, eds. (2001). *Catastrophe and Culture: The Anthropology of Disaster.* Santa Fe, NM: School of American Research.

Perry, R. W., and A. H. Mushkatel. (1984). *Disaster Management: Warning Response and Community Relocation.* Westport, CT: Quorum.

Quarantelli, E. L. (1998). *What Is a Disaster? Perspectives on the Question.* New York: Routledge.

Shaluf, I. M., A. Fakharu'l-razi, and A. M. Said. (2003). "A Review of Disaster and Crisis." *Disaster Prevention and Management* 12, no. 1: 24–32.

Singer, M. (1995). "Beyond the Ivory Tower: Critical Praxis in Medical Anthropology." *Medical Anthropology Quarterly* 9, no. 1: 80–106.

Tobin, G. A., and B. E. Montz. (1997). *Natural Hazards: Explanation and Integration.* New York: Guilford Press.

Tobin, G. A., and L. M. Whiteford. (2001a). *The Role of Women in Post-Disaster Environments: Health and Community Sustainability. Technical Report.* Tampa, FL: Center for Disaster Management and Humanitarian Assistance, 968.

———. (2001b). "Children's Health Characteristics under Different Evacuation Strategies: The Eruption of Mount Tungurahua, Ecuador." *Papers of the Applied Geography Conferences* 24: 183–91.

———. (2002a). "Community Resilience and Volcano Hazard: The Eruption of Tungurahua and Evacuation of the Faldas in Ecuador." *Disasters: The Journal of Disaster Studies, Policy and Management* 26, no. 1: 28–48.

———. (2002b). "Economic Ramifications of Disaster: Experiences of Displaced Persons on the Slopes of Mount Tungurahua, Ecuador." *Papers of the Applied Geography Conferences* 25: 316–24.

White, G. F., ed. (1974). *Natural Hazards: Local, National, Global.* New York: Oxford University Press.

Whiteford, L. M., G. A. Tobin, C. Laspina, and H. Yepes. (2002a). *In the Shadow of the Volcano: Human Health and Community Resilience Following Forced Evacuation.* Technical Report. Tampa, FL: Center for Disaster Management and Humanitarian Assistance, 548.

———. (2002b). *A la sombra del volcán: Salud humana y capacidad de recuperación comunitaria después de una evacuación forzosa.* Community Report. Tampa, FL: Ecuadorian Government Officials and Community Leaders in Ecuador, 16.

Zelinsky, W., and L. A. Kosinski. (1991). *The Emergency Evacuation of Cities: A Cross-National Historical and Geographical Study.* Lanham, MD: Rowman & Littlefield.

13

Social Illegitimacy as a Foundation of Health Inequality: How the Political Treatment of Immigrants Illuminates a French Paradox

DIDIER FASSIN

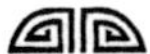

AS FAR AS HEALTH IS CONCERNED, France presents a remarkable paradox, yet one that is seldom recognized. Whereas the World Health Organization rated it in 2000 as the country with the world's best health care system—a rating that was, however, disputed—data produced in the same year by the European Union task force on socioeconomic inequalities showed it to be the country with the widest gaps in Western Europe between male mortality rates measured by socioprofessional category (Leclerc, Fassin, Grandjean, Kaminski, and Lang 2000). As in the biblical parable, the first seems therefore to be the last. In more general terms, one can conclude that the efficiency of a health policy is no guarantee of its justice. While the French celebrate the fact of having one of the world's highest life expectancy rates at birth—75 for men and 82 for women—they deplore a nine-year difference in the life expectancy of engineers compared to unskilled workers at the age of 35.

The explanation for this discrepancy is twofold (Doyal and Pennell 1979). First, the health care system itself can generate health inequalities through inferior access to or quality of care for socially underprivileged groups. In this respect, although France has progressively developed a broader and more universal system of social protection against risk of disease, especially since World War II, this has not eliminated de facto disparities (Murard 1996). Second, the health care system is often powerless to remedy health inequalities resulting from working, housing, income, and general living conditions. From this angle, France is one of the Western countries in which income disparities are the most profound and tend to increase fastest (Piketty 1997). These are the two hypotheses explored in this chapter. Considering the issue from the health care system point of view, one can talk of actively produced inequalities, in the first instance, and of passively induced inequalities, in the second. But in both cases, these inequalities result from political choices reflected in health and social policies regarding the distribution of wealth between citizens and the treatment of the most fragile groups (Sen 1992)—choices, in other words, of what is fair, or rather of what is morally or socially acceptable as a degree of injustice.

From an anthropological perspective, inequalities can be understood in terms of the way in which societies treat their most vulnerable members. One can thus grasp, at its extremes, the nature of the social contract that binds human beings in a given space and defines their sense of politics (Arendt 1995). Immigrants and foreigners seem thus to be the paradigmatic group of greatest liminality since they belong neither to the community of origin nor to that of the nation (I have adopted the distinction usually made in France between immigrants, biographically characterized by their place of birth, and foreigners, defined legally by their nationality). Yet they are still members of the society to which they contribute through their work, culture, and sociability, and whose solidarity they put to the test by forcing it to define the extent of its duties (Noiriel 1988). It is through the prism of this social category that the present chapter illuminates the paradox described above in more general terms. First, I will show that the constructed illegitimacy of a category of the population tends to produce restricted access to its social rights, including in the domain that enjoys the greatest legitimacy: health care. Second, I will demonstrate that this illegitimacy tends to generate inequalities in all sectors of social activities, such as employment or housing, the consequences of which impact decisively on health, and I will illustrate this point through an exemplary case study: child lead poisoning. This twofold production of inequality is, however, largely unperceived in France, as I will discuss in the last section of the chapter, due to a politics of negation of differences and assertion of equity, in the name of which there has been a refusal to see what is considered unspeakable.

Political Variations on the Theme of Immigration

The legitimacy of immigrants and foreigners can never be taken for granted; it always has to be established (Sayad 1991). Most often, it is their economic function that justifies their presence, primarily through their contribution to the production of wealth as an undemanding and unorganized labor force. Even political asylum is subordinated to it (Noiriel 1991). As soon as there is a risk of an economic slump or an increase in unemployment, they become unwanted. The history of French society in the past half-century is a perfect example of this pattern.

During the first three decades after World War II, the labor needs of national reconstruction and industrial development were huge. At the time, immigration from Southern Europe and later North Africa was encouraged by business and endorsed by the government to the extent that immigrants holding a work contract could easily obtain a residence permit (Weil 1991). Some, mostly families, were gradually integrated into the most popular fringes of French society, usually in large low-cost housing complexes that, in the fifties and sixties, served to reduce the most glaring urban poverty, that of the shantytowns; while others, mostly men who had come to France alone, were concentrated in workers' hostels on the outskirts of towns. Even though their contribution to the national wealth as a labor force was recognized, these immigrants constituted the most underprivileged section of the working population.

In the early seventies, following the oil crisis, foreign manpower became far less useful under the combined effects of the modernization and restructuring of industry. In 1974, the first measures were taken by the government to curb immigration (Viet 1998). Only foreign workers' spouses and children were allowed to join them on the grounds of family reunification. In 1984 this so-called populating immigration, which replaced the previous labor immigration, started to be seen as a demographic and economic burden. Gradually, all forms of access to a residence permit—asylum, marriage, studies—were blocked or became suspect, and increasingly restrictive laws were passed. Their effect was to make immigration more difficult, but also to produce growing numbers of foreigners in an illegal position because they were unable to obtain or renew their residence permit. In 1994 this new configuration resulted in what is known as the *mouvement des sans-papiers*, the undocumented migrants' movement, a collective protest expressed through hunger strikes, street demonstrations, and the occupation of churches (Siméant 1998) that has enjoyed a current of sympathy in public opinion as well as support from associations, intellectuals, and artists.

Thus, immigrants and foreigners, who are constantly in a vulnerable position because they are perceived as outsiders to the community, and who share neither its origins nor its nationality, have gradually lost everything that could justify their presence (Sayad 1999). Economically useless, they have also become socially undesirable. Within a few years, the issue of their presence has become a major political challenge around which public debate has been constructed and far-right-wing parties have been formed (Hargreaves 1995). Their loss of value as a labor force has thus contaminated all other forms of recognition, starting with political asylum, which has been increasingly challenged (Julien-Laferrière 2002), as attested by the fact that six times fewer people obtained refugee status in the late 1990s than in the previous decade.

Yet talking of immigrants and foreigners, or even of refugees, in general terms is inadequate to account for the specific reality to which these words refer. The people targeted by the restrictive laws and disparaging judgments are mostly from the Third World, primarily North Africa (Algerians and Moroccans) and sub-Saharan

Africa (Malians and Congolese), but also more recently from Central Asia (Kurds and Afghans) and the Far East (Chinese). Their illegitimacy therefore also relates to a more radical difference, one that is often interpreted as cultural but is in fact racial (Taguieff 1987). Europeans are clearly not subject to the same depreciation as people that political correctness names *extra-communautaires* (i.e., coming from outside the European Union). Migrants from developing countries and more particularly from former French colonies are the main victims of inequalities as a result of a long historical process (Cooper and Stoler 1997). This is reflected, significantly, in the fact that discrimination does not affect only immigrants or foreigners, but also their children, many of whom are now, under the law, French citizens born in France (De Rudder, Poiret, and Vourc'h 2000). Hence, through an accumulation of economic and racial factors linked to present and past realities, disqualifying and ranking processes within immigrant and foreign groups are at work. For those who have no residence permit, the loss of their legality is simply the logical conclusion to their loss of legitimacy. It is therefore hardly surprising that these processes are translated into the way in which rights are exercised, including in the health domain.

The Moral Economy of Access to Health Care

All societies determine the scope of the solidarity they implement by defining who has a right to what. French social protection operates in two modes. The first, insurance-based, functions by distribution of employee and employer contributions as needed for health care: that is social security. The second, assistance-based, functions through taxes intended for people who do not benefit from social security because they are jobless and have no income: that is social aid (Join-Lambert 1997). Since World War II, in the health domain, these two systems have been conjugated toward the extension of rights to all persons living in French territory legally and stably, irrespective of origin or nationality. After a series of regulations all aimed in the same direction, the 1999 law on "universal health coverage" clearly endorsed this orientation, generalizing and unifying social protection (Borgetto 2000). A foreigner living in France has the same right to health care—at least curative health care—as any native French citizen. Only undocumented migrants do not qualify, but under the state medical aid scheme they are entitled to free care in hospitals. With this law, a certain degree of overlap between the two modes—insurance-based and assistance-based—has been developed, since people with very low incomes fall under the general social security scheme, as well as complementary health insurance, therefore qualifying for free access to the medical system.

Thus, in its spirit and its form, solidarity in the health domain progressively constructed in France can be characterized as follows. First, everyone residing usually and legally in French territory is entitled to social security on the same terms. Second, below a certain income threshold everyone has a right to free health care, either in terms of universal coverage for those who are affiliated or in terms of state medical aid for those who are temporarily in France or whose legal papers are not in order. In contrast to other contexts (Rylko-Bauer and Farmer 2002), these are certainly generous regulations: people formerly excluded from health care are now granted access (half those who benefit by the new measures say they had previously given up trying to obtain care) and, what is more, on an egalitarian basis (including for immigrants and foreigners). This extension of the right to health care is particularly remarkable in the case of the latter two groups, for it stretched over a quarter century in a context of increasingly restrictive legislation concerning immigration with decreasing social tolerance toward foreigners (Fassin 2001).

However, generosity and equality need to be relativized in two respects. First, although almost every resident in France enjoys social coverage, it is only partial: a large proportion of medical costs still have to be paid by patients, except for the poorest households, and some types of care are hardly covered at all, such as dental care and optic correction. Second, since the income level giving right to free care is low, corresponding more or less to one half of the minimum legal wage, many households belonging to the working poor do not benefit from this measure. The phenomenon is known as the threshold effect. These two factors of disparity are nevertheless common to all people resident in France, irrespective of their origin and nationality (at least according to the law).

Actual practices give a different picture, however. Immigrants and foreigners clearly do not have access to all the care to which they are entitled. Of the 25,000 people seen annually in free health clinics provided by the NGO Médecins du monde, over 85 percent are foreigners, although they account for only 6 percent of the population resident in France. There are thus 14 times more foreigners than French citizens who use this humanitarian service supposedly intended for patients not entitled to the state medical system (Drouot and Simonnot 2002). The reasons for such high numbers of people using services provided by charitable organizations are complex. They can, of course, be interpreted—as the agents themselves do most of the time, thus excluding their own responsibility—in cultural terms, by claiming that immigrants are simply ill-informed or less inclined to turn to the formal health care system, or else in functional terms, by noting that administrative services have organizational reception problems and that social workers lack knowledge on certain complex aspects of the regulations. Although they are not unfounded, these explanations give a poor phenomenology without affording a real analysis.

In order to understand why immigrants and foreigners, especially those with no legal status in France, tend not to use state facilities, one needs to look at their illegitimate position in the social sphere. This illegitimacy is internalized by them, often leading them to consider that because they are undesirable they have no rights. Many who consult a doctor only at an advanced stage of their disease or when the pain has become unbearable say they thought they were not entitled to any care. Their illegitimacy is also perceived and sometimes affirmed by certain social workers who, in contravention of the law, assure foreigners that they are entitled to nothing, especially when they are in an irregular situation. Testimonies of these illegally imposed limits abound (Fassin 1997). They sometimes result from ignorance of the legislation, sometimes also from personal disagreement with regulations considered too generous. Applicants for political asylum are refused universal medical coverage, to which they are entitled, because certain civil servants anticipate a negative decision by the authorities concerning their refugee status and assume that they will soon be in an illegal position. Certain doctors often reject patients when they feel that state medical aid should not have been granted, a reasoning that the authorities themselves seem to recognize by establishing lists of private physicians willing to see these patients (Fassin, Carde, Ferré, Kotobi, and Musso-Dimitrijevic 2002). The law is thus infringed daily in the name of a restrictive representation that agents have of who can legitimately claim the right to what, and through which they express prejudices found throughout French society and its elite.

In the dialectic generating tension between a more or less illegitimate population (immigrants and foreigners that the country claims not to need) and an increasingly legitimate domain (access to health care, considered as an unalienable right), it is the agents themselves who are often in the position of having to deal with individual situations, either in a pragmatic way by doing their best within the limits of their prerogatives, or in an ideological one related to their personal convictions, imbibed either with xenophobia or progressivism. Instead of applying the law, the decisions of this "street-level bureaucracy" reflect the hesitations and contradictions of the social world (Lipsky 1980). Although unjust, these failures to observe the ethical rules of professions believed and said to be devoted to others have, however, relatively limited effects on the physical state of immigrants or foreigners, since medicine only contributes marginally to morbidity and mortality rates. In a country like France, the harm done by these restrictive practices should then be thought of in terms of rights rather than health. But the same cannot be said for the consequences of illegitimacy in other areas of human activity, where it results in inequalities inscribed in the bodies of the poor and marginalized.

The Political Economy of Infantile Plumbism

Health disparities are caused far more by living conditions than by access to care. Findings of a study in Paris and surrounding areas show that the proportion of poor households is six times greater among non-European foreigners than among French-born inhabitants. Compared to European foreigners, it is still triple (Espinasse 2002). Infantile plumbism is a classic but meaningful illustration of the effects of poverty on health, with specific elements relating to the history of immigration in France. Lead poisoning in young children was first described in North America in the early twentieth century (Fee 1990). Its noxious effects on the nervous system, leading to possible coma and even death, were well identified, but insidious effects on the cognitive functions and learning abilities have been known for only two decades. Whereas contamination by the ingestion of flakes of old paint such as ceruse was fully recognized, the mechanism of passive inhalation of particles of that same paint became known only recently. The absence of curative treatment is still a major constraint in combating the disease, since detoxification by chelation eliminates only small quantities of lead circulating in the body without any effect on the metal that has accumulated in the tissues and remains there throughout the person's life. The only efficient measures consist in removing the children from their environment, either by rehabilitating the building or by housing them elsewhere, yet for a long time pediatricians in French hospitals were content to diagnose the intoxication and to apply palliative measures before sending the children back home where the contamination continued.

Limited to the dilapidated and insalubrious housing into which poor families are crowded, infantile plumbism can be considered as a paradigm of diseases of inequality. In France it concerns almost exclusively children of foreign parents, mainly of African origin. Of the serious cases recorded in Paris in the early nineties, 85 percent were children whose parents came from sub-Saharan Africa. This singularity had health authorities perplexed (Fassin and Naudé 2004). Interpretations of a more or less exotic nature abounded in the search for cultural particularities from the use of ink on prayer tablets, of which Muslim marabouts were suspected, to the consumption of clay by pregnant women, whose geophagy was said to be passed down to their children. These are, however, very slim hypotheses if we consider that in the United States the children concerned are mostly African Americans or Latinos (Sargent et al. 1995). Rather than their culture, what these groups have in common is the social status they have in their host society, with the consequent living and housing conditions.

In the case of France, the frequency of intoxication among children of African families results from the historical conjunction of two policies. Firstly, immigration policies have been increasingly restrictive during a period in which the migratory flows originated primarily in sub-Saharan Africa. These more recent immigrants have joined the ranks of undocumented foreigners, who are obviously the most fragile part of the population (Fassin and Morice 2001). Secondly, social housing policies, based on the idea that the proportion of foreign families in the publicly funded estates was becoming a problem, have applied discriminatory measures making their access to this type of housing particularly difficult. African immigrants have thus been easy prey for unscrupulous private owners who rented them dilapidated apartments, often at high rates, that their legal precariousness forced them to accept (Simon 1997). Situated at the bottom of the scales implicitly established through laws on the entry and residence of foreigners in France, but also through the reactivation of racial prejudices, these immigrants, mostly from former French colonies, had to settle for what others did not want in terms of housing as well as jobs. Their illegitimacy, and sometimes their illegality, thus became the most powerful generator of the inequality of which they were victims.

Nevertheless, in 1998 the so-called fight against social exclusion law listed infantile plumbism as a national priority. It provided for the screening of intoxicated children in insalubrious neighborhoods and for owners of contaminated apartments to undertake the necessary renovations or face prosecution. This legislation, the result of large-scale mobilization by civil society associations, especially the main French humanitarian organizations but also professional bodies, notably municipal health services, recognized the reality of the problem for the first time and provided tools to deal with it. Yet four years later the results were very poor, as noted in reports to the Health Ministry and open letters to the press. Of the estimated 85,000 children with lead poisoning, only about 1 percent have benefited from effective rehabilitation or rehousing measures (Inserm 1999). For many commentators, this relative disinterest, compared to other programs conducted far more energetically, for example the prevention of bovine spongiform encephalopathy, was merely due to the lack of legitimacy of the victims of plumbism.

The history of this disease clearly illustrates just how much an individual's or group's health depends to a very limited degree on medical factors (Wilkinson 1996). One can have an excellent system of pediatric care with ample diagnostic and therapeutic resources, yet very poor results regarding the health of certain categories of children, as is the case with those seriously intoxicated by lead. Physicians' efficiency is reduced here to palliative treatments and, in the final analysis, one could say that their most effective intervention against plumbism has not been in relation with their clinical skills, but with the political mobilization some of them have managed to trigger or support through humanitarian and professional organizations. It is the physical environment and the material conditions, as well as the social relationships that determine them, that account for the frequency and distribution of infantile plumbism (Warren 2000). The illegitimacy that affects certain social categories, such as African immigrants in France, explains why these disparities are tolerated. First, these people are sufficiently undesirable for many to find their situation acceptable (everything is already too good for them) and for those who want to intervene feel they have little authority to do so (especially if the bill is to be footed by the national or local authorities). Second, immigrants themselves (having partially internalized their social position) consider they have no right to complain or make demands, especially when they are already in an illegal position (because they have no residence permit). In the present case, fighting against social inequalities in health therefore implies intervening on immigration policies and acting against discrimination. As much as their dilapidated housing, it is the very image of immigrants, and especially of Africans, that has to be rehabilitated.

Blindness of Policies, Invisibility of Problems

Health inequalities affecting foreigners and people of foreign origin are so often overlooked by decision makers and public opinion in France because an official policy of selective blindness exists in this respect, leading to the same kinds of injustice and contradiction as has been analyzed in other contexts (Singer, Baer, and Davison 1995). Nationality is rarely taken into account in French statistics, origins are never mentioned, and what the state is blind to soon becomes invisible to all. For a long time, no one wanted to say what all the local actors already knew: that infantile plumbism, and especially its most serious forms, affects almost only African families. Similarly, it took nearly two decades for the first figures to be published on AIDS in the foreign segment of the population, thus masking huge inequalities not only in the incidence of the infection but also in access to screening and treatment (Fassin 1999). The reasons for this blindness are complex and deeply rooted in the political history of France.

The Republican model regarding the treatment of immigrants is based on two principles: equality and integration. Underlying these principles is an ideal: universalism. Equality primarily concerns social rights from education to health, and assumes that everyone is treated in the same way under the protective wing of the state (De Swaan 1988). Integration is guaranteed in the short term by minimizing cultural differences and in the long term by the predominance of the right to nationality based on one's place of birth rather than one's parentage (Schnapper 1990). Universalism is the humanistic ideal inherited from the Enlightenment that places humans' similarities above their differences. French political life is thus founded on democratic bases dating back to the French Revolution and the Universal Declaration of Human Rights. The times when these values were flouted are the darkest and most tragic in the nation's memory, especially the period under the Vichy regime during World War II. Consensus is therefore broad, at least as far as the stated principles are concerned, for in practice gaps in tolerance levels are wide. Although the French model has had some noteworthy results regarding equality and integration, French citizens and authorities have reassured themselves too quickly, while spatial segregation and economic precariousness have been steadily growing. Universalism has consequently been challenged not so much by community-oriented policies, which is constantly held up as a specter coming from North America, as by social inequalities and racial discrimination manifested in all areas of daily life (Fassin 2002). It is this failure—at least relative failure—that French society and its intellectual and political elite have had so much difficulty acknowledging.

This explains why health inequalities between French citizens and foreigners and, even more so, between the French themselves depending on their origins are so difficult to grasp. A collective symbolic investment was made in the establishment of a system of social protection and medical care based, as we have seen, on principles of fairness and equality precisely because health seemed to be a universal good that needed to be preserved. Consequently, not only was nothing done for a long time to produce data through which these disparities could be objectified; but when they did become apparent, there was a refusal to analyze their real meaning. The inequalities revealed were said to be disappearing within similar socioprofessional categories. Yet this mathematical hypothesis was simply a rhetorical clause, for inequalities based on origins were significant in the distribution within socioprofessional categories as well. Just like in many other historical contexts, race and class were closely linked.

In fact, the contradictions into which the public authorities' blindness locked them became untenable when the state, rather than allowing itself the means to address problems specific to immigrants, started to withdraw by financing nongovernmental organizations responsible for implementing its health and social policies, and by supporting interventions defined on cultural or ethnic grounds, on the fringe of common law. An extreme example of this trend is a famous publicly funded ethno-psychiatric center near Paris that became the reference not only for the care of immigrants' psychological problems, but also for the qualification in cultural and ethnic terms of a set of social problems faced by foreign families, from delinquency of youngsters to the excision of girls (Fassin 2000). The state and its representatives in the public health domain, renouncing their universalist project, thus abandoned immigrants and their children to therapists who based their practice on particularism. Social inequalities and racial discrimination could thus be expressed in much more acceptable terms of cultural difference and ethnic origin.

If we now revert to the paradox presented in the introduction, our analysis of the limited but exemplary case of immigrants and foreigners is illuminating. The French health care system may be highly efficient, but is not constructed as a tool at the service of social justice. Although it is based on formal principles of equality, the practical effects of those principles are undermined by the threefold mechanism described here. First, the agents concerned may fail to observe the legal and even ethical norms due to tension, in the daily management of problems, between their perception of a population group they consider socially disqualified and their evaluation of a system they see as being too generous. Second, irrespective of its accessibility and quality, health care has only a limited effect on individuals' health compared to the far more decisive consequences of their living conditions, determined by their place in society. Third, the gap between the stated ideal and the observed reality has led to a series of arrangements designed to make disparities less visible, either by removing them from available statistics or by interpreting them in terms of cultural determinism. In all three processes, it is illegitimacy that gives meaning to inequality and moral judgments that underlie social injustice.

Acknowledgments

The text was translated by Liz Libbrecht and revised by the author. Research on racial discrimination in access to health care was conducted with Estelle Carde for a project funded by the French Direction of Population and Migration. Investigation on lead poisoning in children was carried out with Anne-Jeanne Naudé through a grant from the French Ministry of Health.

References

Arendt, H. (1995). *Qu'est-ce que la politique?* Paris: Seuil. (Originally published in 1993.)

Borgetto, D. (2000). "Brèves réflexions sur les apports et les limites de la loi créant la CMU." *Droit social* 1: 30–38.

Cooper, F., and A. L. Stoler, eds. (1997) *Tensions in Empire: Colonial Cultures in a Bourgeois World.* Berkeley: University of California Press.

De Rudder, V., C. Poiret, and F. Vourc'h. (2000). *L'inégalité raciste. L'universalité républicaine à l'épreuve.* Paris: Presses Universitaires de France.

De Swaan, A. (1988). *In the Care of the State.* London: Polity Press—Basil Blackwell.

Doyal, L., with I. Pennell. (1979). *The Political Economy of Health.* London: Pluto Press.

Drouot, N., and N. Simonnot. (2002). *Rapport 2001 de l'Observatoire de l'accès aux soins de la mission France.* Paris: Médecins du monde.

Espinasse, M. T. (2002). "Pauvreté et précarité des étrangers." In *Les travaux de l'observatoire national de la pauvreté et de l'exclusion sociale,* edited by ONPES, 325–47. Paris: La Documentation française.

Fassin, D. (1997). "La santé en souffrance." In *Les lois de l'inhospitalité: La société française à l'épreuve des sans-papiers,* edited by D. Fassin, A. Morice, and C. Quiminal, 107–23. Paris: La Découverte.

———. (1999). "L'indicible et l'impensé. La 'question immigrée' dans les politiques du sida." *Sciences sociales et santé* 17, no. 4: 5–36.

———. (2000). "Les politiques de l'ethnopsychiatrie. La psyché africaine, des colonies britanniques aux banlieues parisiennes." *L'Homme* 153: 231–50.

———. (2001). "The Biopolitics of Otherness: Undocumented Immigrants and Racial Discrimination in the French Public Debate. *Anthropology Today* 17, no. 1: 3–7.

———. (2002). "L'invention française de la discrimination." *Revue française de science politique* 52, no. 4: 395–415.

Fassin, D., E. Carde, N. Ferré, L. Kotobi, and S. Musso-Dimitrijevic. (2002). *Un traitement inégal. Les discriminations dans l'accès aux soins.* Rapport d'étude no. 5. Bobigny: CRESP.

Fassin, D., and A. Morice. (2001). "Les épreuves de l'irrégularité." In *Exclusions au cœur de la cité*, edited by D. Schnapper, 261–309. Paris: Anthropos.

Fassin, D., and A. J. Naudé. (2004). "Plumbism Reinvented: The Early Times of Childhood Lead Poisoning in France 1985–1990." *American Journal of Public Health* 94, no. 9.

Fee, E. (1990). "Public Health in Practice: An Early Confrontation with the 'Silent Epidemic' of Childhood Lead Paint Poisoning." *The Journal of the History of Medicine and Allied Sciences* 45: 570–606.

Hargreaves, A. G. (1995). *Immigration, "Race" and Ethnicity in Contemporary France.* London: Routledge.

Inserm. (1999). *Plomb dans l'environnement: Quels risques pour la santé?* Paris: Editions de l'Inserm.

Join-Lambert, M. T. (1997). *Politiques sociales.* Paris: Presses de la Fondation nationale de sciences politiques-Dalloz.

Julien-Laferrière, F. (2002). *Le droit d'asile en question, Problèmes politiques et sociaux.* Paris: La Documentation française.

Leclerc, A., D. Fassin, H. Grandjean, M. Kaminski, and T. Lang, eds. (2000). *Les inégalités sociales de santé.* Paris: INSERM-La Découverte.

Lipsky, M. (1980). *Street-Level Bureaucracy: Dilemmas of the Individual in Public Services.* New York: Russell Sage Foundation.

Murard, N. (1996). *La protection sociale.* Paris: La Découverte.

Noiriel, G. (1988). *Le creuset français: Histoire de l'immigration XIXe-XXe siècles.* Paris: Seuil.

———. (1991). *La tyrannie du national: Le droit d'asile en Europe 1793–1993.* Paris: Calmann-Lévy.

Piketty, T. (1997). *L'économie des inégalités.* Paris: La Découverte.

Rylko-Bauer, B., and P. Farmer. (2002). "Managed Care or Managed Inequality? A Call for Critiques of Market-Based Medicine." *Medical Anthropology* 16, no. 4: 476–502.

Sargent, J. D., M. J. Brown, J. L. Freeman, A. Bailey, D. Goodman, and D. H. Freeman. (1995). "Childhood Lead Poisoning in Massachusetts Communities." *American Journal of Public Health* 85, no. 4: 528–34.

Sayad, A. (1991). *L'immigration ou les paradoxes de l'altérité.* Brussels: De Boeck Université.

———. (1999). "La double absence." *Des illusions de l'émigré aux souffrances de l'immigré.* Paris: Seuil.

Schnapper, D. (1990). *La France de l'intégration: Sociologie de la nation en 1990.* Paris: Gallimard.

Sen, A. (1992). *Inequality Reexamined.* Oxford: Oxford University Press.

Siméant, J. (1998). *La cause des sans-papiers.* Paris: Presses de la Fondation nationale de sciences politiques.

Simon, P. (1997). "La gestion des discriminations raciales et ethniques par les politiques publiques: l'exemple des politiques de l'habitat." *Etudes et recherches,* Iseres 158: 119–29.

Singer, M., H. Baer, and L. Davison. (1995). *Critical Medical Anthropology.* Amityville, NY: Baywood.

Taguieff, A. A. (1987). *La force du préjugé: Essai sur le racisme et ses doubles.* Paris: Gallimard.

Viet, V. (1998). *La France immigrée: Construction d'une politique 1914–1997.* Paris: Fayard.

Warren, C. (2000). *Brush with Death: A Social History of Lead Poisoning.* Baltimore: Johns Hopkins University Press.

Weil, P. (1991). *La France et ses étrangers.* Paris: Calmann-Lévy.

Wilkinson, R. G. (1996). *Unhealthy Societies: The Afflictions of Inequality.* London: Routledge.

The Indian Health Transfer Policy in Canada: Toward Self-Determination or Cost Containment? 14

KRISTEN M. JACKLIN AND WAYNE WARRY

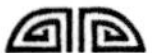

FOR DECADES, ARGUABLY CENTURIES, Aboriginal[1] people have experienced poorer health status than the majority of Canadians. Substandard living conditions, poor access to medical care, and assimilationist policies have contributed to the poor state of health of Aboriginal communities. The ill health of this population raises questions about the nature of Aboriginal health policy and policy making in Canada. We argue that federal policies regarding Aboriginal health have been conflicting, confusing, and arbitrary. We focus specifically on the implementation and evaluation of the Health Transfer Policy. The goals and objectives of this initiative are to enhance Aboriginal self-determination in health care by providing First Nations with increased control over the design, delivery, and administration of health services. However, when the health policies affecting Aboriginal people are examined from a critically applied medical anthropology perspective, the motivation for this policy becomes questionable. The critical medical framework situates the local reality of how health is experienced in the broader framework of macrolevel influences such as political and economic factors (Singer and Baer 1995:62). To critically examine this health policy, we briefly review (1) the historical developments leading up to the Health Transfer Policy, (2) the principles and objectives of the policy, and (3) the process of Health Transfer in the Aboriginal community of Wikwemikong, Ontario.[2] Although the policy has been marketed as a mechanism for healing and self-determination, its formation has been guided primarily by political-economic factors, and as a result there have been very limited benefits at the local level.

Part of the rational for changing Aboriginal health policy has been the recognition that, despite biomedical interventions (and later health promotion), this population continues to be unhealthy (Young 1984:263; Gilmore 1979:92). The

Report on the Health of Canadians (Health Canada 1996a, 1999a, 1999b) recognizes the poorer than average health of Aboriginal people. The report attributes their poor health to crowded living conditions, unemployment, poor educational experiences, and poverty. All of these factors are exacerbated for those who live on reserves. Concurrent research carried out by the First Nations and Inuit Regional Health Survey (FNIRHS 1999) supports these findings.

Historical Developments in Aboriginal Health Policy

Currently, the First Nations Inuit Health Branch (FNIHB) of Health Canada, formerly Medical Services Branch (MSB), administers Aboriginal health policy in Canada. Responsibility for the health care of Aboriginal people has been very poorly defined. The federal government has never admitted to its constitutional responsibility for health care for Aboriginal people.[3] They have provided care for various reasons: to limit the spread of disease to the non-Aboriginal population, and on humanitarian and economic grounds (Graham-Cumming 1967:117).

The overview of the major economic and policy trends in Canadian health care in Table 14.1 provides a national context for the changes to Aboriginal health policy. In general there was a shift toward devolution of responsibility for health care to the provinces and, prior to the Health Transfer Policy, an agenda to transfer Aboriginal health care responsibility to provincial governments. The undercurrents of the economic motivation for this shift are self-evident. The Aboriginal policy shifts are highlighted in gray.

Historically, the Canadian government has, for the most part, assumed an assimilationist policy regarding Aboriginal people. There have been several attempts to offload the responsibility for providing health care for Aboriginal people to the provincial governments. None of the policies of the twentieth century equalized health status of Aboriginal people living on or off reserve. The late 1970s and early 1980s saw some government recognition that Aboriginal community healing will succeed only with the participation of the people living in those communities. It was further recognized that Aboriginal self-determination would foster community growth and development. In this context, the Canadian government offered the Indian Health Transfer Policy in 1986. The new policy was, and continues to be, met with suspicion given the national government's focus on offloading, cost-containment, and deficit fighting.

This Health Transfer Policy allows First Nations south of the 60th parallel to assume administrative control over certain aspects of their health care (Gregory, Russell, Hurd, Tyance, and Sloan 1992:214). In April 1986, an Interim Report from the Sub-Committee on the Transfer of Health Programs to Indian Control was distributed to the First Nations. In this report, Health Transfer was made to

Table 14.1. Time Line of Policy and Economic Trends in Canada

Year	*Event*
1961	Hall Commission recommends that the federal government cost-share a universal medical insurance program with provinces (Deber and Vayda 1992:4).
1968	Federal government adopts the Medical Care Act providing universal medical insurance for Canadians (Deber and Vayda 1992:4).
1969	The federal government's White Paper proposes the discontinuation of special services for Aboriginal people and the assimilation of Aboriginal people into Canadian society (Health Canada 1999d). It also proposes that Aboriginal people receive health services from provincial governments (Young 1984:262).
1970	The Red Paper is released by the Chiefs of Alberta, demanding their right to receive health care (Young 1984:262).
1974	The Lalonde Report is released by the federal government. It suggests a broader definition of health (Lalonde 1974:31).
1974	The proposed Indian Health Policy is released, proposing (again) the transfer of Aboriginal health services to provincial governments (Speck 1989:196).
1977	Bill C-37—Federal—Provincial health care cost-sharing is replaced with block funding (Deber and Vayda 1992:5).
1978	Proposal to reduce non-insured health benefits (e.g., dental benefits, prescription medicines, and eye care) for Aboriginal people (Gilmore 1979:87).
1978	Funding allocated for health promotion at federal level Health Promotion Directorate (Health Canada 1997:2).
1979	New Indian Health Policy created based on the Lalonde Report and the World Health Organization's (WHO) Declaration of Alma Ata (Young 1984:263; Waldram et al. 1995:235).
1980s	Block funding for provincial health care is limited (Deber and Vayda 1992:15), and more money is invested into Health Promotion (Health Canada 1997:4).
1981	A proposal to transfer services to Aboriginal communities is approved (Frideres 1998:178).
1983	The Penner Report is released, calling for administration and policy reforms within current legislation to enhance the movement toward self-government (Canada 1986:6).
1985	The Neilson Report repeats the tenets of the White Paper and reiterates that the priority of the federal government is to fight the deficit (Weaver 1993:92).
1986	The Indian Health Transfer Policy is announced (Speck 1989:198).
1988	The Indian Health Transfer Policy is approved by cabinet (Health Canada 1999d).

(continued)

Table 14.1. Time Line of Policy and Economic Trends in Canada *(continued)*

1990s	All federal funding is reduced in order to fight the deficit (Health Canada 1997:10, 27).
1996	Health Canada adopts the Population Health Model, which focuses on economic development as a means to better health (Health Canada 1996a).
1999	The Health Transfer Policy is revised (Health Canada 1999c).
2001	The Communities First: First Nations Governance Initiative, proposing changes to the Indian Act, is announced (Indian and Northern Affairs [INAC] 2001).

appear very desirable. It stated, "The Branch is proposing a developmental approach to transfer centred upon the concept of self-determination in health" (Canada 1986:ii). It was stated that communities would determine their own needs and make decisions about how services were to be developed and managed, and would be free to take into consideration their own cultural, traditional, and practical circumstances (Canada 1986:6).

The final policy was not as comprehensive and flexible as suggested in the interim report. It did not include noninsured health benefits (NIHB), dental, environmental health,[4] or training for Transfer, but did include a "no enrichment" clause; that is, First Nation budgets were frozen at the time of transfer (Speck 1989:200). In light of the rhetoric of self-determination that was part of the development and marketing of the Health Transfer, it can be argued that the policy has, in fact, enhanced local capacity in health governance and administration and, in so doing, has assisted in the initial steps toward self-determination in health care (Jacklin and Warry 2000; Warry and Sunday 2000; Warry 2000). This is particularly true if one has a long-term, incrementalist view of self-government, a position that the federal government assumes. However, as we now show, there remains great dissatisfaction with the Health Transfer Policy at the local level, disenchantment at the unwillingness of bureaucrats to recognize the need for traditional approaches to care, and considerable frustration with the federal government's unwillingness to acknowledge the need for enhanced services given the poorer than average health status of Aboriginal communities. Thus, the degree of "administrative control" that First Nations have assumed in daily decision making in no way disguises the structural constraints placed on First Nations or the degree of power and control retained by the federal government.

The Health Transfer Process in Wikwemikong

Wikwemikong Unceded Indian Reserve is situated on Manitoulin Island on the North Shore of Lake Huron, Ontario. It is the largest of the seven reserve communities and larger than the non-Aboriginal towns on Manitoulin Island. The residents of Wikwemikong are Ojibwe, Odawa, and Potawatomi. Wikwemikong faces similar health and social issues to other First Nation communities in Canada. It has a young and rapidly increasing population, high levels of disease burden and projected disease burdens, and high rates of suicide, depression, and other mental health concerns. Wikwemikong is also unique in many of its characteristics: it has a larger than average geographic and population size, a lack of housing that forces many residents to live off reserve in nearby towns, emergency medical services that are 40 minutes to an hour away, 49 percent of the reserve population living in rural satellite villages and dependent on potable water and septic systems, a majority of the "elder" population living in the rural villages, and three distinct cultural and language groups making the delivery of "culturally appropriate"[5] services challenging.

The Wikwemikong leadership has pursued an agenda for self-government for many years. Attempts to regain and retain control over the lives of the Band members began in 1862 when the Chiefs of Wikwemikong would not agree to sign the Manitoulin Treaty. In 1968, the Wikwemikong Chief and Council passed a resolution indicating that the Band wished to control all services that are delivered to the community. In 1986, several steps were taken toward the goal of self-determination; for example, the Wikwemikong Band assumed control of its education, and they began to construct a new Health Centre, which would incorporate a traditional healing lodge. Also in 1986, the Band had the opportunity to begin the process to take control of its health services when the Health Transfer policy was introduced. At that time, the Band passed a motion (#1723-86) that "the Band wished to pursue the Transfer of health services, initiated by Health and Welfare Canada" (Wikwemikong Community Health Plan [WCHP] 1989).

The Goals and Objectives of Health Transfer

When the idea of Health Transfer was initially introduced to Wikwemikong, it was described as an opportunity to move toward self-government (Canada 1986). Subsequent information contained in the 1992 Health Transfer Handbooks (Health and Welfare Canada 1992) described the principles of Health Transfer as follows: "Centered on the concept of self-determination in health, the transfer process has been developed in response to the individual circumstances of each community" (Health and Welfare Canada 1992:3). The Transfer Objectives were

> to enable Indian communities to design health programs, establish services and allocate funds according to community priorities; to strengthen and enhance accountability of Chiefs and Councils to community members; and to ensure public health and safety is maintained through adherence to mandatory programs (Health and Welfare Canada 1992). (WCHP 1989)

Health Transfer handbooks released in 1999 (Health Canada 1999c) omitted the emphasis on self-determination, but the objectives remain very similar. In the 1999 handbooks, self-government is an option that is separate and distinct from the option of Health Transfer. These changes reflect the federal government's retreat from a progressive policy that sees health (or other social) policy as a key component of the self-determination process.

The Wikwemikong Reserve also developed their own goals for the process of Health Transfer in their community. The main goals for the Community Health Plans (WCHP 1989, 1994, 2001) included the provision of wholistic health care and the integration of traditional and western medicines leading to improved community health. It is in the context of the goals and objectives of both the community health plans and the government policy that we evaluate the effectiveness of this health policy for Wikwemikong.

Self-Determination and Empowerment

Much like policy development, power over policy implementation is concentrated in the hands of the government. In Wikwemikong, both the initial agreement process (1988 to 1994) and the more recent agreement renewal process (1999) have been frustrating, stressful, and at times disempowering.

The process of transferring health services was documented by the community in their 1989 and 1994 Community Health Plans. The period between 1987 and 1994 consisted of what is termed the pre-transfer planning stage. This stage includes negotiating for short-term contracts to conduct a community needs assessment and the writing of a community health plan (CHP). Some of the text in this document provides an effective narrative to describe the feelings at the time:

> The initial contract was signed by Health and Welfare Canada to run from December 1, 1986 to March 31, 1987. As a result of Health and Welfare's bureaucratic WHITE TAPE, seven (7) contracts were signed between Health and Welfare Canada and the Wikwemikong band, for a twenty four (24) month duration to complete the Comprehensive Community Health Plan.

The WCHP (1989) attempted to strike a balance between Wikwemikong's needs and the requirements of the policy:

> Health Care is our *Right*, and as such is the responsibility of both the individual and of the community as a whole. The Comprehensive Community Health Plan is based on our belief, concepts, perceptions, attitudes, culture, and way of life, that is constantly undergoing change to meet the needs and demands of our people. It is now time to change our health care delivery once again to meet the new demands of our People. We must also meet the demands of the bureaucratic health systems of the Federal and Provincial Governments as they attempt to deliver "their" services to our people.

Despite a long and involved process, Wikwemikong signed its first Health Transfer Agreement in 1994. Health Transfer Agreements are renegotiated every three to five years, depending on the specific contract. In 1999, Wikwemikong was entering into negotiations for a new Health Transfer contract. There are no guarantees that contracts will be renewed—renewals are subject to "appropriation of funds by parliament" (Wikwemikong Health Transfer Renewal Agreement 2000). The lack of any guarantee that the agreements will be renewed has been a concern and criticism of the policy since its inception (Speck 1989:202). While the first Health Transfer contract was anticipated with high expectations and a sense of community ownership over the process, the 1999 negotiation, which followed a successful evaluation of transferred services, was quite different.

The *Health Transfer Evaluation Report* (Jacklin and Warry 2000), despite making recommendations for changes to health governance, was highly favorable, and attested to high levels of community satisfaction with services and to the effectiveness of health services being delivered through the Health Centre. The community expected that with a favorable evaluation in hand, the renewal process would be an opportunity for them to enhance funding to improve programming. They felt that the increase in their population, their increased needs, and the fact that they serviced many off-reserve Band members would situate them in a favorable position during these talks. But although the policy is intended to increase participation, empowerment, and control, the 1999 talks resulted in feelings of defeat and disempowerment. Those present recalled that the MSB representatives corrected the community in thinking of the talks as negotiations; they were in fact, according to MSB, renewals. These contract renewals contained changes to the contracts by MSB—changes in wording, elimination of items, and addition of clauses—but the community could not make any changes. Despite Health Canada reports in 1996 and 1999 (Health Canada 1996a, 1999b) showing increasing rates of disease and population growth on Aboriginal reserves, there was no new program money offered, only a 3 percent increase for wages.

Speaking to visiting policy analysts in July 2000, a Wikwemikong Health Centre manager stated his frustration with the renewal process:

> We were told we could not negotiate, we could only renew and could only get a 3% increase. It is very difficult to run programs on this funding. There are more community members accessing services, budgets are locked and we have no access to money.

The response to his comment was that "the 3% you received reflects pressures on funding in general, the Regional Officer is taking direction from above." Further comments from the Health Director at the Wikwemikong Health Centre support the sentiment of the managers:

> With Health Transfer Policy when there are changes, there is never any input from the community level, it is always just this is what you are getting, that's it, that's all, just sign here. You know, there is really no renewal process because there is always something that changed, and there is no negotiations there, so we are more or less handcuffed, that might be the term to use—communities are handcuffed into signing if they want to receive any dollars.

Medical Services Branch did make several changes to the "renewal" agreement in 1999.[6] One of the most important changes to the Transfer contract, in the eyes of the community, is the inability to negotiate the contract terms. The First Wikwemikong Agreement from 1994 reads:

> Notwithstanding the termination date of this Agreement, it is intended by both parties to renew this Agreement *through negotiations* at its term subject to appropriation of funds by Parliament. Negotiations for renewal shall commence at least six (6) months prior to the termination date of this agreement. (Emphasis added.)

The same clause in the 1999 Wikwemikong Agreement reads:

> Notwithstanding the termination date of this Agreement, it is intended by both parties to renew it at its term subject to appropriation of funds by Parliament. Discussions for renewal shall commence at least six (6) months prior to the termination date.

Other changes to wording in the agreements included the omission of references to self-government found in the 1994 Agreement. When these issues were brought to the table in a subsequent meeting in July 2000 with the Regional Director of MSB, the representative from MSB stated that "it was a renewal, the changes to the clauses were explained to the community at the time."

Key to the process of self-determination and empowerment is the ability to have control over decisions that affect you. Yet the Wikwemikong experience confirms earlier criticisms of the Health Transfer policy citing continued external control over the decision-making process. While the policy makers purport that the objective of Health Transfer is power sharing, the actual decision-making system is still hierarchical. Communities are responsible for the administration of the programs, yet have little to no say in policy formation and implementation (Stout 1990:1).

The lack of participation in policy making is evident in the communication with First Nations regarding the current proposed revisions to Health Transfer agreements across the country. Following a report from the Auditor General of Canada regarding accountability in the Transfer agreements, First Nations are expected to sign new agreements that include stricter reporting requirements (Auditor General of Canada 2000).[7] Until this communication, the Regional Directors for FNIHB had given First Nations some leeway in reporting requirements; that is, deadlines were often extended for annual reports, community health plans, evaluations, and sometimes even renewal negotiations (Health Canada 2001). This flexibility was necessary as the Health Centre attempted to operate with minimal administrative support. The expectation to reopen contracts and revise them to include stricter reporting requirements does not come with any new administrative dollars and is viewed by First Nation Health authorities as onerous and punitive. First Nations will be required to accept this new policy and adhere to these new requirements if they wish to continue to receive Health Transfer funds. Commenting on the process of communication with FNIHB, the Health Director notes:

> Any new policies that come out, we are usually the last to find out. There is no input or consultation with First Nations, it is usually from FNIHB and that's it. When they are called upon to verify which Aboriginal people they consulted with, they can never come up with any names, you know, it is almost like a slap in the face. This happened at our last meeting when we met about dental issues and chiropractic care, when they were called upon they couldn't give us any names, they just say it's our Aboriginal group. We asked, could you at least give us one name, and they couldn't even do that.

Clearly there is ineffective communication of policy between First Nations and the government, and a clear disregard on the part of FNIHB for the principle of consultation or collaboration with the First Nations in policy making. Because of the "no enhancement" provisions of Health Transfer and the increased costs of basic health services such as NIHBs, the government has increased the financial burden on First Nations. The Long-Term Evaluation of Health Transfer (Health Canada 1995:16) recommended changes to the area of policy formation to reflect more consultation and input from First Nations, yet no changes have been made that address the recommendations in this report.

The continuing unilateral and paternalistic relationship between the federal government and First Nations is lamented by community members, who were asked to comment in their health surveys (2000) whether or not they felt the government understood their needs. Many residents took the time to respond to this question, and their comments can be divided into three key themes: they feel government bureaucrats are not in the community and so have no way of understanding people's needs, they have an "Indian is Indian attitude" and are not seeing the uniqueness in each Aboriginal community, and they fail to provide adequate funding when needs are obvious.

It can be seen from this discussion that a policy implemented by the government with little to no input from the communities (or, at best, superficial input) cannot foster a sense of self-determination. While the policy does allow for communities to make certain administrative decisions, they must do so within the specifications of the policy. Warry (1998:96) observed that Health Transfer did not result in true community control in the case of his experience with the North Shore Tribal Council; that the community was still answering to MSB, which continued to make all final decisions. Speck (1989:197) points out that Health

Transfer policy simply puts Aboriginal people in the lowest levels of health care administration in the Canadian health care system. From our perspective of external evaluators charged with assessing the effectiveness and efficiency of health services delivered under the Transfer Policy, it appears that the FNIHB is using the evaluation requirements merely to seek assurances that First Nations can competently deliver services. Yet the FNIHB is disregarding recommendations from the evaluations that might require them to reconsider the "no enhancement" provisions. Thus, even when presented with an independent assessment of First Nations services and health governance, and evidence of the effectiveness of community-based services, the FNIHB seems unwilling, or incapable, of building on this success by developing policies that would recognize enhanced Aboriginal capacity in health care.

While no one interviewed in Wikwemikong used the term "disempowering," a feeling of defeat and disempowerment was evident in the management group during the fieldwork period. Terms used such as "handcuffed" and "slap on the hand" support the contention that Transfer continues under old paternalistic models and that the power is still concentrated in the hands of the government. It is fair to say that the Health Transfer process has been equally frustrating for the community. This suggests that what was once considered a cutting-edge policy and a point of departure from paternalism in Aboriginal health care in Canada has become stale and has fallen back into paternalistic postcolonial relationships.

The Impact of the Policy

Beyond the deficits of the process itself are the impacts of the policy after implementation. In Wikwemikong, there is no doubt that the community and Health Centre staff take pride in their success in administering health services.

> Prior to Health Transfer MSB was calling the shots, they were running everything. Now, we can do what we want with these dollars, which is good, providing we adhere to the immunizations, communicable disease reports, and annual reports and financial, as long as we provide these items they're happy. It has given us the freedom to address a lot of the concerns in the community (Health Director, Wikwemikong Health Centre).

One of the FNIHB's objectives is to have communities define their needs and then move funds into those areas. Wikwemikong's goals included the delivery of wholistic health services and the revitalization and integration of traditional medicine. However, Health Transfer will not fund traditional medicine or mental health programming. Much of Health Transfer funding is used to deliver mandatory programs, and to support underfunded FNIHB programs, such as NIHB and

Environmental Health, so that the amount of money available to initiate and run community health programs based on needs is limited.

A 1988 needs assessment identified a variety of other service needs for the new Health Centre including programs focused on obesity, arthritis, diabetes, heart problems, nutrition, on-reserve medical transportation, family healing programs, and mental health programs. Many of these same needs continued to be identified by the community in 2000.[8] Some of these needs, like diabetes programming, are met through stand-alone programs funded by a provincial organization. This program is highly successful, in part because managers and workers have been given leeway to deliver a culturally appropriate program for the community. The Health Centre also provides a Traditional Indian Medicine program, which works closely with the diabetes program and operates the healing lodge found in the Health Centre. This program operates with a minimum budget, which draws on Health Centre's global budget. Despite the demonstrated success of the program and its designation as a priority need from the community's perspective, FNIHB continues to refuse to support traditional medicine programs. A representative from MSB addressed the issue during the July 2000 meeting:

> I hear your arguments about traditional medicine, but there is no money for this. You have to move your own funds into it—because of the liability factor we can't say we are funding any traditional medicine program in any First Nation, even though we believe in it.

The FNIHB argument is that they are unwilling to assume malpractice liability risks they feel are associated with delivering traditional medicine services. However, Health Transfer requires First Nations to acquire insurance coverage and submit proof of that coverage to FNIHB as part of the Community Health Plan. Coverage for traditional medicine liability is available in Canada and has been purchased by the Wikwemikong Reserve. Despite the explanation provided by the regional director above, there is no liability factor for FNIHB.

Mental health issues such as suicides, violence, and depression were all found to be community concerns in the 2000 needs assessment. The lack of a mental health strategy or funding initiative from FNIHB has made the delivery of these services in a culturally appropriate manner very difficult. The federal government provides patchwork funding to mental health through Health Transfer and other initiatives, such as the Aboriginal Healing Foundation (AHF). The result is a mental health system that is heavy in administration and light in workers. The lack of a mental health strategy from FNIHB was discussed at the July 2000 meeting between FNIHB and Wikwemikong leaders. The following question was addressed to the MSB representative by one of the mental health administrators: "Why isn't there a mental health policy developed at the federal level? Because they would have to then fund it?" The

MSB representative stated, "Mental health remains an issue, but there is no money. There is crisis money available—this is a proposal driven process." As with other "one time funding," the proposal-driven process increases the administrative dollars necessary to run the Health Centre. Further, this "crisis"-driven approach has been universally criticized by Chiefs at the national level, who argue that they are placed in a position of watching their children die before being able to apply pressure to the government to provide funds for crisis intervention or prevention programs.

What is common throughout these examples is the expressed need for more funding and the inability to negotiate for it. Health Transfer funding is based on the on-reserve population size at the time of signing the contract (Warry 1998). At the time of the 1988 needs assessment, the on-reserve population in Wikwemikong was reported to be 2,385. By 1999, the population on reserve had grown to 2,729, an increase of 345—more than the population of many First Nation reserves. Yet there was no provision in the 1999 agreement for the population growth.

In addition to the problems with servicing an increasing population with the same base funding, the no-enrichment clause also limits First Nations' ability to develop new programs to respond to increasing rates of disease or to respond to new reporting requirements. Beyond these financial burdens, there is also the possibility of new health needs or threats arising. For example, for Bands transferring 5–10 years ago, HIV/AIDS may not have been a priority.

The experience in Wikwemikong has shown that Health Transfer does not provide funding to meet the needs of the community. With no enrichment available, Wikwemikong is not able to use the funding to meet the goals and objectives of the policy, namely, needs-based and culturally appropriate programming. The Health Director has put forward the argument to the regional director that their health promotion efforts have been working, "The community is now at the point where they want the services, they want the healing. Transfer is not enough to meet the need."

The Health Director makes an interesting point; an emphasis on health promotion in the early years of Health Transfer has in fact increased awareness of prevention and intervention in the community. However, without enhancement to the agreements, the Health Centre is unable to provide many of the intervention or treatment services that they have been advocating. Some 15 years after the Health Transfer process began, the former Grand Chief of the Assembly of First Nations, Matthew Coon Come, stated:

> Many First Nations are served by clinics that are woefully understaffed and ill equipped. Non-aboriginal communities of comparable size have modern multi-bed hospitals with fully equipped emergency services and operating rooms. It is pitifully easy to demonstrate that medical services for First Nations are inadequate (Matthew Coon Come 2001).

His point is experienced in Wikwemikong where over 2,700 people live without a hospital; yet two regional (Island) hospitals are located in two much smaller, non-Aboriginal communities.

Conclusions: The Rhetoric of Self-Determination

Perhaps it should not be expected that a policy such as Health Transfer will have an impact on how health is experienced in a community; but it is worthwhile to note that there have not been any improvements in health status in Wikwemikong since the introduction of the policy. The pretransfer rates of some chronic illnesses have increased since the 1988 needs assessment; for example; the percent of community members reporting they have diabetes increased by 5 percent, chronic respiratory disease/lung problems by 6 percent, and obesity by 30 percent; those reporting they smoke has increased by 13 percent (now standing at 60 percent of the community members).[9] Health promotion activities such as screening and workshops may explain some of the increase; that is, more people may now be aware that they have a disease than were aware before transfer. However, given the general trends for First Nations, this is not a surprising finding. Wikwemikong continues to realize increasing rates of most diseases, higher rates of disease than the general Canadian population, and, in fact, higher rates of most diseases than the average rates for First Nations (FNIRHS 1999).

First Nations need action now; the health of the communities cannot wait for further policy debates.

> This is not the time to listen to Justice Canada lawyers who claim that health services are not treaty rights. We cannot continue to live with substandard treatment facilities while we argue about offloading to provincial health authorities, or transfers to aboriginal health authorities that are not receiving the funding required to provide decent health services. . . . We will no longer tolerate the enormous gap that separates the state of our health, the health of First Nations people form the rest of Canada (Coon Come 2001).

Shortly after the Health Transfer Policy was created, the Assembly of First Nations (AFN) criticized the policy as assimilationist, as a means for the federal government to relinquish its responsibility for health, and as a strategy to cut costs associated with Aboriginal health care (1988, cited in Gregory et al. 1992:220). This view was supported by the Union of Ontario Indians (Waldram et al. 1995:238). Yet despite these criticisms, the vast majority of First Nations in Canada have participated in the transfer process over the past decade. The question this chapter poses is whether Health Transfer Policy is truly an attempt to foster the movement of First Nations toward self-government or, rather whether the government simply uses this rhetoric to disguise a policy of cost-containment. George

Erasmus, the former co-chair of the Royal Commission on Aboriginal Peoples (RCAP) and former Grand Chief of the Assembly of First Nations, has stated that a key strategy of the federal government in recent years has been to "use our language, but not the concepts they are meant to convey in program and policy formation" (Erasmus 1986:60).

Even having eliminated references to self-government in the Transfer policy, the government clings to the rhetoric of self-determination. It has been argued that movement toward models of self-government occurred during a time when the federal government, faced with a fiscal crisis (national debt), was looking for ways to reduce long-term spending on Aboriginal people. Using the rhetoric of self-government legitimizes their actions to the public (Angus 1991:32).

> Too often, Ottawa has appeared willing to appropriate the rhetoric of change, distort it to suit political purposes, and put "token" aboriginals in positions of "power" to legitimate the reform process in the eyes of the public (Fleras and Elliot 1992:53).

What has been argued elsewhere regarding self-government in general (Angus 1991:33) is applicable to the debate over whether Health Transfer Policy actually recognizes the need for self-determination in health care. If Health Transfer truly represents a movement toward self-government, funding would need to increase in relation to community-identified needs and the demonstrated ability to delivery effective health services. Self-government requires resources, and in the case of First Nations, resources are extremely limited. Poor economic conditions and unhealthy communities mean that there is little opportunity to develop self-sustaining resources or a tax base in the foreseeable future. In reference to self-government, Angus (1991:33) writes: "Given the conditions in most Native communities, Native people will be left with little more than the responsibility for administering their own poverty." What is necessary, as the RCAP report has argued (1996), is for the federal government to pursue a course of long-term investment in Aboriginal communities until such time that improved health, decreased welfare reliance, and increased employment are realized.

The inability of Wikwemikong to secure funding for traditional medicine and mental health limits the degree to which the First Nation can truly base programming on community needs. The process of Transfer "renewal" or nonnegotiation was, if anything, disempowering for those involved. Paternalism prevailed during those talks as well as in subsequent discussions on funding. Is the policy assimilationist, as the Aboriginal critics have suggested? Managers frequently comment on the fact that they are still following someone else's policies and that the lack of administrative funding makes it difficult for them to develop their own policies to reflect their own culture and beliefs. Certainly, the failure to fund wholistic and traditional approaches to health and mental health limits the ability of First Nations to achieve culturally appropriate health care systems.

Communities such as Wikwemikong are faced with increasing pressures as current health care funding has been calculated based on an assessment of need and population figures from six or more years ago, yet the disease burden of communities has increased and will continue to increase in the future. First Nations are faced with new and increasingly onerous contractual obligations if they are to continue to receive federal dollars. And while the financial and administrative difficulties associated with the Transfer Policy are increasingly evident, the changes to the principles of the policy are equally damaging to community morale. The removal of the First Nations' ability to negotiate these agreements and the explicit omission in the new policy of any recognition that agreements might serve as a tool to work toward self-determination have created a process that is now disempowering communities.

Given the limited scope of Health Transfer Policy, it is clear that it cannot and was not intended to address self-determination in health care. It appears as though the Government of Canada is providing funds only to meet the original commitment to health as stated in the Indian Act: to control the spread of disease and provide sanitary conditions. It also appears that the policy does not have the potential to improve the health of First Nations, as the major causes of poor health among Aboriginal people are beyond the mandate of Health Transfer. Further, First Nations have little control over meaningful decision-making processes—ultimate responsibility remains with FNIHB. And, although it has been over six years since the government-sponsored evaluation of transfer recommended a mechanism for community involvement in policy formation (Health Canada 1995), policies are still developed and imposed by the government. Wikwemikong has shown the capability and desire to participate in policy formation, but they are held back by a bureaucratic process that restricts them to old paternalistic relationships.

The Health Transfer policy was introduced during a time when the Canadian government was attempting to reduce spending and fight deficits. In the years prior to the implementation of the policy, the government had made many attempts to offload health care responsibility to the provincial governments. It is clear that despite the rhetoric, self-determination is not what is motivating the government's support of the Health Transfer Policy. If the government were truly serious about implementing a policy that would work to reduce disease, heal communities, and foster self-determination, then the policy would have been updated to reflect evaluation recommendations. There would also be recognition, in the form of enhanced funding, of the various national and community reports documenting the increasing levels of disease and population counts on reserves. But the existence of a policy cloaked in the rhetoric of self-determination allows the government to claim that they are acting progressively in the area of health care. Indeed, it can be suggested that by assuming the rhetoric and ideal of self-determination, the government becomes more impervious to criticism. And it is precisely because some administrative control over health care has been relinquished at the local level that deeper relations of power can be sustained. The historical review of the major policy events suggests that the formation of Health Transfer Policy was guided by political-economic factors, as opposed to a true recognition of Aboriginal rights to self-determination in health or a commitment to improving the lives of Aboriginal people in Canada.

The fact that the communities are experiencing so many difficulties in implementing this Health Transfer Policy suggests that better planning and consultation, collaborative policy making, and improved financing of this program are necessary in order to increase its credibility and, ultimately, its effectiveness. As it stands, Health Transfer Policy appears to be nothing more than a superficial bureaucratic solution to the very real and deeply rooted sociocultural problems facing First Nations in Canada.

Acknowledgments

This research would not have been possible without the generosity of the Wikwemikong people. Chi Miigwetch to everyone who took the time to share their knowledge with us. Special thanks to the Wikwemikong Health Centre staff, managers, health boards, and committees who took time for research discussions and helped ensure that the research process worked for all involved. This research was supported by the Social Sciences and Humanities Research Council of Canada and by the School of Graduate Studies at McMaster University.

Notes

1. Following the Royal Commission on Aboriginal People Report (RCAP 1996), whenever possible the terms "Aboriginal" and "First Nation" are used for the first inhabitants of Canada. On some occasions prior terminology, "Native" and "Indian" are used to refer to a specific policy name: for example, the Indian Health Transfer Policy.

2. The authors were involved in Health Transfer Evaluation research in Wikwemikong and other Manitoulin First Nations in 1999 (Jacklin and Warry 2000). Jacklin began Ph.D. field research at the Wikwemikong Health Centre in January 2000. Her research is carried out under the principles of participatory action research and the Seven Grandfathers teachings. Her work closely parallels what Singer has termed "community-centred praxis," incorporating the principles of PAR and CMA (Singer 1993, 1994). Ethnographic methods employed include key informant interviews, document review, participant observation, and a community members needs-assessment survey.

3. The responsibility for Indian health is not clearly defined in the British North American Act (1867) or the Indian Act (1874). Yet, paragraph 73 of the Indian Act gives the Minister power to control the spread of disease, provide medical treatment and services, promote sanitary conditions on reserve, and force hospitalization and treatment for infectious disease (Young 1984:258). Aboriginal people view federal responsibility for health care as a right deriving from treaties. As we discuss below, the degree of provincial intervention in Indian health varies greatly.

4. One area not discussed due to space limitations is environmental health, a program area originally proposed as part of Transfer, but that for many years was under a moratorium as the MSB continued to administer the services. Environmental health is a very important area for First Nations; clean water and sanitary living conditions are basic to a healthy life. Wikwemikong is particularly disadvantaged in its ability to provide environmental health services given its size, as federal policies do not take geographic circumstances into consideration.

5. The term "culturally appropriate" met with resistance during this research. It is generally felt that the term is being used without an appreciation for the cultural diversity present in the community, and that what some feel is culturally appropriate, others would not.

6. Despite calling this a renewal and not a negotiation, the government added a total of seven new clauses in the sections: Financial Sections, Annual Reporting to the Minister, Authority of the Minister to Conduct Audit, Community Health Plan, Termination, Special Provisions, and Applicable Laws; reworded four clauses; and omitted four clauses (Wikwemikong Transfer Renewal Agreement 1994, 2000).

7. Notification to this effect was sent to Bands in a letter from the assistant deputy minister of Health Canada in a March 16, 2001, letter (Health Canada 2001). The letter stated,

> Over the next few weeks, my senior managers from the FNIHB across the country will be in touch with you to share with you the revised standardized agreement documents. These documents reflect the new Treasury Board policy and responds to a number of important observations made by the Auditor General to the department last year.

8. The 2000 needs assessment identified funding needs for the traditional medicine program, diabetes program, and mental health programs. In addition, it recognized the need to decrease smoking rates (a shift in attitude from the 1988 survey) and an increased emphasis on health promotion.

9. Health status indicators are drawn from self-reported data in the 1988 and 2000 community members needs assessments. These two needs assessments were conducted by different researchers using different methodologies; while both are valid and reliable sources of information, comparisons of the data should be interpreted cautiously.

References

Angus, M. (1991). *"And the Last Shall Be First": Native Policy in an Era of Cutbacks.* Toronto: NC Press.

Auditor General of Canada. (2000, October). "Health Canada–First Nations Health Follow-Up." In *Report of the Auditor General of Canada to the House of Commons,* chapter 15. Cat. no. FA1-2000/2-15E. Ottawa: Minister of Public Works and Government Services Canada.

Canada. (1986). *Interim Report: Subcommittee on the Transfer of Health Programs to Indian Control.* Ottawa: Medical Services Branch.

Coon Come, M. (2001, February 25). Speech given at National Health Conference: First Nations Health: Our Voice, Our Decisions, Our Responsibility. Assembly of First Nations.

Deber, R., and E. Vayda. (1992). "The Political and Health Care Systems of Canada and Ontario." In *Case Studies in Canadian Health Policy and Management,* vol. 1, edited by R. B. Derber, 1–15. Ottawa: Canadian Hospital Association Press.

Erasmus, G. (1986). "NSR Comment: Indian Policy in the New Conservative Government, Part III: The Neilson Task Force in the Context of Recent Policy Initiatives by Sally Weaver." *Native Studies Review* 2, no. 2: 53–63.

First Nations and Inuit Regional Health Survey (FNIRHS). (1999). *First Nations and Inuit Regional Health Survey, National Report.* Ottawa: First Nations and Inuit Regional Health Survey National Steering Committee.

Fleras, A., and J. L. Elliot. (1992). *Aboriginal-State Relations in Canada, the United States, and New Zealand.* Toronto: Oxford University Press.

Frideres, J. S. (1998). *Aboriginal Peoples in Canada: Contemporary Conflicts.* Scarborough, Ontario: Prentice Hall Allyn and Bacon Canada.

Gilmore, A. (1979). "Indian Health Care: What the Dispute Is All About." *Canadian Medical Association Journal* 121: 87–94.

Graham-Cumming, G. (1967, February). "Health of the Original Canadians, 1867–1967." *Medical Services Journal*: 115–66.

Gregory, D., C. Russell, J. Hurd, J. Tyance, and J. Sloan. (1992). "Canada's Health Transfer Policy: The Gull Bay Experience." *Human Organization* 51, no. 3: 214–22.

Health and Welfare Canada. (1992). *Transfer (Health Transfer Handbook).* Ottawa: Health and Welfare Canada.

Health Canada. (1995). *Long Term Evaluation of Transfer: Final Report.* Ottawa: Institute for Human Resource Development.

———. (1996a). *Report on the Health of Canadians: The Federal, Provincial and Territorial Advisory Committee on Population Health.* Ottawa: Minister of Supply and Services Canada.

———. (1996b). *Your Environmental Health Program.* Cat. no. H34-67/1995E. Ottawa: Minister of Supply and Services Canada.

———. (1997). *Health Promotion in Canada: A Case Study.* Ottawa: Minister of Public Works and Government Services Canada.

———. (1999a). *Statistical Report on the Health of Canadians: The Federal, Provincial and Territorial Advisory Committee on Population Health.* Ottawa: Minister of Supply and Services Canada.

———. (1999b). *Toward a Healthy Future: Second Report on the Health of Canadians: The Federal, Provincial and Territorial Advisory Committee on Population Health.* Ottawa: Minister of Supply and Services Canada.

———. (1999c). *Transferring Control of Health Programs to First Nations and Inuit Communities, Handbooks 1 to 3: Program Policy.* Ottawa: Health Canada, Transfer Secretariat and Planning Directorate, Medical Services Branch.

———. (1999d). Ten Years of Health Transfer First Nations and Inuit Control. Cat. No. H34-104/2000. Ottawa: Minister of Public Works and Government Services Canada.

———. (2001). Letter to Wikwemikong Health Centre from assistant deputy minister of health Canada. File number 01-103124-100. Ottawa: Health Canada.

Indian and Northern Affairs (INAC). (2001). *About Governance: Communities First: First Nations Governance.* Ottawa: Indian and Northern Affairs Canada.

Jacklin, K., and W. Warry. (2000). *Wikwemikong Unceded First Nation Health Transfer Evaluation Report.* Northwind Consultants, prepared for the Wikwemikong Health Board. (Unpublished community report held at the Wikwemikong Health Centre.)

Lalonde, M. (1974). *A New Perspective on the Health of Canadians: A Working Document.* Ottawa: Minister of Supply and Services Canada.

Royal Commission on Aboriginal People (RCAP). (1996). *Volume 3: Health and Healing.* Ottawa: Minister of Supply and Services Canada.

Singer, M. (1993). "Knowledge for Use: Anthropology and Community Centred Substance Abuse Research." *Social Science and Medicine* 37, no. 1: 15–25.

———. (1994). "Community-Centred Praxis: Toward an Alternative Non-Dominant Applied Anthropology." *Human Organization* 53, no. 4: 336–44.

Singer, M., and H. Baer. (1995). *Critical Medical Anthropology.* Amityville, NY: Baywood Publishing.

Speck, D. C. (1989). "The Indian Health Transfer Policy: A Step in the Right Direction, or Revenge of the Hidden Agenda?" *Native Studies Review* 5, no. 1: 187–213.

Stout, M. D. (1990). "The Role of Participation in First Nations Health Development: Is Transfer an Empowering Process?" *Synergy* 3(2/3): 1–3.

Warry, W. (1998). *Unfinished Dreams: Community Healing and the Reality of Aboriginal Self-Government.* Toronto: University of Toronto Press.

———. (2000). *Mnaamodzawin Health Services Health Transfer Evaluation Report.* Northwind Consultants, prepared for the Mnaamodzawin Health Board. (Unpublished community report held at the Mnaamodzawin Health Centre.)

Waldram, J. B., D. A. Herring, and T. K. Young. (1995). *Aboriginal Health in Canada: Historical, Cultural, and Epidemiological Perspectives.* Toronto: University of Toronto Press.

Warry, W., and J. Sunday. (2000). *M'Chigeeng Health Services Health Transfer Evaluation Report.* Northwind Consultants, prepared for the M'Chigeeng Health Committee. (Unpublished community report held at the M'Chigeeng Health Centre.)

Weaver, S. M. (1993). "The Hawthorn Report: Its Use in the Making of Canadian Indian Policy." In *Anthropology: Public Policy and Native Peoples in Canada,* edited by N. Dyck and J. B. Waldram, 75–97. Montreal: McGill-Queen's University Press.

Wikwemikong Community Health Plan (WCHP). (1989). *Wikwemikong Community Health Plan (WCHP).* (Unpublished community report held at the Wikwemikong Health Centre.)

———. (1994). *Wikwemikong Community Health Plan (WCHP).* (Unpublished community report held at the Wikwemikong Health Centre.)

———. (2001). *NAHNDAHWEH TCHIGEHGAMIG Wikwemikong Community Health Plan,* vols. 1–2. (Unpublished community report held at the Wikwemikong Health Centre.)

Young, T. K. (1984). "Indian Health Services in Canada: A Sociohistorical Perspective." *Social Science and Medicine* 18, no. 3: 257–64.

Land and Rural New Mexican Hispanics' Mistrust of Federal Programs: The Unintended Consequences of Medicaid Eligibility Rules

15

SARAH HORTON

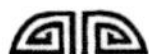

THIS CHAPTER EXAMINES why rural Hispanics continue to be underrepresented on the Medicaid rolls in northern New Mexico even as the state and federal government have attempted to extend the reach of health care benefits. In 1997, the state of New Mexico implemented Medicaid managed care, which theoretically would "mainstream" Medicaid recipients by extending the benefit of primary care to each Medicaid recipient enrolled. At the same time, the federal government developed a new policy of "presumptive eligibility," which accelerated the Medicaid enrollment process for individuals who appeared to meet income qualifications. Both of these reforms were part of federal efforts to reduce the number of uninsured Americans and to expand the reach of Medicaid to individuals who qualified for them but were not enrolled.

Despite these efforts, a gulf remains between the number of New Mexican Hispanics presumed eligible for Medicaid and those enrolled. New Mexico first attracted national concern in 1995, when it came to light that 24 percent of the state's children were uninsured, compared to 14 percent of children nationwide. An estimated 86 percent of these uninsured children were eligible for but not enrolled in Medicaid (New Mexico Health Policy Commission 1998). While presumptive eligibility outreach efforts have since reduced the number of unenrolled children, many eligible persons remain without benefits. New Mexico continues to lead the nation with 22 percent of its population uninsured in 2000. Sixty percent of adults who reported that they were unable to afford health care coverage in 1998 in fact met state income criteria for Medicaid eligibility and thus would be eligible if they had dependent children. Hispanics are overrepresented among the uninsured; in 1998 they comprised 43 percent of the uninsured but only 30 percent of the state's population (Reynis and Alcantara 2000:20).

Scholars have pointed to a number of factors contributing to the underutilization of welfare benefits, ranging from cultural barriers to obstacles in the enrollment and eligibility process. This chapter examines the cultural factors that have contributed to rural New Mexican Hispanics' reluctance to receive Medicaid benefits. I show that many rural Hispanics view the welfare system as an extension of the American legal system that had historically dispossessed them of their land. This case study illustrates that policy change must be not only community driven, but also attentive to the broader historical context of oppression, of which such policies may be perceived as a logical extension.

Methods

The findings presented here are part of a broader University of New Mexico ethnographic study on the effects of Medicaid managed care (MMC) on the health care safety net in one rural and one urban New Mexican county.[1] Researchers were onsite to observe the startup of New Mexico's Salud! program in July 1997 and returned to conduct additional phases of study at three subsequent nine-month intervals. Over this period, we conducted over 1,300 hours of fieldwork at 15 different health care sites, including nonprofit community health centers, hospitals, and welfare agencies.[2]

Because our study was multisited and used a longitudinal approach, our findings were able to illuminate the changing strategies of health care safety net providers as they responded to the financial pressures of Medicaid managed care (Horton, McCloskey, Todd, and Henriksen 2001). The experiences of Medicaid managed care that emerged most from this study were those of health care providers and staff, the employees charged with putting health care policies into practice. As critical medical anthropologists, however, a primary research concern of ours was the effects of this health care reform on Medicaid patients. How could we better give voice to the "submerged, fragmented, and largely muted subcultures of the sick" (Scheper-Hughes 1990:189)—or, at least, illuminate the experiences of rural Hispanics with the health care system?

To do this, I conducted fieldwork at La Luz,[3] a rural nonprofit community clinic, about Hispanics' experiences with the health care and welfare system. La Luz is a Federally Qualified Health Center (FQHC) that was established in 1971 in order to improve health care access for medically underserved residents in Rio Arriba County. At the clinic, I conducted over 60 interviews with three important sets of informants: (1) providers, (2) clerical workers, and (3) patients. I supplemented these with interviews with those knowledgeable about rural Hispanics' experiences with the health care and welfare system, including (1) workers in a well-known county social services agency, and (2) workers at the state Income

Support Division, the agency that certifies individuals' eligibility for welfare and Medicaid benefits.

This chapter follows the critical medical anthropological tradition of exploring the macrosocial and macropolitical forces that affect the health care access of specific groups. Providing a valuable corrective to public health's emphasis on the individual's responsibility for his or her own health status, critical medical anthropology has instead illuminated the way that prevailing structures of inequality profoundly affect the health status of minority groups. Following Baer, Singer, and Johnsen (1986:95), then, I present here a "dialectical examination of contending forces in and out of the health arena that impinge on health and healing." Baer et al. (1986) call for an examination of how processes of power operating at multiple levels in the health care system—at the macrosocial level, the level of the health care institution, that of the doctor-patient relationship, and finally the individual level. Due to space constraints, this chapter will dwell on the macrosocial level, illustrating the way that historical processes of colonization have left a legacy of rural Hispanic mistrust of federal programs.

The Rural Context

Rio Arriba County, the focus of this study, is a poor, predominantly Hispanic county. Hispanics comprise 73 percent of the county's population. Twenty-three percent of families with children under 18 were living at or below poverty level in 1999 (U.S. Census 2000). Meanwhile, 21.5 percent of county residents did not have health insurance in 1998, compared to roughly 15 percent nationwide (Reynis and Alcantara 2000). Contributing to the region's poverty is its colonial past. Spanish colonists first settled the region in the sixteenth and seventeenth centuries and created a "homeland of continuous settlement." Yet following the U.S. annexation of New Mexico in 1848 and its linking to the East by railroad, Anglo settlers expropriated Hispanic land through outright theft, swindle, and legal sleight of hand (Montoya 2002). Residing on a dramatically diminished land base, rural Hispanics have been the focus of sporadic national concern due to their "underdevelopment" and resistance to attempts to change their rural lifeways.

Under the Balanced Budget Act of 1997, the federal government phased in a number of health care and welfare reforms intended to increase health care access while reducing spiraling health care costs. First, the state allowed qualified community outreach workers to temporarily qualify women and children for Medicaid based on "presumptive eligibility"—or the preliminary determination of eligibility based on a declaration of family income below the state's Medicaid income eligibility guidelines. This reform moved eligibility determination from welfare offices to social service workers conducting outreach, helping mitigate low-income families' fears of an arduous Medicaid application process. As a General Accounting Office report (1991) put it, determining eligibility on the spot "conveys a message of inclusion rather than exclusion early in the application process." This reform was intended to recapture eligible Medicaid recipients who had fallen off the rolls in the wake of the welfare reforms of 1996.[4]

Secondly, the government also allowed states to mandate that Medicaid recipients participate in MMC. Under MMC, the state turned its budget for the Medicaid population over to three for-profit managed care organizations (MCOs) who in turn "manage" the services received by Medicaid patients. Once a patient has chosen an MCO, he or she selects from that MCO's list of approved primary care providers (PCPs), who are solely responsible for that patient's care. By assigning each Medicaid patient a PCP who serves as a "gatekeeper," MMC would in theory reduce unnecessary referrals and emergent care. Thus, MMC's proponents argue that the reform would reduce health care costs while improving health care access and continuity of care (Eichstaedt 1996).

However, health care analysts have questioned whether managed competition would work in a rural context due to a lack of health care services and of a dense population base (Kronick, Goodman, Wennberg, and Wagener 1993; Slifkin, Hoag, Silberman, Felt-Lisk, and Popkin 1998). Lack of transportation, long distances to access care, as well as cultural and literacy issues complicate patient access in rural areas. Moreover, analysts have pointed to the discrepancy between the number of those eligible for welfare benefits and those enrolled as indicative of both cultural and systemic obstacles to the utilization of Medicaid benefits (Ellis and Smith 2000; Urban Institute 2001). Rio Arriba County is one such site in which welfare benefits have historically been underutilized. What explains rural Hispanics' underutilization of welfare benefits? How might welfare and health care policies themselves contribute to the low numbers of Hispanics enrolled?

Cultural and Systemic Obstacles to Medicaid Eligibility

Lack of Familiarity with Primary Care

A predominantly rural and poor colonized region, northern New Mexico has historically been medically underserved. It was not until the 1970s when the federal government made grants available to create community health clinics in medically underserved areas that residents could access a stable source of primary care. Because of the scarcity of medical care, most rural Hispanics are not only unfamiliar with the concept of primary care, but also view it as a luxury.

Interviews with rural patients at La Luz revealed the broader context that has bred this lack of familiarity with primary care. Estevan, one Hispanic man who visited the La Luz clinic, explained that a "country doc" had been the sole provider of health care for the population of the remote rural village of Chama when he was a child during the 1960s. The Cumbres-Toltec Railroad, which first entered northern New Mexico in the late 1880s, later brought this "country doctor" to the area to care for its employees. Because he was the only doctor administering to Hispanics and Anglos in the area, this man acquired the status of a folk hero. "Dr. Dunham delivered everybody in that town," Estevan explained. "He delivered me, my mom, and my dad. I know for sure he delivered at least four generations."

Through such "country doctors," Hispanics had access to only the most rudimentary primary care. Medical supplies were scarce and visits to the doctor reserved for circumstances of dire need, Estevan recalled. "If a kid came in and was sick, he'd either give him penicillin or sulfur. If it didn't require that, you wouldn't get good medical care. . . . He had his whole clinic in a bag about this big," he said, pointing to his wife's purse. Even the county's seat and largest city, Española, offered a choice of only three doctors during the 1950s. Rather than resort to receiving care from an unfamiliar institution, rural Hispanics have instead traditionally relied on folk healers such as *curanderas* and *sobadoras,* who heal with herbs and ritual, and usually know the patients they serve.

Not only do many Hispanics remain unfamiliar with primary care, but they also view the American health system as foreign and suspect. This is especially true for an older generation that is less accustomed to trusting physicians with their care. For example, Linda, a Hispanic woman in her 40s, remembered that her mother had seen the same doctor at a community clinic in Española for 12 years. "Then one day, she walked into the clinic for an appointment, and he wasn't there. She'd come in for a checkup, and they asked her to see another doctor. She wouldn't. She absolutely wouldn't. She said, no, I'll come back when he gets back." One of her mother's primary concerns was that she would have to undress for this new physician, a stranger.

Because of the historical lack of medical resources as well as this mistrust of Western medicine, even many Hispanics in a younger generation remain quick to dismiss their need for routine preventive care. "I never get sick," one Hispanic man without insurance explained. The last time he had been to a doctor was when he needed a physical to play sports in high school—at least 12 years ago, he said. Linda explained that Hispanics of her generation had little familiarity with the concept of preventive medicine. "When I was little, I never knew what a doctor was. If you had whooping cough, you'd go to the doctor. If you had an earache or something, you'd stay home. You'd only come in when you were really sick. I mean, not the sniffles. More like when you were in dire need," Linda said.

Medicaid Regulations and Fluctuating Eligibility

The introduction of Medicaid managed care in Rio Arriba County has only created further obstacles to Hispanics' access to health care. Hispanic patients I interviewed found that MCO and state regulations were difficult to negotiate and created further obstacles to accessing health care. The opacity of such regulations and the remoteness of these agencies contributed to patients' feeling disempowered and unable to manage their own health status.

Complicated eligibility rules under Medicaid led to patients' fluctuating Medicaid eligibility, constituting obstacles to continuity in patient care. The federal government recently made it easier for medically underserved populations like those in Rio Arriba to qualify for Medicaid and welfare through "presumptive eligibility" outreach and enrollment. As a result of aggressive public education efforts and expedited enrollment processes, outreach workers across the nation have been able to enroll more and more individuals on Medicaid. However, at the same time, highly regulated eligibility rules mean that a majority of those newly enrolled are later disenrolled within one year (Carrasquillo, Himmelstein, Woolhandler, and Bor 1998).

In Rio Arriba County alone, outreach workers qualify an estimated 500 to 1,000 new individuals for Medicaid each month, said Darren Griego, the director of the Rio Arriba Families and Children Network (RAFCN), a county provider of social services. At the same time, however, Medicaid eligibility rules that disqualify patients for not providing additional paperwork within a designated window of time have caused many Medicaid recipients to later be disenrolled. Thus, patients who had been assured that they may receive benefits under Medicaid show up at health clinics only to find that they have been disqualified. Griego said,

> The Medicaid system is so highly regulated that it's been very easy for an individual to be disenrolled. . . . We kind of missed the boat in thinking that the problem was simply identifying people and getting them enrolled. It's not just identifying people, it's *keeping* them enrolled.

Presumptive eligibility assumes that individuals qualify for Medicaid on a temporary basis and allows them to receive services before their eligibility is processed and verified by the state welfare office. Since qualifying for Medicaid requires proof of individual and household income, residency, children's births, and household size, many enrollees find that they must return to present additional information. However, if some paperwork necessary for the verification of the enrollee's application is missing, the enrollee will be disqualified within 45 days of application. Moreover, once an individual has been disqualified for want of submitting additional documentation, he or she must wait from three to six months to reapply.

Furthermore, individuals who are eligible for Medicaid benefits because they qualify for welfare find that they must face an even more rigorous scrutiny of their eligibility. Those who receive both Medicaid and welfare benefits must provide documentation reverifying their eligibility at least every three months. "Because it carries cash with it, that one requires more aggressive reporting from clients. Sometimes we recertify them on a monthly basis, sometimes we do it every three months," explained one welfare office employee.

Eligibility for welfare is calculated based on the household's gross monthly income. If the household's income is no longer within federal guidelines for welfare, the applicant must wait three months before reapplying. As a result, some Medicaid recipients find their eligibility fluctuating each time it is recertified. "Let's say you apply this month for that child's Medicaid. And you qualify. The following month, if you work overtime, when you bring in your pay stubs your income could be so high that it disqualifies you," the welfare office employee explained.

As a result of such Medicaid eligibility rules, many patients "fall off" the Medicaid rolls from month to month. Such "fluctuating eligibility" has proven a thorn in the side of health care providers and patients, many of whom have been unaware that their health care benefits had been terminated. Ironically, although one of the state's intended goals in implementing MMC was to improve continuity of care, its highly regulated eligibility rules have led to fluctuating eligibility and discontinuous care. Patients faced with negotiating this highly regulated system frequently receive a message of disempowerment. "The message these patients walk away with is that the system is not negotiable, and there is little they can do to improve their health care status," one Hispanic health care activist commented.

Medicaid Eligibility Rules and the Value Placed on Land

Finally, Medicaid eligibility rules pose an additional problem for the region's Hispanics because they neglect the cultural value of land to northern New Mexicans. The value of land must be placed within the context of New Mexican Hispanics' dispossession at the hands of Anglo colonists. For rural New Mexican Hispanics, family land is a symbol of their deep history in the region and their prior settlement. Because of this legacy, many Hispanics regard Medicaid eligibility rules regarding valued cultural resources, such as land, with suspicion.

Over the course of my fieldwork, many Hispanics I interviewed expressed mistrust and suspicion about the Medicaid enrollment process. "Well, one of the big problems is that if people apply for Medicaid, they have to give up their family land," one Hispanic employee at La Luz confided to me in hushed tones. According to this employee, federal dependency went hand in hand with relinquishing one's valued possessions. As one Hispanic health care activist in Rio Arriba explained, this regulation especially worried those with plots that had been passed on for generations:

> I know that (dispossession) was always a concern of families. Their concern was that if they apply for a public benefit, the government may have access to their land. And this was especially a concern for Hispanic families with deep roots on family land.

Although many Hispanics qualify, many are hesitant to apply for Medicaid because of a fear that it will entail giving up inherited family land. The eligibility rules that the federal government has established for Medicaid disqualify individuals who own land worth at least $1,500 and do not occupy that land themselves. As a worker at the state's welfare office, the Income Support Department (ISD), explained regarding this rule, "If you have a resource of that worth, and your home is not on it, then the state assumes that resource could be sold before you seek assistance."

Analysis of Hispanic attitudes toward the welfare system in northern New Mexico must be placed in the context of Hispanics' oppression by Anglos and the federal government. New Mexico has long formed a "Hispanic homeland" upon which Anglo encroachment has been relatively recent. It was not until the 1920s that the introduction of ranching and mining undermined the self-sufficiency of such Hispanic villages, forcing them to depend upon a new Anglo-dominated economy for their survival (Deutsch 1987). Land has remained a potent symbol of this process of ongoing expropriation. Under the Treaty of Guadalupe Hidalgo concluding the Mexican-American War in 1848, the U.S. government legally ratified the land grants deeded Spanish settlers by the governments of Spain and New Spain. However, following the American occupation of the Southwest, Anglo settlers slowly consolidated Hispanic landholdings through legal sleight of hand, swindling, and debt (Deutsch 1987; Montoya 2002).

The heirs of the original land grants deeded their forebears by the governments of Spain and New Spain—many of whom still occupy small parts of such grants—continue to press Congress for the full restoration of their lands. In 1967, Hispanic activist Reyes Lopez Tijerina staged a raid on the county courthouse in Tierra Amarilla as a dramatic protest. Tijerina's action was motivated, in part, by the federal government's recent revocation of Hispanic farmers' permits to graze livestock in Carson National Forest, part of the historic Tierra Amarilla land grant deeded Hispanic settlers in the seventeenth century. In Tierra Amarilla, a billboard by the highway reminds visitors that the town's Hispanic residents have not forgotten these historic fights. Showing the face of Emiliano Zapata, it reads, "Tierra O Muerte," or "Land or Death."

Because of this past, rural Hispanics tend to view federal programs—the health care system among them—with mistrust and suspicion. Such programs have historically attempted to alter rural Hispanics' livelihoods or to teach them middle-class Anglo behavior and cultural values while contributing little to their overall well-being. For example, historians Suzanne Forrest (1989) and Sarah Deutsch (1987) have shown how the region's present-day poverty and dependence are in part the legacy of New Deal programs of the 1930s. While these programs were ostensibly designed to "preserve" rural Hispanics' traditional lifestyle, they simultaneously aimed to "modernize" them by transmitting Anglo middle-class economic behavior norms (Forrest 1989:16). Hispanics in turn viewed such programs with "varying degrees of skepticism, cynicism, or guarded optimism in direct proportion to the extent that past experiences have led them to expect injury or help" (Forrest 1989:181).

Thus, many Hispanics regard government benefit programs such as welfare and Medicaid with a similar skepticism. "People would think it's a handout, and they say nothing is free," said one La Luz employee. Simply put, many Hispanics in Rio Arriba feared that they would fall victim to the ongoing process of Hispanic dispossession simply by applying for public benefits.

Conclusions and Implications

What are the implications of this case for other health policies—both nationally and internationally? First and foremost, this case illustrates the way that the implementation of new health policies must be complemented by attention to the historical and social context of the populations they affect. Policy analyses of Medicaid and welfare reform have neglected how such "one-size-fits-all" policies may ill suit particular populations and regions. The federal government's efforts to increase health care access would likely be more successful if its welfare eligibility rules were to take into account the historical value of family plots of land to Hispanics. This case points to the way that anthropological analyses of local attitudes to the welfare and health care system may help public health initiatives be more responsive to community needs.

Secondly, this case study highlights the need for anthropologically grounded analyses of how policy reforms work in practice. The underutilization of welfare benefits in northern New Mexico must be placed within the context of Hispanics' skepticism toward federal intervention in the region. Moreover, grounded fieldwork may uncover the unintended effects of reforms, effects that policy analyses often overlook. While presumptive eligibility welfare policies may help extend benefits to more welfare recipients, they must also attend to the more difficult issue of keeping recipients enrolled. If the federal government were to simplify the recertification process by allowing greater time to lapse between recertification, the extension of welfare benefits to greater numbers of recipients would indeed be a meaningful accomplishment.

Acknowledgments

I am grateful to Caroline Todd, a member of the University of New Mexico ethnographic team, for her help with my understanding of, and locating statistics regarding, Hispanics' underutilization of welfare benefits.

Notes

1. The ethnographic team was based in the Department of Anthropology and the Division of Community Medicine at the University of New Mexico and was led by Principal Investigators Louise Lamphere and Howard Waitzkin. Our research was made possible by a grant from the Agency for Healthcare Research and Quality (1RO1HS09703), on which Howard Waitzkin was the principal investigator.

2. This particular chapter is based on over 130 hours of fieldwork conducted at La Luz.

3. All sites and individuals will be referred to by pseudonyms.

4. The presumptive eligibility clause was part of a federal response to concerns regarding the high number of uninsured children, as well as the number of former Medicaid recipients who fell off the rolls following the welfare reforms of 1996. The 1996 Personal Responsibility and Work Opportunity Act (PRWOA) repealed the Aid to Families with Dependent Children program and replaced it with block grants to the states, ending the linkage between eligibility for cash assistance (Temporary Assistance for Needy Families, or TANF) and Medicaid. While most states have policies in place ensuring that TANF recipients are automatically enrolled in Medicaid, gaps in the recertification process caused a number of low-income individuals exiting the welfare system to be disenrolled from Medicaid benefits as well; see Ellis and Smith (2000).

References

Baer, H. A., M. Singer, and J. H. Johnsen. (1986). "Introduction: Toward a Critical Medical Anthropology." *Social Science and Medicine* 23, no. 2: 95–98.

Carrasquillo, O., D. U. Himmelstein, S. Woolhandler, and D. H. Bor. (1998). Can Medicaid Managed Care Provide Continuity of Care to New Medicaid Enrollees? An Analysis of Tenure on Medicaid. *American Journal of Public Health* 88, no. 3: 464–66.

Deutsch, S. (1987). *No Separate Refuge: Culture, Class, and Gender on an Anglo-Hispanic Frontier in the American Southwest, 1880–1940.* Oxford: Oxford University Press.

Eichstaedt, P. (1996). "Medicaid's Price Tag: New Mexico's Search for a Cure." *Albuquerque Journal,* December 15, A1.

Ellis, E. R., and V. K. Smith. (2000). *Medicaid Enrollment in 21 States: June 1997 to June 1999.* Washington, DC: Kaiser Family Foundation.

Forrest, S. (1989). *The Preservation of the Village: New Mexico's Hispanics and the New Deal.* Albuquerque: University of New Mexico Press.

General Accounting Office. (1991). *Prenatal Care: Early Success in Enrolling Women Made Eligible by Medicaid Expansions.* Washington, DC: GAO.

Horton, S., J. McCloskey, C. Todd, and M. Henriksen. (2001). "Transforming the Safety Net: Responses to Medicaid Managed Care in Rural and Urban New Mexico." *American Anthropologist* 103, no. 3: 733–46.

Kronick, R., D. C. Goodman, J. Wennberg, and E. Wagener. (1993). "The Market Place in Health Care Reform: The Demographic Limitations of Managed Competition." *New England Journal of Medicine* 328: 142–52.

Montoya, M. E. (2002). *Translating Property: The Maxwell Land Grant and the Conflict over Land in the American West, 1840–1900.* Berkeley: University of California Press.

New Mexico Health Policy Commission. (1998). *Health Care in New Mexico: Quick Facts.* Santa Fe: New Mexico Health Policy Commission.

Reynis, L. A., and A. Alcantara. (2000). *Health Care Coverage and Access in New Mexico: An Analysis of the 1999 Health Policy Commission Statewide Household Survey of Health Care Coverage.* Albuquerque: University of New Mexico.

Scheper-Hughes, N. (1990). "Three Propositions for a Critically Applied Medical Anthropology." *Social Science and Medicine* 30, no. 2: 189–97.

Slifkin, R. T., S. D. Hoag, P. Silberman, S. Felt-Lisk, and B. Popkin. (1998). "Medicaid Managed Care Programs in Rural Areas: A Fifty-State Overview." *Health Affairs* 17, no. 6: 217–27.

Urban Institute. (2001, July 2). "Parents' Reasons for Not Obtaining Public Health Insurance for Children More Complex than Once Thought." Urban Institute Press Release. Washington, DC: Urban Institute.

U.S. Census. 2000. *Census of the Population.* Table GCT-P14. "Income and Poverty in 1999." Summary File 3 (SF3)—Sample Data.

The Death and Resurrection of Medicaid Managed Care for Mental Health Services in New Mexico

16

CATHLEEN WILLGING, HOWARD WAITZKIN, AND WILLIAM WAGNER

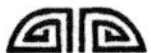

FOLLOWING NATIONAL trends toward privatization of physical and mental health services, state governments have increasingly turned to managed care for their Medicaid programs (Lewin and Altman 2000). There is a pressing need for critical anthropological work assessing the implementation and impact of this major policy reform on health services for the poor (Rylko-Bauer and Farmer 2002; Maskovsky 2000). Recent ethnographic studies suggest that such reform is fundamentally transforming the fiscal, ethical, and professional contexts of contemporary mental health practice (Hopper 2001; Donald 2001; Robbins 2001; Ware, Lachicotte, Kirschner, Cortes, and Good 2000), while often resulting in decreased quality of care and access problems for low-income populations (Maskovsky 2000). Such problems are exacerbated in medically underserved rural areas (Waitzkin et al. 2002).

The social and demographic conditions of rural states intensify the challenges of implementing managed mental health services (Silberman, Poley, James, and Slifkin 2002; Slifkin and Casey 1999). Rural populations comprise a disproportionate share of the uninsured and are at greater risk for mental illness than the general population (Wolff, Dewar, and Tudiver 2001). Geographical isolation, transportation, stigmatization, confidentiality, and limited availability of psychiatric services are common problems in rural areas (Roberts, Battaglia, and Epstein 1999).

In 1997, the Centers for Medicare and Medicaid Services (CMS), a federal body that oversees state Medicaid programs, granted the largely rural state of New Mexico a waiver to implement a fully capitated Medicaid managed care system for physical and mental health services. Despite opposition from providers, patient advocates, and Medicaid recipients, who believed that mental health services should remain separate from managed care, the state established an "integrated" delivery system. In October 2000, after an onsite review prompted by the reporting of serious system deficiencies, CMS required the removal of mental health services from the new program. However, in an unprecedented action, CMS later reversed its decision.

As part of a multimethod study of Medicaid reform in New Mexico (Waitzkin et al. 2002), we conducted in-depth interviews and onsite observations at mental health safety-net institutions—organizations that historically have provided services to the poor. These organizations included inpatient hospitals, residential treatment centers, and outpatient clinics located in one urban county and one rural county. Sixty-five interviews were conducted with staff, clinicians, and patients at these sites, and with behavioral health organization administrators and state officials. We also reviewed program monitoring data and documents pertinent to New Mexico's Medicaid reform. In this chapter, we report our ethnographic findings to illustrate the reform's impact on mental health safety-net institutions and examine the implications of CMS's atypical decisions for the accountability of federal oversight in state Medicaid programs.

New Mexico Context

Rates of poverty, unemployment, alcohol and drug deaths, and suicides in New Mexico rank among the highest in the nation (Waitzkin et al. 2002). Twenty percent of 1.8 million residents receive Medicaid. In 1994, during Democratic Governor Bruce King's administration, the state legislature had mandated the creation of a Medicaid managed care program in an effort to curtail expenditures for public sector health services. King's administration had favored a "carve-out" approach to managed care, in which mental health services would have been funded and administered separately from the physical health portion of a non-profit Medicaid program.

The course of health policy in New Mexico shifted when Republican Governor Gary Johnson took office in 1995. The Johnson administration advanced an "integrated" managed care program in which three for-profit managed care organizations competed for contracts to provide physical and mental health services to Medicaid recipients. Inexperienced in the provision of mental health care, the managed care organizations contracted separately with behavioral health organizations to deliver such specialty services. As corporate entities based in states other than New Mexico, these organizations then contracted with local mental health organizations, referred to as regional care coordinators, adding another administrative and financial layer to the system. Finally, the regional care coordinators contracted with direct service providers.

In July 1997, the new program was officially instituted for all Medicaid recipients, except those in nursing homes or on Medicare. Unless they formally "opted out" of the program, Native Americans on Medicaid were automatically enrolled. The state government mandated the inclusion of the chronically mentally ill at the inception of the program, although most other states first targeted the healthier segments of the Medicaid population (Waitzkin et al. 2002). The new Medicaid program was "rolled out" first in urban areas, allowing three months before its implementation in rural areas, where greater access problems were anticipated. In most other states, such programs began and remained in urban areas; when rural areas were included, participation was voluntary for Medicaid recipients (Slifkin and Casey, 1999).

Ethnographic Findings

Administrative responsibilities and reimbursement. Administrative work at mental health safety-net institutions increased after Medicaid reform, as providers interacted with multiple managed care entities. Urban and rural safety-net institutions sustained financial expense in complying with credentialing, paperwork, and utilization review requirements, without which behavioral health organizations would delay or withhold service authorizations and payments.

All safety-net personnel whom we interviewed underscored the link between paperwork and reimbursement. One administrator said:

> [The behavioral health organizations] all have different forms to fill out. If you don't fill them out correctly, they can refuse payment. They'll [often] tell you that there's a problem with your paperwork and send it back. You do the changes on the paperwork and send it in. Then they tell you that there's another problem and they send it back. The whole time they're waiting to send you the payment.

By increasing the complexity and number of actions required to deliver mental health services, and by creating administrative obstacles to receiving reimbursements, Medicaid managed care markedly augmented administrative work at safety-net institutions while diminishing revenue.

Stress, turnover, and quality of care. The increased workload resulting from managed care contributed to stress and burnout for some mental health clinicians. A social worker, who had reluctantly returned to work at a rural residential treatment center, disclosed:

> I was working here for two years when I decided to quit. I couldn't take it any more. I was working a minimum of 50 hours a week and being paid for less than 40. I was trying to be a therapist. I ended up doing more case management and secretarial work than therapy. . . . I quit this job recently because of managed care's hassles. . . . The center is perpetually understaffed these days. It means that I have to pick up the slack.

The informant explained that deteriorating morale in the workplace and organizational changes prompted by Medicaid reform contributed to the shortage of clinicians in the rural county. A licensed professional clinical counselor at another rural residential treatment center stated:

> I am barely making a living because of Medicaid. I can hardly meet my expenses with the salary that I am making and the workload is incredible. It is such a hard job. To do it well you need to have skills as a therapist, a case manager, and as a bureaucrat. You have to be good at working the system if you want to be an advocate for these patients. On top of it, the supervision here isn't very good because experienced clinicians don't last very long in this system. I have had more than five supervisors in the past two years.

The frustration conveyed in these comments was common among the providers we interviewed.

The frustration that pervaded clinical settings did not deter state officials and behavioral health organization administrators from their belief that Medicaid managed care was essential for ensuring that providers practiced responsibly. Under the fee-for-service system, these officials and administrators claimed, Medicaid patients were placed in costly institutional environments—especially residential treatment—for prolonged periods, even though their conditions did not necessarily warrant such intensive treatment and providers did not demonstrate that the patients benefited from these services. As a result of Medicaid reform, behavioral health organizations undertook the task of utilization review, which involved authorizing requests from providers for residential treatment and all requests for services made on the behalf of Medicaid recipients.

State officials and behavioral health organization administrators professed their commitment to services that enhance familial involvement in the care of the mentally ill without separating patients from their communities. Conventional residential treatment, they argued, undermined this commitment. Through utilization review, providers were encouraged to rely on less expensive services purportedly available within local communities, including outpatient therapy, day treatment, and case management. They considered these forms of care to be in accordance with best practices and more effective than residential treatment. However, the shift to community-based care was not accompanied by the redirection of funding for those services.

In spite of their attempts to abide by utilization review processes, clinicians feared that they could not adequately serve Medicaid recipients because behavioral health organizations did not authorize required levels of care for appropriate lengths of time. One psychiatrist no longer participated in Medicaid managed care because it was "fundamentally unethical." Allotted eight minutes per clinical consultation, she felt unable to assess patients' clinical status. A second psychiatrist, complying with his ethical standards of clinical practice, continued services without reimbursement for a suicidal Medicaid recipient after the behavioral health organization denied outpatient therapy. Consequently, he started "cherry-picking," scrutinizing referrals for Medicaid recipients, weighing the financial risks they posed, and seeing only those in need of minimal intervention. Psychiatrists also expressed concern that managed care limited them to medication management, while formulary restrictions prevented Medicaid patients from filling prescriptions.

Continuity of care and access. When Medicaid managed care was first implemented, many patients continued to use their prior providers. Continuity of care for some patients was compromised when their providers ceased participation in Medicaid because of work-related stress and low reimbursements. One parent in the urban county commented on the difficulties of securing outpatient services for her son, a minor:

> I watched the news. I heard the talk about Medicaid managed care. I paid attention because my son was on Medicaid. He saw this therapist for five years. She turned us away when managed care came in. As did his psychiatrist. They weren't taking Medicaid kids anymore. . . . I didn't actually have a clear understanding until he was turned away.

Another parent in the urban county disclosed what his family experienced as they sought inpatient care for his son, also a minor. Against the advice of a psychiatrist, the boy was turned away from three separate hospitals because staff members presumed the behavioral health organizations were unlikely to agree that his illness episode required intensive treatment:

> My son was in a crisis period. . . . We took him to a psychiatrist, who strongly recommended that we get him into a hospital. . . . We took him to one hospital. They said, "Is he suicidal? Has he threatened to hurt himself or others? Is he hearing voices? Is he actively psychotic?" I said, "No." They wouldn't take him. . . . Three days later we were in acute crisis. We went to a second hospital. . . . They said, "Is he trying to hurt himself? Is he trying to hurt others? Is he psychotic?" . . . They wouldn't take him. We took him to a third hospital. They told me the same thing verbatim. . . . "It's not our criteria," they said. It was the insurance companies that controlled quietly the fact that my kid couldn't get into the hospital because he wasn't suicidal or homicidal.

This parent sought help from an elected state official, who worked with the family and was finally able to obtain care for the son.

Case management. Case management involves coordinating health and social services for mentally ill individuals residing within community settings. Behavioral health organizations intended to rely on case management as an alternative to residential treatment. For example, one behavioral health organization administrator concurred that case management is essential to the care of patients diagnosed with chronic mental illnesses. He stated, "In this office, there're almost no restrictions on how much case management we'll authorize for a person."

Ironically however, as inpatient services in New Mexico became less accessible under Medicaid managed care, case management positions became harder to fill due to large caseloads and low wages. A social worker in the urban county commented:

> Case management isn't a glamorous job, but it's important to the New Mexico Medicaid population. . . . At the level that I'm working with my clients, it's obvious that they aren't going to improve their situations by themselves, but there's no one willing to do case management for what behavioral health organizations pay.

Reductions in case management, particularly in rural regions, increased the workloads of clinicians caring for Medicaid recipients. As case management decreased, coordination of health and social services fell to clinicians or was neglected entirely. Respondents reported a similar lack of coordination of care between physical health providers and mental health clinicians.

Legal actions and investigations. Several legal actions called into question the system for mental health services. In 1998, plaintiffs in a lawsuit argued that the new system failed to meet the needs of children with chronic mental health conditions (Shapiro et al. 1998). One year later, a legal audit commissioned by the state's attorney general revealed that the system lacked adequate appeal processes and protections of patients' rights, assurances of timely and appropriate referrals, and assurances that managed care contractors fairly represented the services they delivered (Office of the Attorney General 1999).

In 2000, the state Medicaid agency investigated behavioral health organization utilization review practices. It uncovered serious problems in chart documentation of clinical case files, including improper denials and poor discharge planning. This report verified that Medicaid recipients were being placed in lower levels of care than their conditions warranted (Medical Assistance Division 2000). Reports by regional care coordinators also confirmed decreased access to services in rural areas (Martinez 2000; Rio Grande Behavioral Health Services 2000).

Medicaid managed care changed the environment for safety-net institutions sufficiently that their capacity to provide services to Medicaid recipients was jeopardized. Sixty child and adolescent mental health programs closed between 1998 and 2001 (Waitzkin et al. 2002). Many agencies that remained open reduced services because of economic constraints. During the year after the reform's onset, a psychiatric hospital in Albuquerque reported a 33 percent decrease in revenues. Hospital administrators attributed this decline to the reform. In an attempt to conserve financial resources, they terminated the hospital's adolescent residential treatment program.

Fewer clinicians served Medicaid recipients under managed care. There was a net decline of seventeen child psychiatrists in New Mexico since 1997. Of forty-seven licensed child psychiatrists, nine did not accept Medicaid (Legislative Finance Committee 2000). Eighty-six percent of psychologists accepted Medicaid before managed care's implementation; only 34 percent did so afterward (New Mexico Psychological Association 1998). Due to the decline in clinicians and services, mental health safety-net institutions assumed heavier work burdens, while recipients of Medicaid experienced longer waits for care. The weakening of the state's mental health care infrastructure led recipients, providers, and patient advocates to declare that Medicaid reform in New Mexico had created to a crisis of severe consequence, especially for the safety-net institutions.

Federal Intervention

CMS's changing decisions. Key events that occurred during our research underscore the controversies surrounding Medicaid managed care for mental health services in New Mexico. During the summer of 2000, CMS considered the state government's request to renew the Medicaid program's waiver. The state government downplayed indications that the reform had compromised mental health services. However, recipients, providers, and advocates organized to change the mental health portion of the system, garnering support from the state's bipartisan congressional delegation in the process. Citing documents reviewed above, these groups argued that behavioral health organizations were out of compliance with Medicaid contracts and that the state was not imposing appropriate sanctions. They argued that managed care had hurt residential treatment centers in New Mexico because numerous facilities had closed. Especially in rural areas, advocates reported increasing shortages of both residential and outpatient mental health services.

In September 2000, responding to mounting public pressure and intervention from the congressional delegation, CMS conducted an onsite review of the Medicaid program. CMS representatives met with Medicaid recipients, providers, and patient advocates for three days. These groups articulated concerns about access to services and argued that CMS should reconsider the mental health portion of the Medicaid program. The Legislative Finance Committee (2000), which had audited Medicaid mental health services at the request of state legislators, shared its findings with the CMS review team. While CMS requires state governments to provide evidence that their Medicaid programs are cost-effective, the committee's audit demonstrated a disproportionate diversion of financial resources to administrative services, as only 55 percent of Medicaid managed care funds earmarked for mental health services in 1999 were distributed to providers.

As a result of the review, CMS revoked the state's waiver on October 19, 2000, and gave New Mexico 90 days to transition the mental health portion of its Medicaid program into a fee-for-service structure. State officials expressed an intention to appeal CMS's decision after the inauguration of President George

W. Bush. Governor Johnson stated in a letter to Tommy Thompson, incoming secretary of the Department of Health and Human Services, that reversal of CMS's decision was "my only request from his [President Bush's] new administration when I met him at his Crawford ranch on January 6, 2001" (Johnson 2001). All of the state's congressional representatives urged Secretary Thompson to acknowledge the "devastating problems" caused by Medicaid managed care as he considered nullifying the denial (Waitzkin et al. 2002).

On February 16, 2001, in an unprecedented move, CMS retroactively approved the state government's request to provide mental health services under the extant service delivery model. This approval was contingent upon a list of conditions, which included the implementation of mechanisms to act upon patients' concerns and complaints and intensive monitoring procedures. CMS also required the creation of an advisory committee composed of recipients, providers, and other stakeholders to redesign mental health services under Medicaid.

Medicaid managed care since CMS's decisions. The state government modified the delivery of mental health services under Medicaid managed care. In July 2001, the state government eliminated the behavioral health organization contracts; managed care organizations were required to contract directly with providers. In May 2002, the state government sanctioned one managed care organization for inadequate delivery of mental health services to Medicaid recipients. This event marked the first occasion in the five-year history of Medicaid managed care in New Mexico that sanctions were applied to pressure managed care organizations to improve their performance. However, in the effort to sustain their profit margins, such corporations are increasingly terminating Medicaid managed care contracts in less lucrative rural settings (Silberman et al. 2002). Given this context, New Mexico faces the prospect that managed care organizations will withdraw from the Medicaid marketplace if state oversight becomes too exacting (Fossett et al. 1999).

Discussion

The impact of Medicaid managed care on safety-net institutions has raised significant concern nationwide (Lewin and Altman 2000). In New Mexico, such reform affected access to and quality of mental health services and adversely impacted safety-net institutions, particularly in rural areas. While the reform was intended to improve mental health practice, the new system led to administrative burdens, payment problems, and stress among clinicians. It diminished incentives to care for the poor and exacerbated access problems for Medicaid recipients. The state's mental health care infrastructure was downscaled by 60 programs. Our data indicate that the advantages of fully capitated Medicaid managed care programs for cost control, access, and quality assurance may be diminished in medically underserved states with large rural populations. Because our study focused on a single state, additional research is needed to compare the impacts of Medicaid managed care in states with differing policies, populations, and urban versus rural characteristics. Evidence from other rural states indicates that problems resemble those observed in New Mexico (Silberman et al. 2002; Chang et al. 1998).

The federal government's role in overseeing Medicaid waiver programs also warrants close monitoring. CMS's decision not to renew New Mexico's waiver was based on the acknowledgment of serious system deficiencies and illustrates the capability of local groups and federal agencies to hold state governments and managed care organizations accountable for corporate expansion in the public sector. CMS has required corrective action in mental health services delivery under Medicaid managed care in other states, particularly Tennessee (Chang et al. 1998). Nevertheless, the decision to withdraw a waiver was unprecedented. CMS's reversal of this decision calls into question its willingness and ability to implement its regulatory responsibilities. The U.S. General Accounting Office (2003) has confirmed that CMS is not providing consistent oversight of state waivers. The intervention of the Bush administration in support of New Mexico's Medicaid policies for mental health services further suggests that CMS's capacity to monitor state Medicaid programs with local input has become more restricted.

Acknowledgments

This work was supported by grants from the Agency for Healthcare Research and Quality (IR01 HS09703) and the National Institute of Mental Health (IR03 MH65564). The authors thank Sarah Horton, Louise Lamphere, Cindy Foster, and Rafael Semansky for their helpful comments.

References

Chang, C. F., L. J. Kiser, J. E. Bailey, M. Martins, W. C. Gibson, K. A. Schaberg, et al. (1998). "Tennessee's Failed Managed Care Program for Mental Health and Substance Abuse Services." *JAMA* 279: 864–69.

Donald, A. (2001). "The Wal-Marting of American Psychiatry: An Ethnography of Psychiatric Practice in the Late 20th Century." *Culture, Medicine & Psychiatry* 25: 427–39.

Fossett, J. W., M. Goggin, J. S. Hall, J. Johnston, C. Plein, R. Ropper, and C. Weissert. (1999). *Managing Accountability in Medicaid Managed Care: The Politics of Public Management.* Albany, NY: Nelson A. Rockefeller Institute of Government.

Hopper, K. (2001). "Commentary: On the Transformation of the Moral Economy of Care." *Culture, Medicine & Psychiatry* 25: 473–84.

Johnson, G. (2001). *Letter to Tommy Thompson.* Santa Fe: State of New Mexico Office of the Governor.

Legislative Finance Committee. (2000). *Audit of Medicaid Managed Care Program (SALUD!) Cost Effectiveness*. Santa Fe: State of New Mexico Legislative Finance Committee.

Lewin, E., and S. Altman. (2000). *America's Health Care Safety-Net: Intact but Endangered.* Washington, DC: National Academy Press.

Martinez, L. (2000). *Trends in Community-Based and Day Treatment Services.* Santa Fe, NM: Presbyterian Medical Services, Behavioral Health Network Service Center.

Maskovsky, J. (2000). "'Managing' the Poor: Neoliberalism, Medicaid HMOs, and the Triumph of Consumerism among the Poor." *Medical Anthropology* 19: 121–46.

Medical Assistance Division. (2000). *Salud! On-Site Program Integrity Review.* Santa Fe: State of New Mexico Human Services Department.

New Mexico Psychological Association. (1998). *New Mexico Survey of Salud! Managed Care Programs.* Albuquerque: New Mexico Psychological Association.

Office of the Attorney General. (1999). *The Law and Health Issues in New Mexico.* Santa Fe: State of New Mexico Office of the Attorney General.

Rio Grande Behavioral Health Services. (2000). *Evaluation of Access to Care.* Las Cruces, NM: Rio Grande Behavioral Health Services.

Robbins, C. (2001). "Generating Revenues: Fiscal Changes in Public Mental Health Care and the Emergence of Moral Conflicts among Care-Givers." *Culture, Medicine & Psychiatry* 25: 457–66.

Roberts, L. W., J. Battaglia, and R. S. Epstein. (1999). "Frontier Ethics: Mental Health Care Needs and Ethical Dilemmas in Rural Communities." *Psychiatric Services* 50: 497–503.

Rylko-Bauer, B., and P. Farmer. (2002). "Managed Care or Managed Inequality? A Call for Critiques of Market-Based Medicine." *Medical Anthropology Quarterly* 16: 476–502.

Shapiro, D., C. Bettinger, P. Cubra, P. Gaddy, B. Hall, and D. Ely. (1998). *Taylor v. Johnson,* no. 98-09776, Second Judicial District County of Bernalillo, State of New Mexico.

Silberman, P., S. Poley, K. James, and R. Slifkin. (2002). "Tracking Medicaid Managed Care in Rural Communities: A Fifty-State Follow-Up." *Health Affairs* 21: 255–63.

Slifkin, R., and M. Casey. (1999). "State Laws and Programs that Affect Rural Health Delivery." In *Rural Health in the United States,* edited by T. I. Rickets, 95–100. New York: Oxford University Press.

U.S. General Accounting Office. (2003). *Federal Oversight of Growing Medicaid and Home and Community-Based Waivers Should Be Strengthened.* Washington, DC: General Accounting Office.

Waitzkin, H., R. L. Williams, J. A. Bock, J. McCloskey, C. Willging, and W. Wagner. (2002). "Safety-Net Institutions Buffer the Impact of Medicaid Managed Care: A Multi-Method Assessment in a Rural State." *American Journal of Public Health* 92: 598–610.

Ware, N. C., W. S. Lachicotte, S. R. Kirschner, D. E. Cortes, and B. J. Good. (2000). "Clinical Experiences of Managed Mental Health Care: A Rereading of the Threat." *Medical Anthropology Quarterly* 14: 3–27.

Wolff, T., J. Dewar, and F. Tudiver. (2001). "Rural Mental Health." In *Textbook of Rural Medicine,* edited by J. P. Geyman, T. E. Norris, and L.G. Hart, 181–84. New York: McGraw Hill.

Sugar Blues: A Social Anatomy of the Diabetes Epidemic in the United States

17

CLAUDIA CHAUFAN

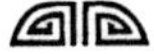

The Social Construction and Production of Disparities in Diabetes

On September 27, 2000, the *San Francisco Chronicle* announced the discovery of a gene, first reported in *Nature Genetics* (Horikawa et al. 2000), that appeared to explain why Mexican Americans are at high risk of type 2 diabetes (Maugh 2000:A1).[1] Earlier that same year, the *Los Angeles Times* had given a different account of risk disparities for this and other diseases: Mexican Americans were at disproportionately higher risk when compared to non-Hispanic whites because of a "startling lack of health insurance" that "forced them to miss out on the benefits of early detection" (*Newsday* 2000). Yet another perspective on risk disparities appeared in the *New York Times* almost exactly a year later, reporting a study from the *New England Journal of Medicine* (Tuomilehto et al. 2001) that provided "convincing evidence" that obesity and a sedentary lifestyle account for a high risk for diabetes, and that better diet and exercise can delay or prevent the disease (Nano 2001).

Whether explanations about disparities in diabetes rely on genes, access to health care, or lifestyle, experts agree that the variety known as type 2 is increasing worldwide in epidemic proportions. In the United States, it affects close to 16 million women, men, and children, killing close to 400,000 people every year (American Diabetes Association 2001). It has been pointed out that diabetes affects people of any age, gender, or nationality, "including all races and ethnic groups, the rich and the poor" (Permanent Subcommittee on Investigations of the Committee on Governmental Affairs 1999:5). It has also been claimed that "prosperity" has produced the perfect environment for diabetes to flourish (Bernstein 2000). Yet these claims are not the whole story behind this epidemic. First, while diabetes *may* affect all groups, it is not an "equal opportunity disease." Among African Americans, Hispanics, and Native Americans, the risk of suffering from diabetes is approximately 2, 2.5, and 5 times higher, respectively, than among non-Hispanic whites. Nor are the complications of diabetes distributed equally. End-stage renal disease (ESRD), a major complication of poorly managed diabetes, is 4 times higher among African Americans, 4 to 6 times higher among Mexican Americans, and 6 times higher among Native Americans than among non-Hispanic whites (American Diabetes Association 2001). Second, diabetes is not, at least not unambiguously, a "disease of prosperity." The World Health Organization has suggested that in the next 30 years cases of diabetes are likely to increase by 200 percent in developing countries, yet only by 45 percent in developed countries. Within the latter, diabetes is likely to strike harder at the socially disadvantaged. Thus it is the poor, not the prosperous, who will bear "the brunt of the diabetes epidemic in the 21st Century" (Jervel 1998:6).

Now, the word "prosperity" here does not refer to *all* wealth, but merely to wealth of a particular kind: availability of calories, which, as the history of famines has shown, is not to be taken for granted. But prosperity so measured is enjoyed by all social groups affected by diabetes, so while it may explain the overall increase in rate, it can't explain the disparities. Furthermore, it is perfectly compatible with, and tends to conceal, other forms of social deprivation. The poverty dimension of diabetes is further concealed by the biological mechanisms underlying this and other noncommunicable diseases (NCD)—among which diabetes is paradigmatic—as they emerged as the "new epidemics" in the twentieth century. At the turn of this century, changes in fertility and mortality rates throughout the nineteenth century, resulting from some combination of improved hygiene, sanitation, and nutrition, and the actions of the "medical police" had boosted the world population. This *demographic transition* was accompanied by a *health transition*—a change in patterns of population health—the key factor of which was the reduction of infectious disease (McMurray and Smith 2001). When antibiotics were introduced later into the twentieth century, it seemed that humanity had finally got rid of the scourge of infection, which up to that moment had been the paradigm of disease (Porter 1997).[2]

Yet poorly understood changes—related to rapid industrialization and urbanization—were setting the stage for new ills of an entirely different nature, ills that did not seem to call for, or respond to, the public measures that had effectively controlled infectious disease. Epidemics of smallpox or cholera had necessitated broad-based interventions—immunization, treatment, or isolation—if all, or most, social groups were to be spared. In contrast, with new emerging diseases, the fact that some people were affected seemed irrelevant to whether others were or not. What protected from these diseases were by and large "save oneself" strategies and personal resources. As in the past so today, the poor have been ill-equipped to gather the resources necessary to avoid those "unhealthy lifestyles and behaviors of the industrialized world" such as "inadequate physical activity [and] unsatisfactory diets" (Jervel 1998:6), that lead to diabetes and other diseases.

While poverty has rarely been subjected to the same scientific scrutiny as, say, insulin resistance, in most research on the diabetes epidemic in America, many theories have sprung up to explain the rapidly increasing rate of diabetes and its disparities, most of them linking lifestyle with some gene or genes (Bernstein 2000). There are powerful reasons to believe that lifestyle is an important factor in the causation of diabetes type 2—even more so than genes. After all, it is more plausible that changes in the lifestyle of American youth account for the dramatic rise in the last ten years of cases of type 2 diabetes among youth and children than any substantial change in the genetic pool of this population, where, interestingly, disparities are appearing along clear social categories even as the "new epidemic" emerges in front of our eyes (Kaufman 2002). Furthermore, sound empirical evidence has shown that diabetes can be delayed, if not prevented, through lifestyle changes (Tuomilehto et al. 2001), and at any rate, no single gene or genes have been pinned down as *the* mark for the disease, at least so far.

Yet the causal role of lifestyle is an important truth only to the extent that people have actual control over their lives. If lifestyles are constrained by larger structural and political arrangements, as much sociological theory suggests, then this fact about diabetes would be a rather shallow truth, and an overemphasis on it would leave the larger problem unresolved at best. At worst, it would lead, as it often does, to a narrow understanding of causality that views disease "as the price (paid) for excesses of diet and 'life-style' (resulting from) weakness of the will or a lack of prudence" (Sontag 1988:11) and to the blaming, albeit subtle, of those affected.

Yet another problem that in my view obscures the understanding of the structural mechanisms underlying the diabetes epidemic is the many referents of the word "environment," depending on the unit of analysis and on the theoretical framework adopted. In a narrowly defined biomedical sense, environment refers to that which surrounds the gene, and thus what individuals do (i.e., their health-related behaviors) becomes the environment for that gene or genes. This is how the diabetes medical literature uses "environment." A journal article illustrative of this approach and discussing risk factors in diabetes refers to eating and exercise habits as "obesity-promoting environments" and to health care professionals encouraging patients to voluntarily modify these habits as "therapeutic approaches focused on the environment" (Filozof and Gonzales 2000). The environmental health literature, which points to the *physical* environment surrounding human beings (in the totality of their genes, behaviors, and psyche), examines the causal role of the environment so defined in many medical conditions (Brown 2000). Complementing this latter use, the sociological literature broadly understands "environment" as encompassing the principles underlying the distribution of social resources, such as institutional arrangements, power relations, and formal and informal normative structures (Fitzpatrick and LaGory 2000).

When arguments about disparities in diabetes, as well as in health more generally, point to the environment as the culprit (the nature-nurture debate), they may be referring to different things depending on the theoretical/explanatory framework adopted. Explanatory frameworks matter because societies shape their public policies and decide the use of resources depending on what they see as the source and cause of their problems. And when social resources are limited, as they usually are, support for certain measures often means neglecting others. Thus scarcity may demand that a society choose either to concentrate on features of individuals at risk or to implement societal changes to protect all social groups as if "everybody were at risk." As it has been suggested, in the best of all worlds "the whole society" would lead a healthy lifestyle (Hirsh 2002b), clearly an impossible pursuit unless the *physical and social environments* are conducive to it.

In contrast to *modern risk factors epidemiology*—which looks at features of and within individuals to explain disease in human populations—studies in the tradition of *social epidemiology* have theorized about mechanisms causally connecting disease with social stratification. The fundamental difference between these two epidemiological traditions lies in where they place the emphasis in the chain of disease causation. Because disease is not randomly distributed across social groups and because disparities stubbornly persist through time despite changes in the knowledge of, and intervention upon, particular risk factors (proximal causes of disease), it follows that none of these factors per se can account for this historical persistence. It also follows that eliminating any *particular* risk factor may eliminate disparities in a *particular* disease, yet it is unlikely to erase overall health disparities across social groups. Even if it did, new risk factors pointing to new "diseases" may be "discovered" in the future and result in new disparities.

When history is factored into the equation, it appears that money, power, access to knowledge, and social connections have enabled those who are better off, in the past as well as today, to gather whatever resources are available at a particular time, place, and state of knowledge to secure conditions to stay healthy, and that individual pathways (i.e., individual risk factors) mediating the relationship are less important than the totality of socioeconomic location itself (Link and Phelan 2000). This line of studies is rare in the diabetes literature—it provides poor material for a "scientific breakthrough." Whenever *rates* of morbidity in diabetes—a social fact in a Durkheimian sense—differ among social groups, the causes are assumed to lie within "risk factors"—features of individuals such as their culture, their behaviors, their genes—in a classic case of "individual fallacy," a sort of "ecological fallacy" in reverse (Brown 2000).

Why a social anatomy of the diabetes epidemic in the United States? Why such analysis in the context of current health policies? As a diabetes clinician, I am perfectly aware of the role of lifestyle and genes in the proximal causation of diabetes. However, social inequality and poverty are increasing in America (Krugman 2002; Clemetson 2003), setting clear limits on people's actual choices and, as I have suggested, undermining the lifestyle argument.[3] Therefore, I contend that a sociological analysis of diabetes epidemic is overdue, especially because the widespread acceptance of the "genes plus lifestyles" theory of diabetes has major policy implications, as I try to illustrate throughout this essay. My social anatomy of this epidemic in the United States draws from a variety of sources: two (unpublished) studies presented at professional conferences (Chaufan 1999, 2001), where I examined barriers to treating diabetes from the perspective of patients and the portrayal of risk for diabetes in the lay and medical literature; ethnographic work as a participant observer of, and professional experience as a diabetes educator for, a Latino community in northern California (Chaufan 2000a); close to ten years of work as a clinical diabetologist in my home country, Argentina; and over 30 years of living with type 1 diabetes. The shortcomings of my empirical data limit their generalizability and reliability, yet the existence and persistence through time of disparities in a host of health conditions—whether acute or chronic—along well-defined social categories provide good reasons to believe that my conclusions, albeit their limitations, may illuminate the diabetes epidemic in America. The overall argument is no "big" news—almost unimpressive—but the mounting belief that "spotting" genetic markers of complex and multifactorial health conditions is the way to eliminate disparities in these conditions, by making it possible to "target" interventions to those "at risk" (Vedantam 2003; Wade 2003), I think, makes a case for this argument all the more urgent.

Accounts of diabetes type 2 that emphasize individual risk factors as the main "causes" of health disparities, to the relative neglect of social/structural factors, operate as a "smoke screen," and turn even the best intentioned interventions into subtly victim-blaming ones, lead to an uncritical placement of medical and behavioral research at the top of the political agenda, depoliticize the epidemic, and diminish the social, political, and moral choices that an alternative construction would entail. To the claim that "intensified biomedical research" will help "conquer diabetes" (Diabetes Research Working Group 1999:1), I counter that the diabetes epidemic is better viewed as resulting from social and political factors—poor medical practices, commodification of health care, "unhealthy" health and social policies, and broader social inequalities. These can only be changed by sounder policies backed up by committed political will leading to "healthier" physical and social environments. While it might be naïve and hopelessly futile to claim that only social and economic justice can "control" the diabetes epidemic, at least aspects of this epidemic can be improved by improving health policies and practices. I now turn to a summary of mainstream accounts of diabetes and its disparities.

Genes and Lifestyle as the "Source" of Disparities in Diabetes: The Official Story

Most medical studies today agree that diabetes type 2 "runs in families"—a claim that tends to be understood as entailing that some gene or genes must be implicated. Yet so far the search for *the* gene has been elusive (Harris 1998; American Diabetes Association 2001). The *genetic/hereditary* approach gives strong support to biomedical research. For instance, a study conducted by the Center for the Advancement of Genomics in Duke University suggests that the screening for genetic predisposition for major diseases such as diabetes, heart disease, or cancer will enable to determine "individualized risk for disease or response to therapy" and better target interventions (Wade 2003:A20). While this view has recognizable strengths in increasing the arsenal against disease, its weakness resides in the way it oversimplifies its etiology.

The *lifestyle* approach suggests that those having the "right" genes (for diabetes) increase their risk of triggering the expression of these genes by choosing the "wrong" lifestyles (i.e., overeating and being sedentary; Diabetes Research Working Group 1999; Lochhead 2000; Pimentel 2000). This approach tends to support behavioral research and public health campaigns aimed at raising awareness about diabetes, particularly among high-risk communities (National Diabetes Information Clearinghouse (NDIC) Diabetes Mellitus Interagency Coordinating Committee 1993; National Diabetes Education Program 2000). Its limitation is that "increasing awareness" may be taken as sufficient to encourage those at risk to make the "right" lifestyle choices.

Motives underlying human behaviors are another area of inquiry. Thus, the *psychological approach* separates psyche from behaviors for the purpose of analysis and examines, among others, coping mechanisms at different stages of development, stages throughout the course of illness, disease identities, and dependence of these on formal or informal support systems. For instance, inability to cope or inadequate support from the family or the local community may explain differences in the course of diabetes and its complications (Auslander et al. 1993; Philoteou 1997). How historically deprived families or "cultural communities" are to become empowered to provide support is often absent from these debates.

Because it has been recognized that health behaviors and psychological makeup are embedded in culture (Kleinman 1995; Fadiman 1997), the *cultural approach* examines lifestyles and psyche in their cultural contexts. Garro (1995) compares lay and health professionals' explanations of diabetes in three Canadian

Anishinaabe communities and suggests that understanding the differences between patients' and practitioners' worldviews may help design better preventive or treatment interventions tailored to the needs of these at-risk communities. Amir, Rabin, and Galatzer (1990) examine cognitive and behavioral correlates of compliance in ethnic communities and consider their implications in diabetes clinical outcomes. Yet this approach often ignores the effect of structural constraints over diabetes outcomes, which follow a logic that is fairly independent from the circumstances surrounding the patient-provider relationship. For instance, a major problem among Native communities worldwide is the poor quality of health care they have access to, or the sheer distance to community health services, not to mention other forms of social deprivation that they are subject to and that jeopardize their health. Improved patient compliance would certainly have no effect on these structural factors of risk.

Last, the *diabetes educational approach* relates the development of diabetes complications to the education in diabetes and training in self-management of patients (Falvo 1996).[4] Views range from encouraging patients to comply or adhere to medical recommendations, to empowering them to make "informed choices" and to become primary decision makers in their daily diabetes care, setting their own disease management goals. Patient empowerment has challenged traditional doctor-patient roles and seems to accommodate best to the nature of chronic disease (Anderson 1995). However, self-empowerment is embedded in a web of social interactions, and when social circumstances are dire they get in the way of people's ability to make meaningful and empowered choices. All of these are accounts of what triggers diabetes or its complications, yet often directly, and clearly indirectly, they refer to disparities in their *distribution* as well.

Medicalization and Depoliticization: An Alternative Story

The accounts described above have recognizable strengths and may lead to improved clinical outcomes in a very real way, yet there is a sense in which all of them construct the "problem of diabetes" around those who bear [the disease] to the relative neglect of structural factors. By this, I mean that information about the benefits of healthy nutrition does not make healthy foods accessible, nor does it counteract the advertising power of the food industry—both "healthy" and "unhealthy"—that often leads to confusion even as increasingly hard-to-disentangle nutrition labels become more "informative." Public recognition of the benefits of physical activity cannot "fix" neighborhoods that are too unsafe to walk in, or provide public transportation that would enable Americans to decrease the use of cars, or compensate for budget cuts that threaten physical education programs in public schools. Well-intentioned "raising-awareness-about-the-dangers-of-diabetes" campaigns are no substitute for accessible preventive health care. Empowering people to become the protagonists of their diabetes care, to set their own goals, and to demand fair and competent treatment from their health providers cannot change a health care system that at best is ill-equipped to deal with chronic disease, and that at worse leaves vast sectors of the population unprotected, precisely those who are vulnerable because they lack the social capital to make the "right choices" to prevent disease in the first place. The pressures that ensue from a range of social deprivations that lead to disparities in diabetes and elsewhere are unlikely to be eliminated until the sources of those deprivations are addressed. In sum, when the leading assumption is that the "problem" lies *within* individuals or communities "at risk"—and this is a matter of degree—accounts may fall into victim-blaming patterns (Ryan 1976).

In my experience as a diabetes educator in a Latino community, failures in the treatment of diabetes were usually attributed to patients—their lack of compliance or cultural barriers to lead "a healthy lifestyle"—who were referred to me by their physicians to be "educated." The poor medical treatments these patients were receiving and the financial barriers to receiving even these treatments, not to mention the broader social factors that put "healthy choices" out of reach of these patients, were rarely mentioned as "the problem" (Chaufan 2000b), despite evidence on the contrary (Hirsh 1999). In another study, patients reported that the main barriers in their diabetes care were the blame that they were subject to by their health professionals when confronted with "failures" in the treatment (largely failure to comply with a "diabetic diet"), or the stigma surrounding a disease that is supposed to ensue from "unhealthy lifestyle choices," in addition to financial barriers in securing diabetes care and supplies (Chaufan 1999). Examining their stories in detail, and being trained not only as a sociologist but also as a clinician and a diabetes educator, it was clear to me that all too often, poor medical practices or dated recommendations (such as dietary restrictions or insulin regimes not endorsed by any current clinical guideline) were creating the major barriers to the effective management of these patients' diabetes. Inadequate dietary interventions and inflexible insulin regimes only add to the burden of a health care system that is ill equipped to deal with the complexities of diabetes (Hirsh 2002a). Last, in a discourse analysis of lay and expert diabetes literature, *individualistic* and *medicalized* arguments about risk of diabetes prevailed (Chaufan 2001). By this I mean that to varying degrees, the assumption underlying this literature was that disparities emerge from *something about* individuals, and that they may disappear if individuals can be changed to stand up to the challenges of unhealthy social environments and policies. I also mean that the problem was seen as one falling primarily under the jurisdiction of the medical sciences and requiring a medical solution. I will comment on the implications of individualizing and medicalizing social problems in the next few paragraphs.

As an aside, I'd like to point to two recurrent issues within this literature: one is the insistence on aiming at agreed-upon "clinical targets," and the other is that of encouraging "evidence-based medicine" to improve diabetes care. While adequate clinical targets and scientific evidence are recognizably important to guide medical practices, both need to be considered in context and may benefit from a sociological analysis. In the case of clinical targets, as the saying goes, one doesn't fatten cattle by weighing them. Insistence on them alone is of little value if it fails to consider years of scholarship pointing to the social roots of disparities in health, which won't disappear by pushing toward tighter targets in clinical measurements. Regarding the demand that practices be based on evidence, it may turn into a double-edged sword if it operates to the detriment of "softer," hard to "demonstrate" interventions, such as spending time with patients, which are critically important in quality diabetes care. Given the economic and political arrangements underlying the organization of medical practice in America today, which a sociological analysis can illuminate, insistence on evidence may conceal interests that have little to do with its alleged purpose—a concern with patients' welfare or setting limits on medical incompetence or greed. Indeed, it has been suggested that rather than encouraging better practices, this insistence is undermining the ideals of many who chose medicine as a vocation (Hirsh 2001). I now turn to some policy-relevant documents in this discourse analysis that are particularly illustrative of my points.

In the "Epidemiology/Health Services/Psychosocial Research" section of *Diabetes Care,* a leading medical journal geared to diabetes specialists, one article suggesting the direction of policy interventions examined several purported risk factors for diabetes and its complications, and concluded that "(low) socioeconomic status . . . can determine a risk (of diabetic complications) not dissimilar from *hard* clinical variables" (Nicolucci et al. 1998:1439). However, the finding that poverty increases risk resulted in a call to the medical community to "design and implement specific educational interventions, *targeted* to the socially disadvantaged strata of the population" rather than a call for major structural change at best, or underscoring the relation between poverty and disease at a minimum. In *Diabetes Advocacy,* a newsletter produced by and for lay constituents in diabetes (in some sense, "natural advocates" within the community), most issues called for "a cure" and demanded an increase in the budget for intensified medical research, or treated coverage for diabetes care and supplies by the health care insurance industry on a state-by-state, or even plan-by-plan, basis. That in America health care depends largely on the ability to pay was not at the forefront of the calls for change.

In the website of the Department of Health and Human Services, I found an illustrative example of the individualistic view on health disparities in one major document, the *Behavioral Risk Factors Surveillance System* (Bolen et al. 2000). This document pointed in detail to low socioeconomic status and insufficient access to health services as independent variables for disparities in diabetes, while suggesting with its title that what were being tracked were "risk behaviors." The same website provided a link to the well-known document *Healthy People 2010* and to its lofty calls for a redoubling of the efforts to "address barriers and reduce disparities for (vulnerable and at-risk populations)." When sorting barriers to "appropriate preventive care" into three categories—patient's, provider's, and system's—"lack of money to pay for preventive care" was classified under "barriers of patients" (Agency for Healthcare Research and Quality Health Resources and Services Administration 2001). This categorization, one could argue, says far more about the American health care system than about American patients. Extremely illustrative was a document that underscored the strong negative correlation between diabetes and SES and mentioned the woeful situation of the uninsured, yet concluded that the "diabetes epidemic" can only be stopped through "intensified biomedical research" (Diabetes Research Working Group 1999:1).

That social failures appear disguised as personal troubles is already a classic sociological concept (Wright Mills 1959). One of the ways to gloss over these failures is to "socially construct" such issues as "medical problems" (Conrad and Kern 1986). This is not to say that they exist only in the eyes of the beholder or that they have no biological substratum. Disparities in diabetes are verifiable through simple counting, and blindness, kidney failure, or foot amputations provide tangible evidence of the effects of chronic high blood sugar on the body. The notion of *social constructionism* is rather a reminder that classifications are not a simple reflection of how the world is, but rather of ways selected by people to represent it (Searle 1995). They have more to do with choices made by people than with facts of the matter. Indeed, calling something a "medical problem" merely because it affects the body shows a narrow understanding of causation, as much public health research has historically shown (Waitzkin 1989).

Many conditions that affect the body and its functions, such as HIV/AIDS or breast cancer, have been successfully reconceptualized as social problems with a medical dimension and thus deserving of medical intervention (Lantz and Booth 1998; Pollock and Vittes 1993). Now these conditions have affected single, identifiable, "oppressed" social groups that gave sufferers the political impetus to organize and the capacity to shift the emphasis away from the medical dimension of these diseases to their social and political aspects (Epstein 1996). In contrast, diabetes type 2 does not affect a single social category. Racial and ethnic minorities or the poor have multiple problems other than diabetes. Maybe this is why the notion that disparities depend largely on biological/behavioral features *of individuals* has only exceptionally been challenged (Chaufan 2000b; Leichter 2000; Maryniuk 2000; Chaufan 2002). One "dark" side to medicalization is the individualization and depoliticization of social problems (Conrad and Schneider 1992). Disparities in diabetes may well be one such case.

Social Policies and Diabetes: Ecologies of Risk

To summarize, mainstream accounts of the diabetes epidemic do not fail to point to factors of the "environment" (a term that I'm now using in a broad sense that includes its physical and sociopolitical dimensions) and to acknowledge what I have labeled "ecologies of risk" in the genesis of disparities in diabetes type 2. Yet, by and large, these disparities are understood as emerging, in the last instance, from *high-risk individuals*—their genes, their lifestyles choices, or whatever. Most public strategies to "control the diabetes epidemic" are bounded by the structures of the existing market-based health care system, whose features are referred to as "a changing health care environment" (Tobin 2000:370). These boundaries give market interests a disproportionate power over other constituencies, and place research, biomedical or behavioral, at the top of the policy agenda. By and large, health professionals think and act within the constraints of these interests, which often affect their ability to provide quality diabetes and medical care (Hirsh 2001; Kershaw 2003). Even advocates are bounded by these interests, limiting themselves to urge politicians to support research for a "cure" or to demand that insurers include what is considered quality diabetes care in their coverage policies.

While few would doubt that it is better not to have diabetes than to have it, the bottom line is that once people are affected, good diabetes care matters (American Diabetes Association 2002a, 2002b). It can make the difference between a productive and happy life and one constrained by disability. Complications from poorly controlled diabetes drive up health care costs, not to mention costs in human suffering, in no small way. Having a usual source of care makes a difference in diabetes clinical outcomes, and having health insurance is a strong predictor of having a usual source of care (Diamant et al. 2003). In the meantime, under the American health care system, Latinos are more than twice as likely as non-Hispanic whites to lack health insurance. Thirty-three percent of all Hispanic-origin Americans are uninsured, including 27 percent of Mexican Americans, 22 percent of African Americans, and 21 percent of Pacific Islanders, in contrast with 10 percent of non-Hispanic whites (Himmelstein and Woolhandler 1994; Famighetti 2000). When concentrating on income rather than on ethnicity (categories that frequently overlap), only 8 percent of those with a household income of $70,000 per year or higher are without health insurance, as compared with 25 percent or over when income falls under $25,000 a year

(Famighetti 2000:899). Last, it is sadly no news that close to 44 million Americans lack any form of health insurance, a strong predictor of which is inability to pay for it, which puts them "at risk" not just of having no access to *quality* medical care but to *any* health care at all (Harrington and Pellow 2001). Lack of health insurance has been labeled "a serious health risk" that needs to be treated "with the same urgency as not wearing seat belts or drunk driving" (Tanner 2000). Rarely, however, is this risk, which strongly correlates with poverty, examined with the same scientific rigor or addressed with the same political will as lifestyle or genes in the examination of disparities in diabetes.

And yet, I am not suggesting that individual risk factors are unimportant. What people are or do at an individual level *does* affect their individual health and deserves attention, yet won't direct effective public policy (Fitzpatrick and LaGory 2000). Public health debates that center on genes or lifestyle choices ignore the very complex ways in which genetic predisposition interacts with environmental context and the dependence of choices on life circumstances, a classic theme in the sociological literature. Indeed, they overlook the significant social-class gradient in patterns of disease that remains after controlling for individual risk factors (Lawlor, Ebrahim, and Davey Smith 2002; Lynch, Smith, and House 2000; Lynch, Davey Smith, Kaplan, and House 2000; Marwick 2002; McKenzie 2003; Ross et al. 2000; Wolfson, Kaplan, Lynch, Ross, and Backlund 1999). This gradient was already suspected at the turn of the nineteenth century—if not before. Nineteenth-century German physician Rudolf Virchow, his best-remembered book *Cellular Pathology* notwithstanding, emphasized social aspects of disease and underscored researchers' roles in advocating social reform (Waitzkin 2000).

My point is that answers to health disparities, in diabetes and elsewhere, may vary depending on how questions about disparities are asked. Granted, eliminating barriers to health care has failed to fully eliminate socioeconomic disparities in health (Robert and House 2000),[5] and racial and ethnic differences in health outcomes for adults with type 2 diabetes seem to persist when controlling for access to health care (Harris 2001). These studies are perfectly compatible with, and can lead to, two radically different directions of research and of policy. One would "control for" access to care and take a close-up look, yet again, on features of those "at risk" that are either known or to be discovered. The other would follow the leading assumption in social epidemiology that because it is the *totality* of socioeconomic location that strongly predicts disparities in health at any given point in time, "access to quality medical care" is only one among the many factors constituting that totality. Because, as a factor, it is easier to isolate and modify than social inequality at large, it is worth concentrating all health policy efforts on it. The choice of direction, I suggest, is more a matter of worldview and social ethics than of available evidence.

My position within, and contribution to, the diabetes type 2 debate[6] is that *at a very minimum,* as long as medical benefits in America remain tied to employment, to being too old or too poor, or to being solvent enough to afford them, it is unlikely that quality preventive and diabetes care services—that would do much to moderate the effects of the epidemic—will be a "choice" for "high-risk" populations. Employer-paid health insurance provides medical care to those who already are at "lower risk" (for the rather obvious reason that they are employed), and piecemeal approaches targeting "special" populations provide band-aid solutions and a mere illusion of change. Managed care, proposed under the current system to offset the problem of rising medical costs, follows the logic of the market to reduce these costs, while remaining competitive. In the language of business, this means cutting costs *while* making profit. Business cannot be blamed for pursuing what is at its very heart. The real question is whether health care is a market commodity or a social good and, in the latter case, whether it should be left largely to the workings of business.

The strength of a sociological analysis lies in that it goes beyond the appearance of individuals and their attributes and examines the underlying social logic, the logic of organizations and institutions, of power relations, of human interests, and of collective values underlying decisions in the distribution of social resources. I suggest that diabetes research needs to address very explicitly the sociological logic underlying the epidemic. Yet research can only inform, not substitute for, human choice and decisions that depend less on fact than on shared values and interests. Social policies reflect these values and interests that no amount of empirical research can prove right or wrong, and that need to be explicitly included in debates about the diabetes epidemic. Advocates in the community should encourage groups who shape discourses and debates in the public sphere to rethink individual and social responsibilities vis-à-vis the best starting points for better, and "healthier," health policies.

Notes

1. In this chapter, I focus on diabetes type 2, formerly known as adult-onset diabetes. The distinction between types 1 and 2, I think, is relevant to a comprehensive analysis of the disease. Type 1 diabetes (formerly known as juvenile-onset diabetes) and type 2 diabetes share many features, yet their pathophysiologies are distinct. Discussions about the "diabetes epidemic" and about the causal role of lifestyle usually refer to type 2, whose "fundamental etiology," I argue, is structural.

2. A belief undermined by new "plagues" such as AIDS in the 1980s and, more recently, SARS.

3. In turn, the genetic argument is weakened by evidence showing that lifestyle changes can delay or prevent the onset of diabetes type 2, and by the fact that rates are increasing at a pace faster than the possibility of there being any substantial change in the genetic pool.

4. Unlike acute disease, where the scope of the patient's intervention in medical decisions is limited (typically, one does not discuss with doctors the frequency or dose within a course of antibiotics or chemotherapy), the treatment of diabetes requires that patients be trained in complex technical skills to be performed daily. Self-management diabetes care refers to the set of such skills that the patient is in an optimum position to perform and that aims at maintaining near-normal blood sugar levels in order to delay or prevent complications.

5. The problem is that much of this research takes *mortality* as the dependent variable. Yet the relevant dependent variable in chronic conditions such as diabetes is *health-related quality of life*, where modern medical care can make a difference by enhancing this quality (Robert and House 2000).

6. I suggest once again that diabetes type 2 is important not just in itself but as a model to think sociologically about so-called lifestyle-related diseases, more generally, and most chronic diseases as well. A fully developed argument would require clinical considerations of diabetes type 2 and of "coronary risk factors" that are beyond the scope of this chapter.

References

Agency for Healthcare Research and Quality Health Resources and Services Administration. (2001). *Healthy People 2010*. Accessed at www.health.gov/healthypeople/document/html/volume1/01access.htm, April 21, 2004.

American Diabetes Association. (2001). *Diabetes 2001 Vital Statistics*. Alexandria, VA: American Diabetes Association.

———. (2002a). "Implications of the Diabetes Control and Complications Trial." *Diabetes Care* 23: S24–26.

———. (2002b). "Implications of the United Kingdom Prospective Diabetes Study." *Diabetes Care* 23: S27–31.

Amir, S., C. Rabin, and A. Galatzer. (1990). "Cognitive and Behavioral Determinants of Compliance in Diabetics." *Health and Social Work* (May): 145–51.

Anderson, R. (1995). "Patient Empowerment and the Traditional Medical Model: A Case of Irreconcilable Differences?" *Diabetes Care* 18, no. 3: 412–15.

Auslander, W., J. Bubb, M. Rogge, and J. Santiago. (1993). "Family Stress and Resources: Potential Areas of Intervention in Children Recently Diagnosed with Diabetes." *Health and Social Work* 18, no. 2: 101–14.

Bernstein, G. (2000). "1999 Presidential Address: The Fault, Dear Brutus." *Diabetes Care* 23, no. 4: 719.

Brown, P. (2000). "Environment and Health." In *Handbook of Medical Sociology*, edited by C. E. Bird, P. Conrad, and A. Fremont, 143–59. Upper Saddle River, NJ: Prentice Hall.

Bolen, J. C., L. Rhodes, et al. (2000). *State Specific Prevalence of Selected Health Behaviors, by Race and Ethnicity—Behavioral Risk Factors Surveillance System, 1997*. National Center for Chronic Disease Prevention and Health Promotion—Center for Disease Control. Accessed at http://www.cdc.gov/mmwr/preview/mmwrhtml/ss4902a1.htm, December 15, 2000.

Chaufan, C. (1999). "Looking through Patients' Eyes: The 'Other' Barriers to Treatment (Abstract)." *Diabetes Care* 48, supp. 1: A160.

———. (2000a, August). "Sugar Blues: A Social Ethical Approach on Diabetes Care." Paper presented at the annual meeting of the Society for the Study of Social Problems, Washington, DC.

———. (2000b). "To Comply or Not to Comply: In Search of the Real Question." *Clinical Diabetes* 18, no. 1: 46–47.

———. (2001). "Sugar Blues: Diabetes Mellitus, Ethnic Communities, and the Social Construction and Production of Risk." Paper presented at the annual meeting of the American Sociological Association, Anaheim, CA.

———. (2002). "Sugar Blues: The Social (Silent) Side of Diabetes." *Clinical Diabetes* 20, no. 4: 207–10.

Clemetson, L. (2003). "Census Shows Ranks of Poor Rose by 1.3 Million. " *New York Times*, A16.

Conrad, P., and R. Kern, eds. (1986). *The Sociology of Health and Illness: Critical Perspectives*. New York: St. Martin's Press.

Conrad, P., and J. W. Schneider. (1992). *Deviance and Medicalization: From Badness to Sickness*. Philadelphia: Temple University Press.

Diabetes Research Working Group. (1999). *Conquering Diabetes: A Strategic Plan for the 21st Century*. Bethesda, MD: National Institute of Health.

Diamant, A., S. Babey, R. Brown, and N. Chawla. (2003). *Diabetes in California: Findings from the 2001 California Health Interview Survey*. Los Angeles: UCLA Center for Health Policy Research.

Duenwald, M. (2003). "Gene Is Linked to Susceptibility to Depression." *New York Times*, A12.

Epstein, S. (1996). *Impure Science: AIDS, Activism, and the Politics of Knowledge*. Berkeley: University of California Press.

Fadiman, A. (1997). *The Spirit Catches You and You Fall Down: A Hmong Child, Her American Doctors and the Collision of Two Cultures*. New York: Farrar, Straus and Giroux.

Falvo, D. (1996). *Effective Patient Education: A Guide to Increased Compliance*. Gaithersburg, MD: Aspen Publications.

Famighetti, R., ed. (2000). *The World Almanac and Book of Facts*. Mahwah, NJ: World Almanac Books.

Filozof, C., and C. Gonzales. (2000). "Predictors of Weight Gain: The Biological-Behavioral Debate." *Obesity Reviews* 1: 21–26.

Fitzpatrick, K., and M. LaGory. (2000). *Unhealthy Places: The Ecology of Risk in Urban Landscape*. New York: Routledge.

Garro, L. (1995). "Intracultural Variation in Causal Accounts of Diabetes: A Comparison of Three Canadian Anishinaabe (Ojibway) Communities." *Culture, Medicine and Psychiatry* 20, no. 4: 381–420.

Harrington, C., and D. N. Pellow. (2001). "The Uninsured and Their Health: Micro-Level Issues." In *Health Policy: Crisis and Reform in the US Health Care Delivery System*, edited by C. Harrington and C. Estes, 56–60. Boston: Jones & Bartlett.

Harris, M. (1998). "Diabetes in America: Epidemiology and Scope of the Problem." *Diabetes Care* 21, supp. 3: C11–C14.

Harris, M. I. (2001). "Racial and Ethnic Differences in Health Care Access and Health Outcomes for Adults with Type 2 Diabetes." *Diabetes Care* 24, no. 3: 454–59.

Himmelstein, D. U., and S. Woolhandler. (1994). *The National Health Program Book*. Monroe, ME: Common Courage Press.

Hirsh, I. (1999). "Diabetes Education (for Doctors)." *Clinical Diabetes* 17, no. 2: 50–51.

———. (2001). "Evidence-Based or Hassle-Based Medicine?" *Clinical Diabetes* 19, no. 2: 49.

———. (2002a). "The Death of the "1800-Calorie ADA Diet." *Clinical Diabetes* 20, no. 2: 51–52.

———. (2002b). "The Prevention of Type 2 Diabetes: Are We Ready for the Challenge?" *Clinical Diabetes* 20, no. 3: 106–108.

Horikawa, Y., N. Oda, N. Cox, X. Li, M. Orho-Melander, and M. Hara. (2000). "Genetic Variation in the Gene Encoding Calpain-10 Is Associated with Type 2 Diabetes Mellitus." *Nature Genetics* 26, no. 2: 163–75.

Jervel, J. (1998). "Early Malnutrition and Diabetes: Why Is Type 2 Diabetes (NIDDM) Becoming so Common in Developing Countries?" *IDF Bulletin* 43, no. 2: 6–7.

Kaufman, F. (2002). "Type 2 Diabetes in Children and Young Adults: A 'New Epidemic.'" *Clinical Diabetes* 20, no. 4: 217–18.

Kershaw, S. (2003). "In Insurance Cost, Woes for Doctors and Women." *New York Times on the Web*. Accessed at www.nytimes.com, June 3, 2003.

Kleinman, A. (1995). *Writing at the Margin: Discourse between Anthropology and Medicine*. Berkeley: University of California Press.

Krugman, P. (2002). "For Richer, Part 1." *New York Times on the Web*. Accessed at www.nytimes.com, October 20, 2002.

Lantz, P. M., and K. M. Booth (1998). "The Social Construction of the Breast Cancer Epidemic." *Social Science and Medicine* 46, no. 2: 907–18.

Lawlor, D. A., S. Ebrahim, and G. Davey Smith. (2002). "Socioeconomic Position in Childhood and Adulthood and Insulin Resistance: Cross Sectional Survey Using Data from British Women's Heart and Health Study." *BMJ* 325, no. 7368: 805–809.

Leichter, S. (2000). "The Business of Diabetes: The Silent Standards in Diabetes Care: Millman and Robertson." *Clinical Diabetes* 18, no. 3: Accessed at http://clinical.diabetesjournals.org, December 1, 2000.

Link, B., and J. Phelan. (2000). "Evaluating the Fundamental Cause Explanation for Social Disparities in Health." *Handbook of Medical Sociology*, edited by C. E. Bird, P. Conrad, and A. Fremont, 43. Upper Saddle River, NJ: Prentice Hall.

Lochhead, C. (2000). "This Country's Obesity Crisis." *San Francisco Chronicle*. Accessed at http://sfgate.com/cgi-bin/article.cgi?file=/chronicle/archive/2000/07/09/SC74632.DTL, July 9, 2000.

Lynch, J., D. Smith, and J. House. (2000). "Income Inequality and Mortality: Importance to Health of Individual Income, Psychosocial Environment or Material Conditions." *BMJ* 320: 1200.

Lynch, J. W., G. Davey Smith, G. Kaplan, and J. House. (2000, April 29). "Education and Debate: Income Inequality and Mortality: Importance to Health of Individual Income, Psychosocial Environment, or Material Conditions." *BMJ* 320: 1200–1204.

Marwick, C. (2002). "Uninsured Americans Are More Likely to Die Prematurely." *BMJ* 324, no. 7349: 1296.

Maryniuk, M. D. (2000). "The New Shape of Medical Nutrition Therapy." *Diabetes Spectrum* 13, no. 3: 122.

Maugh, T. H., II. (2000). "Mutated Gene Tied to Diabetes in Some Groups." *Los Angeles Times*, A-1.

McKenzie, K. (2003). "Racism and Health." *BMJ* 326, no. 7380: 65–66.

McMurray, C., and R. Smith. (2001). *Diseases of Globalization: Socioeconomic Transitions and Health.* London: Earthscan Publications.

Nano, S. (2001). "Exercise May Thwart Diabetes." *New York Times on the Web.* Accessed at www.nytimes.com, May 2, 2001.

National Center for Chronic Disease Prevention and Health Promotion. (1996). *Building Understanding to Prevent and Control Diabetes among Hispanics/Latinos: Selected Annotations.* Atlanta: U.S. Department of Health and Human Services.

National Diabetes Education Program. (2000). *Making a Difference: The Business Community Takes on Diabetes.* Accessed at http://ndep.nih.gov, May 30, 2001.

National Diabetes Information Clearinghouse (NDIC) Diabetes Mellitus Interagency Coordinating Committee. (1993). *Diabetes in Hispanic Americans: Current Research and Education Programs.* Bethesda, MD: NIDDK, 107.

Newsday. (2000). "No Insurance Puts Latinos at Risk." *Los Angeles Times*, S-7.

Nicolucci, A., F. Carinci, and A. Ciampi. (1998). "Stratifying Patients at Risk of Diabetic Complications: An Integrated Look at Clinical, Socioeconomic and Care-Related Factors." *Diabetes Care* 21, no. 9: 1439–44.

Permanent Subcommittee on Investigations of the Committee on Governmental Affairs. (1999). *Conquering Diabetes: Are We Taking Full Advantage of the Scientific Opportunities for Research?* Congressional hearing. Washington: DC: U.S. Government Printing Office, 1–156.

Philoteou, A. (1997). "Educating the Adolescent with Diabetes." *IDF Bulletin* 42, no. 2: 18–20.

Pimentel, B. (2000). "Growing Obesity Risk Seen in State's Children Study Finds Unhealthy Eating Habits Flourishing." *San Francisco Chronicle*, A3.

Pollock, P. H., III, and M. Vittes. (1993, March 1). "On the Nature and Dynamics of Social Construction: The Case of AIDS." *Social Science Quarterly* 74: 1220–35.

Porter, R., ed. (1997). *Medicine: A History of Healing: Ancient Traditions to Modern Practices.* New York: Marlowe & Company.

Robert, S. A., and J. S. House. (2000). "Socioeconomic Inequalities in Health: An Enduring Sociological Problem." In *Handbook of Medical Sociology*, edited by C. E. Bird, P. Conrad, and A. Fremont, 79–97. Upper Saddle River, NJ: Prentice Hall.

Ross, N. A., M. C. Wolfson, J. Dunn, J. Berthelot, G. Kaplan, and J. Lynch. (2000, April 1). "Relation between Income Inequality and Mortality in Canada and in the United States: Cross Sectional Assessment Using Census Data and Vital Statistics." *BMJ* 320: 898–902.

Ryan, W. (1976). *Blaming the Victim.* New York: Random House.

Searle, J. R. (1995). *The Construction of Social Reality.* New York: Free Press.

Sontag, S. (1988). *Illness as Metaphor and AIDS and Its Metaphors.* New York: Anchor Books. (Originally published in 1978.)

"State-Specific Prevalence of Selected Health Behaviors by Race and Ethnicity-Behavioral Risk Factors Surveillance System, 1997." Surveillance Summaries, Centers for Disease Control and Prevention, /49(SS02); 1–60. Accessed at http://www.cdc.gov/mmwr/preview/mmwrhtml/ss4902a1.htm, March 24, 2000.

Tanner, L. (2000). "High Numbers of Uninsured Not Getting Proper Medical Care, Study Says." New York: Associated Press. Accessed at http://archive.ap.org, February 5, 2000.

Tobin, C. (2000). "Success." *The Diabetes Educator* 26, no. 3: 370–72.

Tuomilehto, J., J. Lindstrom, and J. Eriksson. (2001). "Prevention of Type 2 Diabetes Mellitus by Changes in Lifestyle among Subjects with Impaired Glucose Tolerance." *NEJM* 344, no. 18: 1343–50.

Vedantam, S. (2003). "Genetic Link with Depression Discovered." *San Francisco Chronicle,* A23.

Wade, N. (2003). "Project Will Seek to Uncover Genetic Roots of Major Diseases." *New York Times,* A20.

Waitzkin, H. (2000). *The Second Sickness: The Contradictions of Health Care in Capitalist Systems.* Lanham, MD: Rowman & Littlefield.

Wolfson, M., G. Kaplan, J. Lynch, N. Ross, and E. Backlund. (1999, October 9). "Relation between Income Inequality and Mortality: Empirical Demonstration." *BMJ* 319: 953–57.

Wright Mills, C. (1959). *The Sociological Imagination.* London: Oxford University Press.

Syringe Access, HIV Risk, and AIDS in Massachusetts and Connecticut: The Health Implications of Public Policy

18

DAVID BUCHANAN, MERRILL SINGER, SUSAN SHAW, WEI TENG, TOM STOPKA, KAVEH KHOSHNOOD, AND ROBERT HEIMER

IN THE CLASSIC PUBLIC HEALTH ACCOUNT, "A Tale of Two States," Fuchs (1974) writes about the health of populations living in Utah and Nevada. He observed that the health of the upright citizens of the Mormon-dominated Utah was far better than the health of the decadent populace in neighboring Nevada. The conclusion of his study is that how people choose to live their lives makes all the difference in the world. We would like to tell another tale of two states now, but it is one in which we draw different conclusions, with different moral and political implications. It is a study of the health implications of public policy regarding access to sterile syringes. Our observations are set in Connecticut and Massachusetts, another pair of states sharing a common border, yet with AIDS epidemics now headed in far different directions.

In many places across the United States and the world, practices associated with injection drug use have become the most prevalent mode of transmission of the human immunodeficiency virus (HIV) as well as the hepatitis B and C viruses. Public health professionals and community advocates are testing different interventions to try to reverse these epidemics and are constantly looking for evidence of their effectiveness. A recent set of editorials in the *American Journal of Public Health* reignited debate about the efficacy of syringe exchange programs (SEPs) in interrupting the transmission of HIV (Collin and Coates 2000; Coutinho 2000; DesJarlais 2000; Moss 2000a, 2000b; Vlahov 2000). In this chapter, we present the results of the Syringe Access, Use, and Discard (SAUD) research project. Because SAUD compares nearby northeastern cities with opposing public policies regarding access to sterile syringes, the results bear directly on the question of the effectiveness of promoting access to sterile syringes in controlling the AIDS and hepatitis epidemics among injection drug users.

Social and Historical Context of Syringe Exchange in Connecticut and Massachusetts

In a continually evolving legal environment, syringe exchange programs operated in an estimated 30 states at the end of 2001, although only ten state legislatures had formally authorized their lawful operation (Centers for Disease Control and Prevention 2001b; Singer and Needle 1996). In Connecticut, in response to the growing epidemic of HIV/AIDS among injecting drug users (IDUs) and mounting scientific evidence of the effectiveness of SEPs, a coalition of AIDS activists in New Haven lobbied for the start of the first legal syringe exchange program in New England in 1990 (O'Keefe 1991; Kaplan 1991). The results of preliminary studies of the New Haven experience led the Connecticut legislature to pass a new law in 1992 that expanded the number of SEPs statewide from one to six and that allowed anyone to purchase up to ten syringes at a time at pharmacies without a doctor's prescription (Heimer, Bluthenthal, Singer, and Khoshnood 1996). A similar mobile exchange program was then initiated in Hartford in 1993 (Singer 1994; Singer, Himmelgreen, Weeks, Radda, and Martinez 1997).

In contrast, in Massachusetts, it is still illegal to purchase syringes without a doctor's prescription. In Massachusetts, injection drug use is now the leading cause of HIV infection, accounting for 52 percent of all new AIDS cases in 2001 (Massachusetts Department of Public Health 2001). Disrupting this mode of transmission thus should be a major public policy objective here.

In 1993, the Massachusetts legislature passed legislation authorizing the initiation of the first pilot syringe exchange program there, with the qualification that startup was contingent upon local approval. In 1994, the legislation was amended to allow a total of ten "pilot" SEPs. The wording of chapter 111, section 215, of Massachusetts General Law holds that the state Department of Public Health is authorized to

> promulgate rules and regulations for the implementation of a pilot program for the exchange of needles in cities and towns within the Commonwealth upon nomination by the Department. Local approval shall be obtained prior to the implementation of the pilot program in any city or town (MGL 1993, c. 111, s. 215).

Significantly, the legislature failed to define what "local approval" meant and localities have interpreted the term differently. Pilot programs were initiated in Boston and Cambridge in 1995 with the approval of their city councils. Northampton started a program in 1996 based solely on the approval of the mayor. Provincetown started a new program in 1997 with the approval of the local board of health and support of the chief of police. There have been no new programs initiated since 1997. There have been a number of popular referenda seeking "local approval" on the issue since 1997, but whenever syringe exchange has been put to a popular vote in Massachusetts, it has been defeated.

The history of syringe exchange in Springfield, Massachusetts—one of our three study sites—reflects the torturous dynamics of class and race in local policy making. The mayor, the director of health and human services, the chief of police, and the Public Health Council have all gone on record in favor of starting a SEP in Springfield. The Public Health Council even declared a public health emergency to expedite its opening, but the city attorney rendered an opinion that "local approval" required a vote of the city council. In 1998, in a close 5–4 vote, the city council initially voted to approve the start of a pilot SEP. However, in response to the city council's vote, a group of neoconservative residents banded together to form a new organization, Citizens against Needle Exchange (CANE), that launched a petition drive to put a measure on the ballot to stop the opening of the SEP. In a further twist of events, the registrar of voters determined that, although they had come close, CANE had not collected the required 10,000 signatures needed to qualify a referendum for the ballot. CANE then lobbied their state representatives, who introduced legislation to exempt the petition from the required minimum number of signatures and thus qualify for the ballot. In a compromise effort, the state representatives urged the registrar to put the question on the ballot as a nonbinding resolution. It was, and in November 1998, the measure asking voters to reject the SEP passed on 55–45 percent popular vote. Subsequently, one city council member changed his vote, so the city council reversed itself, voting against syringe exchange. Local AIDS/public health activists have since worked hard to get the city council to reconsider its vote, but all parties acknowledge that the prospects for passage have worsened since that time. Ten years after the initiation of legal access to sterile syringes in New Haven and Hartford, the health impact of this divergence in public policy is beginning to emerge.

Inequalities in Health

To understand why Springfield has adopted unhealthy health policies, we need to examine the populations affected and their status in society. Springfield (population 150,198) is like many other mid-sized cities across the United States, where the politics of class and race drive local policy making. How have people of color fared in Springfield?

According to the 2000 U.S. Census data, the per capita income in Springfield is $11,584, compared to an average per capita income of $17,224 across Massachusetts. Among blacks in Springfield, the per capita income is $9,128; among Springfield Latinos, it is $5,254. In Springfield, more than 20 percent of the total population lives in poverty (compared to 8.9 percent of all citizens in the state); among Springfield blacks, 25.9 percent live in poverty, and among the Latino population the rate is 36.7 percent. More than one-third (33.8 percent) of all children under 18 in Springfield live in poverty (versus 13.2 percent of all children in Massachusetts). A total of 37.2 percent of all black children—and fully 66.9 percent of all Latino youth in Springfield—are growing up in poverty.

In 2002, the rate of newly diagnosed AIDS cases in Springfield was more than three times higher than the state rate, 43.6 versus 13.9 per 100,000 population (Massachusetts Department of Public Health 2003). Similarly, the prevalence of AIDS is almost three times as high (281.6 versus 110.2) and would be even higher, except for the fact that people with AIDS residing in Springfield are dying at five times the rate of people dying of AIDS across Massachusetts (17.8 versus 3.6 per 100,000). In addition, residents of Springfield are admitted into Department of Public Health (DPH)–funded substance abuse treatment programs at twice the rate of people living elsewhere in Massachusetts, and are twice as likely to be admitted for injection drug use. According to research conducted by the National Development and Research Institute (Friedman et al. in press), estimates of the total number of injection drug users range from 4,000 to 7,500, with an overall best estimate of 6,000 IDUs living in Springfield.

More palpably, the Mason Square area is the center of Springfield's African American community, a tight-knit neighborhood that was once home to a thriving black middle class and a small historic home district. Like many cities of the northeastern rust belt, Springfield had a growing black middle class in the 1950s and 1960s before changes in the economy displaced better-paying manufacturing jobs (Fullilove, Green, and Fullilove 1999). Evidence of this petite bourgeoisie remains in two small strip malls that form the commercial center of Mason Square.

Today, much of the neighborhood has a rundown, neglected appearance. Abandoned buildings are common, and 17 percent of the housing units are substandard (compared to 6 percent citywide). The Winchester Square mall is the primary hangout and illicit drug-copping area for African American IDUs in Mason Square. It has a fast food restaurant, several shops, a library, and a neighborhood health center. Longtime drug users in their late 40s and 50s can be seen hanging out in the parking lot most of the time, weather permitting. An abandoned rail line runs through the center of Mason Square. Informants say that the wooded areas adjacent to the tracks were used as injection sites some ten years ago. Based on our fieldwork, there appears to be little, if any, drug activity in them now.

Closer to the Connecticut River, the North End transitioned from a mixed to a predominantly Puerto Rican neighborhood in the wake of redevelopment programs in the 1960s that displaced many black homeowners. The North End is dominated by Main Street, the main commercial and drug-copping area that runs the length of the neighborhood. Traveling north from downtown, one enters the

North End by passing under a railway bridge and past the Greyhound bus station, a well-known hangout for prostitutes and street pill sellers. Further up Main Street, there are Spanish food stores, car repair shops, restaurants, and rows of brick apartment buildings. The whole neighborhood has a distinctive Puerto Rican flavor, with salsa music blasting, people greeting each other in Spanish, and scents of *bacalao* (fried cod) and *sofrito* (a condiment) in the air. IDUs often buy drugs on Main Street and walk to vacant lots to inject. Vacant lots covered with brush are scattered throughout the North End on the heels of an aggressive city policy of tearing down abandoned buildings that were reported as refuges for the homeless and IDUs (Buchanan, Shaw, Teng, Hiser, and Singer 2003).

Research Methods

The purpose of the Syringe Access, Use, and Discard: Context in AIDS Risk research project was to identify ecological factors that influence risk for contracting HIV and hepatitis C among IDUs in Hartford and New Haven, Connecticut, and Springfield, Massachusetts. With data collection running over a two-and-a-half-year period ending in May 2002, the SAUD project employed ethnographic, epidemiological, and serological research methods to identify risk factors for contracting HIV and hepatitis at the individual, neighborhood, and city levels. The major research hypotheses addressed whether there were differences in microsocial contexts at the neighborhood level (e.g., the presence of a syringe exchange van) that influence patterns of HIV risk. Because it has neither an SEP nor pharmacy access, Springfield served as a control site.

Ethnographic methods included (1) field-based descriptions of target neighborhoods; (2) syringe acquisition interviews, conducted in conjunction with collecting syringes naturalistically in the field, which we subjected to serological analysis; (3) ethnographic field observations of discard sites and injection locales; (4) participant observation during drug injection; (5) IDU diaries recording a week's worth of daily drug use and injection activities; (6) ethnographic "day visits" with IDUs; (7) syringe seller interviews; and, (8) neighborhood-based IDU focus groups to construct social maps of local equipment acquisition and drug use sites (Singer et al. 2000).

For epidemiological data, we conducted structured, largely forced-choice, interviews with 988 active IDUs—approximately 330 from each site—regarding syringe acquisition, use, and discard practices. The questionnaire was adapted from the NIDA AIDS Risk Assessment and administered orally in Spanish or English by field staff in community settings.

There were two outreach workers and one ethnographer at each site. The outreach workers were typically (all but one) people in recovery and were reflective of the race and ethnicity of populations at high risk in these cities. The outreach workers were well known and highly trusted in the neighborhoods where they worked, most having lived in the community all of their lives. In addition to recruitment for research purposes, field staff provided harm reduction materials and education and assistance with securing admission into drug treatment programs. Participants were paid a small stipend in compensation for their time.

Results

Based on ethnographic fieldwork, we found a hierarchy of risk with respect to sources for acquiring syringes. We uncovered six major sources, from most to least safe as follows: (1) SEPs, (2) pharmacies, (3) diabetics, (4) street sellers, (5) other IDUs, and (6) sexual partners. Within categories, a further breakdown in the hierarchy of risk was identified. Among diabetics, IDUs feel that they can trust and are more likely to be sold sterile syringes by diabetics with whom they have a family relationship (e.g., an uncle or in-law) than when they buy from diabetics to whom they are not related. In turn, they trust long-term acquaintances more than other diabetics whom they learn about via word of mouth on the street. In general, they trust people who only sell syringes more than dealers who sell syringes *and* drugs (Stopka, Singer, Eiserman, and Santelices 2003). In situations where IDUs need to acquire a syringe immediately, they will often buy, borrow, or rent syringes from other IDUs. As above, they believe that they are more likely to get a clean unused syringe from a close friend than they are from someone whom they do not know well. Finally, in this research at least, we found a fairly fatalistic sense that when users get their syringe from their lover, they generally seem resigned to the idea that they will get whichever diseases their partner may have. Further compounding the level of risk, IDUs in Springfield are frequently offered the opportunity to purchase either new or *used* syringes, sold as such, from each of these sources.

This research sought to identify the factors that press people to use riskier sources of syringes. In interviews, IDUs in Hartford and New Haven stated that they obtained sterile syringes at SEPs or pharmacies in significantly higher quantities than IDUs in Springfield. That is because the two safest sources of syringes—SEPs and pharmacies—are not available in Springfield. The single most powerful factor determining risk is thus public policy.

When safe sources are available, a large majority of IDUs indicate that they use them. Sixty-four percent of Hartford IDUs and 85 percent of New Haven IDUs stated that they used an SEP or pharmacy to acquire sterile syringes in the last 30 days, whereas only 5 percent of Springfield IDUs have done so ($\chi^2 = 445.66$, $p < .0001$). The small number of respondents in Springfield who stated that they have used a pharmacy or SEP report that they drove down to a pharmacy in Enfield, Connecticut, about ten miles away, or drove up to Northampton, Massachusetts, about 20 miles away, to access the nearest SEP in Massachusetts. When asked about their *usual* source, 69 percent of the Springfield participants stated their usual source of syringes is a diabetic. While diabetics are not without risk, more than 30 percent of IDUs in Springfield acknowledge that they usually acquire syringes from even riskier sources.

Another consequence of public policy is that injection drug users in Springfield live under the constant threat of arrest for syringe possession. The percentage of the respondents who report that they have been arrested for syringe possession is almost three times higher in Springfield (33 percent) than for people living in Hartford (12 percent) ($\chi^2 = 43.04$, $p < .0001$).

Turning to factors influencing risk in the use of syringes, Kaplan and Heimer (1994a, 1994b) have shown that the longer a syringe remains in circulation, the more likely it is that the syringe will become a vehicle for transmitting diseases such as hepatitis and HIV. SAUD data reveal that the average number of times a syringe is used prior to disposal is 16 times among Springfield IDUs, almost twice as high as users report in Hartford (nine times) and four times higher than IDUs in New Haven ($F = 68.64$, $p < .0001$).

In our field research, Springfield IDUs report that the lack of legal access to syringes means that they typically use syringes until they fall apart, since each time they attempt to acquire a new syringe, they expose themselves to the threat of arrest (Stopka, Springer, Khoshnood, Shaw, and Singer 2004). Restrictions on the legal availability of sterile syringes drive up costs, too. Higher costs have created a flourishing market for used syringes sold at a cheaper price. As one might expect, we encountered a lot of scamming about the status of syringes in our fieldwork, with used syringes sometimes being passed off as new. In one instance, after lengthy haggling with a seller, and telling him that we simply did not believe that the syringe for sale was new, he finally admitted that it was used and threw in a bleach kit to go with it. The price of new syringes in Springfield ranged from $2 to $5, with an average cost of $3.60, compared to average costs of less than half that in Hartford. Used syringes in Springfield cost $1 to $3. Notably, used syringes were not found to be sold in Connecticut.

The lack of access to SEPs was also associated with differences in how IDUs dispose of syringes (Singer, Teng, Shaw, Heimer, and Buchanan 2003). IDUs in Hartford and New Haven were much more likely to use a SEP for the safe disposal of syringes: 51 percent of IDUs in Hartford reported that they used a SEP, as did 32 percent of IDUS in New Haven, but only 1.2 percent of Springfield IDUs reported that they used a SEP for the safe disposal of their syringes ($\chi^2 = 201.74$, $p < .0001$).

Conversely, IDUs in Springfield were much more likely to toss their used syringes in an alley or open sewer, or stash them for later use (27.7 percent in Springfield, versus 12.3 percent in Hartford, and 7.2 percent in New Haven; $\chi^2 = 52.54$, $p < .0001$). More syringes discarded in open public spaces means more risk of accidental needle sticks. Because of a hard-line policy of tearing down abandoned buildings in Springfield, we found only two indoor injection locales there during two and a half years of fieldwork. Most injection sites were outdoor sites, mostly vacant lots, areas next to the railroad tracks, and brushy wooded areas next to raised highways. In low-income neighborhoods, these vacant lots were often adjacent to public housing projects, and it was not uncommon to observe young children playing or riding their bikes through them.

Finally, evidence of the cumulative effect of public policy restricting access to sterile syringes is beginning to surface in different rates of infection. Self-report rates of hepatitis C infection are almost 50 percent higher in Springfield compared to the other two sites (40 percent in Springfield versus 30 percent in New Haven and 29 percent in Hartford; $\chi^2 = 10.97$, $p < .01$). With respect to HIV, a similar picture emerges: 32 percent of the respondents in Springfield self-report that they are HIV positive, compared to 23 percent in New Haven and 24 percent in Hartford.

Using data on new AIDS cases reported to the state departments of health over the past two years, we compared rates of AIDS diagnosis in the three cities. In 1999–2000, there were 276 new cases reported in Springfield, 215 in Hartford, and 166 in New Haven (Centers for Disease Control and Prevention 2001b). These numbers translate into rates of 175.8, 153.9, and 127.2 cases per 100,000 residents, respectively. Thus, there is a 13 percent lower rate of new AIDS cases in Hartford and a 43 percent lower rate in New Haven. If a city the size of New Haven were experiencing new AIDS cases at the same rate as Springfield, there would have been 126 AIDS cases attributable to injection drug use over the past two years. Instead, only 71 were reported, a difference of 55 fewer AIDS cases in two years. Conversely, if Springfield had experienced new AIDS cases at the same rate as New Haven, we would have expected 88 new cases. Instead, there were 152 cases, or an excess of 64 new AIDS cases. The difference between Springfield and New Haven has momentous implications, because the legal syringe exchange has been ongoing in New Haven for a decade, long enough to affect the lagging indicator of AIDS cases.

Conclusion

Fuchs (1974) may have been right: how people act does impact their health. But he failed to see how public policy shapes people's behaviors, expanding or constricting the range of options available to them. As the results of the SAUD study demonstrate, when public policy allows access to sterile syringes, people adjust their behaviors accordingly, with striking effects.

When public policy allows, the preponderance of injection drug users use guaranteed safe sites to acquire clean syringes. Conversely, when legal access is restricted, IDUs report that they (are forced to) obtain their syringes from much riskier sources such as diabetics and street dealers. Due to public policy, syringes in Springfield remain in circulation twice as long, placing IDUs at higher risk for HIV and other blood-borne infections. Moreover, the inability to acquire new sterile syringes means that IDUs are inhibited from using other harm reduction practices. As a consequence of public policy, most IDUs in Springfield do not have contingency plans in case their syringe stops working for any reason. Because they face a higher likelihood of police interference, IDUs in Springfield are reluctant to carry a spare, backup syringe, or any other paraphernalia such as bleach kits on their person. When in the throes of withdrawal, they then turn to highly risky sources to obtain syringes immediately. Furthermore, where access to SEPs for safe disposal is unavailable, IDUs report that they are much more likely to discard their used syringes in ways that pose a greater public health threat. Public disposal in dumpsters, alleyways, or vacant lots places noninjectors at greater risk of accidental needle sticks and thereby increases their chances of bacterial or viral infection.

In conclusion, our analysis suggests that policy efforts—instituting syringe exchange and allowing over-the-counter sales of syringes—can have a significant impact on HIV transmission. As seen in the other chapters of this book, public policy, which is enacted ostensibly to improve the public weal, can become the very source of unhealthy behaviors and resulting incidences of disease. The results of our study also demonstrate that medical anthropology has a critically important role to play in public discourse about significant public policy issues. CDC data on infection rates are far too removed from the reality of people's daily lives and the dynamics of local social and political contexts to make a compelling case for the effects of policy initiatives. Medical anthropologists and social scientists have a responsibility to make clear the human consequences of sometimes seemingly abstract ideas and distant government policies. We need to continue to resist efforts to demonize the Other—poor and marginalized people—and clarify the values for which we as a society stand, one in which we hope the brutality of poverty and racism will no longer be tolerated.

Acknowledgments

This study was supported by grant #R01 DA12569, awarded by the National Institute on Drug Abuse, Principal Investigator Merrill Singer.

References

Buchanan, D., S. Shaw, W. Teng, P. Hiser, and M. Singer. (2003). "Neighborhood Differences in Patterns of Syringe Access, Use and Discard: Implications for HIV Outreach and Prevention Education." *Journal of Urban Health* 80, no. 3: 438–54.

Centers for Disease Control and Prevention. (2001a). "Table 4." *HIV/AIDS Surveillance Report* 12, no. 1: 8–9. Accessed at www.cdc.gov/hiv/stats/hasr1201.pdf, April 19, 2004.

———. (2001b). "Update: Syringe Exchange Programs—United States, 1998." *Morbidity and Mortality Weekly* 50, no. 19: 384–87.

Collin, C., and T. Coates. (2000). "Science and Health Policy: Can They Cohabit or Should They Divorce?" *American Journal of Public Health* 90, no. 9: 1389–90.

Coutinho, R. (2000). "Needle Exchange, Pragmatism, and Moralism." *American Journal of Public Health* 90, no. 9: 1387–88.

DesJarlais, D. (2000). "Research Politics, and Needle Exchange." *American Journal of Public Health* 90, no. 9: 1392–95.

Friedman, S. D, B. Tempalski, H. Cooper, T. Perlis, M. Keem, R. Friedman, and P. Flom. (In press). "Estimating Numbers of IDUs in Metropolitan Areas for Structural Analyses of Community Vulnerability and for Assessing Relative Degrees of Service Provision for IDUs." *Journal of Urban Health.*

Fuchs, V. (1974). *Who Shall Live? Health, Economics, and Social Choice.* New York: Basic.

Fullilove, M., L. Green, and R. Fullilove. (1999). "Building Momentum: An Ethnographic Study of Inner-City Redevelopment." *American Journal of Public Health* 89, no. 6: 840–44.

Heimer, R., R. Bluthenthal, M. Singer, and K. Khoshnood. (1996). "Structural Impediments to Operational Syringe Exchange Programs." *Journal of AIDS and Public Policy* 11: 169–84.

Kaplan, E. (1991). "Evaluating Needle Exchange Programs via Syringe Tracking and Testing." *Journal of AIDS and Public Policy* 6: 109–15.

Kaplan, E., and R. Heimer. (1994a). "A Circulation Theory of Needle Exchange." *AIDS* 8, no. 5: 567–74.

———. (1994b). "HIV Incidence among Needle Exchange Participants; Estimates from Syringe Tracking and Testing Data." *AIDS* 7: 182–89.

Massachusetts Department of Public Health. (2001). *HIV/AIDS in Massachusetts: An Epidemiologic Profile, Fiscal Year 2001.* Boston: Massachusetts Department of Public Health.

———. (2003). *Community Health Indicators Program (MassCHIP).* Boston: Massachusetts Department of Public Health. All figures here and text that follows are as of January 1, 2003.

Moss, A. R. (2000a). "Epidemiology and the Politics of Needle Exchange." *American Journal of Public Health* 90, no. 9: 1385–87.

———. (2000b). "For God's Sake, Don't Show This Letter to the President. . . ." *American Journal of Public Health* 90, no. 9: 1395–97.

O'Keefe, E. (1991). "Altering Public Policy on Needle Exchange: The Connecticut Experience." *Journal of AIDS and Public Policy* 6: 159–64.

Singer, M. (1994). "Community Centered Praxis: Toward an Alternative Non-Dominative Applied Anthropology." *Human Organization* 53, no. 4: 336–44.

Singer, M., D. Himmelgreen, M. Weeks, K. Radda, and R. Martinez. (1997). "Changing the Environment of AIDS Risk: Findings on Syringe Exchange and Pharmacy Sale of Syringes in Hartford, CT." *Medical Anthropology* 18, no. 1: 107–30.

Singer, M., and R. Needle. (1996). "Preventing AIDS among Drug Users: Evaluating Efficacy." *Journal of Drug Issues* 26, no. 3: 521–24.

Singer, M., T. Stopka, C. Siano, K. Springer, G. Barton, K. Khoshnood, et al. (2000). "The Social Geography of AIDS and Hepatitis Risk: Qualitative Approaches for Assessing Local Differences in Sterile Syringe Access among Injection Drug Users." *American Journal of Public Health* 90, no. 7: 1049–1056.

Singer, M., W. Teng, S. Shaw, R. Heimer, and D. Buchanan. (2003, April 4). "Factors in Risky Syringe Discard among Injection Drug Users." Presentation for AIDS Science Day, Center for Interdisciplinary Research on AIDS, Yale University, New Haven, CT.

Stopka, T., M. Singer, J. Eiserman, and C. Santelices. (2003). "Public Health Interventionists, Penny Capitalists, or Sources of Risk? Assessing Street Syringe Sellers in Hartford, Connecticut." *Substance Use & Misuse* 38, no. 9: 1339–70.

Stopka, T., K. Springer, K. Khoshnood, S. Shaw, and M. Singer. (2004). "Writing about Risk: Use of Daily Diaries in Understanding Drug-User Risk Behaviors." *AIDS and Behavior* 8, no. 1: 73–85.

Vlahov, D. (2000). "The Role of Epidemiology in Needle Exchange Programs." *American Journal of Public Health* 90, no. 9: 1390–92.

19

Why Is It Easier to Get Drugs than Drug Treatment in the United States?

MERRILL SINGER

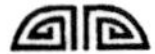

ON THE FRONT PAGE of its Sunday edition on June 8, 2002, the *New York Times* ran an article entitled "Latin American Poppy Fields Undermine U.S. Drug Battle." This article encapsulates one half of the purpose of this chapter, namely documentation of the failure of the War on Drugs to stop the flow of drugs to U.S. cities, towns, and rural areas. As the article notes, amid this long-fought war, drugs are readily available and new users are joining the ranks of illicit drug consumers (Forero and Weiner 2002). If we add to this picture the rapid spread of so-called club drugs, and their movement toward becoming a new wave of street drugs, as well as the domestic production and widespread use of substances like methamphetamine, and under the counter sales of pharmaceutical narcotics and tranquilizers on the street, it is evident that the War on Drugs can claim few real victories: it is still easy to get drugs anywhere in the United States, from down the street from the White House to the least populated county in the country and from inner-city streets to Wall Street suites. Getting into effective drug treatment, on the other hand, remains a major challenge for the many drug users who would like to overcome their drug dependency. In short, a burning question for health policy in the United States is "Why is it easier to get drugs than drug treatment?"

The unhealthy state of policies and strategies enacted in response to illicit drug use is captured in the following anecdote. In response to the AIDS epidemic, I helped develop a study of the role of syringes in HIV infection among drug users (see chapter 18, this volume; see also Singer et al. 2000). The study design called for the collection of syringes acquired on the street by drug users for laboratory testing for the presence of human DNA (to determine if syringes sold on the street are being recycled and are a possible source of infection). Additionally, ethnographers were to visit abandoned buildings or other frequently used illicit drug-injection sites to collect discarded syringes to be tested for HIV and hepatitis C antibodies (indicating that the syringe has been used by an infected individual and that reuse by another individual could transmit infection). While many of the procedures used in this project reflect strategies implemented elsewhere in AIDS prevention research, in Springfield, Massachusetts, one of the three northeastern U.S. cities in which the project was to be implemented—and despite the full support from the local public health department, AIDS prevention programs, and community-based organizations—the local police flatly told the research team that if they were caught in possession of syringes in transit to the laboratory, they would be arrested for violation of state paraphernalia laws. No attempts to explain the public health procedures employed in the project or its HIV risk-reduction goals convinced police officials that arresting AIDS researchers would only retard AIDS prevention and not further the cause of the War on Drugs. At several meetings, the police unswervingly affirmed their commitment to arresting drug users or anyone else that violated a strict reading of existing paraphernalia laws.

This vignette reflects in microcosm the enormous difficulties our society has had in responding effectively and reasonably to the AIDS epidemic in light of prevailing attitudes, laws, and criminal justice practices directed at drug users. As a result of the War on Drugs, every 20 seconds someone in the United States is arrested for a drug violation and, at the rate of one per week, a new prison is completed to house the unprecedented throng of inmates that are now locked up in the world's largest and most populous penal system (Egan 1999). Perhaps the logic of this approach might be defended if it actually achieved its intended goal of stopping the production, distribution, and use of dangerous substances. However, as noted above, there is abundant evidence that the War on Drugs has been an unmitigated failure in achieving its publicly expressed purposes. The War on Drugs continues unabated, presidential administration after administration, one bloated "drug-fighting" annual budget after the other, seemingly headed toward a modern reenactment of the 100 Years' War.

It seems reasonable to ask why this apparently futile war continues. The conclusion reached by a growing number of people concerned with this public health and social issue is that even while the War on Drugs can claim little in terms of achieving its primary goals, it has, in fact, produced enormously useful secondary gains. This chapter argues that the War on Drugs, seen *not* as a war on drug use per se but as a social war on *those who can be classified as drug users (or pushers)*, functions as a well-financed societal control mechanism that redundantly reinforces and reproduces the most overtly inegalitarian features of the structure of American society.

Anatomy of the War on Drugs

The 1960s left an indelible mark on American drug use patterns. Prior to this time, the United States had experienced various waves of drug use, all of which were shaped in their character and composition by distinctive historic forces and prevailing social relationships, but the 1960s marked a significant shift in prevailing patterns. This shift—which can be seen as the ever-widening expansion of illicit drug use from the social margins (e.g., ethnic minorities and other devalued social groups like jazz musicians or beat generation writers) to the mainstream core—provided the initial public motivation for the War on Drugs. This war was publicly declared in 1969 by Richard Nixon early in his presidential term as part of his campaign to restore "law and order" to American society. As Musto (1987:254) notes, "No President has equaled Nixon's antagonism to drug abuse, and he took an active role in organizing the federal and state governments to fight the onslaught of substance abuse." In fiscal year 1969, the antidrug budget was $86 million (Drug Abuse Council 1980). Nixon resolutely declared that illicit drugs were now "public enemy number one" (cited in Chambers and Inciardi 1974:221). The war was on!

Without doubt, drug use had expanded greatly just prior to (and during) the Nixon administration. Survey data from 1971 suggest that as many as 24 million Americans admitted that they had broken with convention and tried marijuana, a drug that had been nationally condemned as a "killer weed" in previous decades. Most notably, among young adults (18–21 years), 40 percent reported having used marijuana. Moreover, so-called hard drug use also was growing. It is estimated that the number of heroin users jumped from a relative handful during World War II to 50,000 by 1960 and to 500,000 a decade later (Domestic Council Drug Abuse Task Force 1975; National Commission on Marijuana and Drug Abuse 1972). By 1972, a Gallup Poll found that drug abuse was seen as the major cause of urban decay (cited in Inciardi 1986), although others would see drug abuse and urban decay as common consequences of social policies and economic practices such as the exportation of industrial production and the federal financing of suburban flight (Baer, Singer, and Susser 2003). With the expressed purpose of turning the tide against the ever-widening circle of drug use, Nixon quickly established the Special Action Office for Drug Abuse Prevention, the Office of Drug Abuse Law Enforcement, and the Office of National Narcotics Intelligence. At all appearances, the Nixon administration seemed quite serious about fighting a full-scale war to extinguish illicit drug use.

A closer look at the oft-cited Nixon opposition to drug abuse, however, suggests a somewhat different understanding of his widely heralded War on Drugs. In his book, *Agency of Fear*, investigative reporter Edward Epstein (1977) argues that Nixon's primary motive in launching new criminal justice and investigative bodies was to gather information on his political enemies. While this allegation has never been verified, it is evident that hypersensitivity to opposition and a willingness to launch covert initiatives characterized the "Nixon years." It is notable that prior to being elected president, Nixon had been (circa 1959), as vice president of the United States, the chief political officer of the National Security Council's (NSC) Special Group, the entity that planned the Bay of Pigs invasion of Cuba by expatriate Cubans in Florida in 1961. Known to its planners as Operation Mongoose, the invasion of Cuba was linked to various other covert operations, including several failed assassination attempts on Fidel Castro. Notably, in 1963, a number of leaders of Operation Mongoose were caught smuggling narcotics into the United States from Cuba (Fresia 1988; Kruger 1976). This event was not unique. Rather, it marks the opening of a continued pattern of using drug money to finance covert (and often illegal) U.S. government–sponsored activities against disliked foreign regimes. For example, as Schultheis (1983:237) reports, from

> the 1950s through the Vietnam War era, the Nationalist Chinese in the Golden Triangle were supplied, even advised, by the CIA; the involvement of the Chinese in the opium and heroin business was excused because of the fact that they carried out paramilitary and intelligence activities along the Burma-Chinese border and elsewhere in the Triangle.

When Operation Mongoose (which had achieved little of its expressed agenda) was shut down in 1965, its director Theodore Shackley and his assistant Thomas Clines were transferred to Laos, where Shackely became the deputy chief of station for the CIA. During this period, Schackley and Clines began working closely with General Van Pao, a Laotian warlord (and former French colonial officer) who was struggling to gain control of the Laotian opium trade. Van Pao repaid Shackley and Clines for their support by using his drug money to train Hmong tribesmen in guerrilla war tactics (including political assassination). By 1969, Van Pao's control of the opium trade had expanded. With help from leaders of the Operation Mongoose team, Van Pao was on his way to becoming "the number one importer and distributor of China White heroin in the U.S." (Fresia 1988:124).

In 1973, Shackley and Clines were sent to Vietnam under the Phoenix Project. Again, Van Pao's drug money was used to finance secret operations, this time against village leaders who were sympathetic to the Viet Cong. During the Vietnam War, one of the biggest markets for Van Pao's opium (some of it processed as heroin) was U.S. troops. The dark irony of this situation is noted by Browning and Garrett (1986:119):

> While the President is declaring war on narcotics and on crime in the streets, he is widening the war in Laos, whose principal product is opium and which has now become the funnel for nearly half the world's supply of the narcotic, for which the U.S. is the chief consumer.

But this fact—that at the time the Golden Triangle was the source of 80 percent of the world's supply of opium, and that the area was controlled by U.S.-backed forces—was never acknowledged by the Nixon administration. Rather, Turkey was pointed to as the primary source of most opium, and the Nixon administration and the Department of Agriculture promoted the development of a biological agent to destroy Turkey's poppy crop, although it was never used for fear that it would spread to other areas (Inciardi 1986). Argue Browning and Garrett (1986:123): "It is no accident that Nixon has ignored the real sources of narcotics trade abroad and by so doing has effectively precluded any possibility of being able to deal with heroin at home."

Similarly, in Burma, which in the mid-1970s was a recipient of U.S. State Department International Narcotics Control (INC) funding to eliminate narcotics production, investigators from the U.S. House Select Committee on Narcotics found "convincing evidence that [the] . . . antinarcotics campaign is [in fact] a form of economic warfare aimed at subjugation of . . . Minority Peoples" (U.S. Congress 1977:225). When not attacking the ethnic minority Kachin, Shan, and Karen peoples, Burmese soldiers were found to be busily engaged in harvesting minority-owned opium fields for their own profit. Ironically, one consequence of the Burmese military campaign against ethnic minorities—including a regular pattern of raping minority girls and women, was the flight of large numbers of women into Thailand where they became ensnared in international commercial sex trafficking, drug use, and the spread of HIV (Singer, He, and Salaheen 2004).

In sum, the War on Drugs, *from the beginning*, was a tainted war characterized by conflicted and, from a public health standpoint, questionable and contradictory subagendas. In fact, Nixon's War on Drugs was not alone in this respect. U.S. federal government, as well as state or even judicial, opposition to drugs before and after Nixon was no less tainted, no less "political" in nature, and no more driven by a primary concern with the health of the nation. Moreover, Nixon's drug suppression, interdiction, and treatment policies are sometimes credited with turning the corner on the heroin epidemic of the 1960s, as Agar and Reisinger, based on their review of the literature, stress (2000:393): "We now see that the war on drugs disrupted the conditions under which the 1960s epidemic had flourished. But the disruption was short-lived, and supply systems and addiction returned after the early 1970s heroin drought in even stronger form."

U.S. opposition to drug use did not begin until the late nineteenth century. Importantly, congressional debate on the first narcotics laws *did not focus on the negative health effects* of drugs like opium and cocaine, nor even on the rising rate of addiction in the U.S. population, but rather was driven in no small measure by concern with America's rising position in international trade. Specifically, Congress's first action against drugs developed in direct response to the fact that the British were gaining an economic bonanza from their forced opium sales (from their Indian colony) to China, profits that enabled England to achieve a competitive edge against U.S. businesses globally.

At this time, public drug use was widespread in the United States as well. Drugs like heroin and cocaine were readily available. A study done in 1888 of the contents of prescriptions purchased from pharmacies in Boston, for example, found that of the 10,200 prescriptions filled that year, 15 percent contained opiates, and that opiate-based proprietary drugs had the highest sales (Eaton 1888). The end result was that during the 1800s, opium use was treated as a "normal" behavior that was both legal and integrated into everyday experience.

Indeed, the only behavior that was labeled as a "drug problem" per se was the smoking of opium in opium dens often located in the Chinese sections of U.S. cities, although not only used by Chinese clients. From this moment on, U.S. societal reactions to drug use and attitudes about particular racial/ethnic groups have been closely intertwined. In the case of Chinese opium smoking, a major underlying factor in social condemnation was the depression that began in the 1860s and the resulting redefinition of the Chinese as surplus labor in the American West. As with opium, attitudes about cocaine also were colored by societal racism. Throughout the American South, a publicly expressed fear developed that if blacks had access to cocaine, they "might become oblivious of their prescribed bounds and attack white society" (Musto 1987:6).

These examples reveal an important aspect of U.S. experience with illicit drugs that is often hidden behind moral, legal, and even public health initiatives like the War on Drugs. As Helmer (1983:27) has argued, "The conflict over social justice is what the story of narcotics in America is about." Thus, assessments of federal actions at the outset of the twentieth century in response to the emergence of a global drug market—in what might be called the first U.S. War on Drugs—including passage of a series of ever-more-draconian laws on drug use, find a central role played by political economic factors (Baer, Singer, and Susser 2003; Musto 1987). Congressional debate around passage of the first federal drug laws did not center on the negative health effects of opium and cocaine, nor on the rising rate of addiction in the U.S. population, but instead was most concerned about international relations and profit. The ultimate social effect of the new federal law, formally known as HR 6282 but generally referred to as the Harrison

Act—which was passed on December 14 and signed by the President several days later on December 17, 1914—was to label the drug user as a criminal. In the aftermath of this labeling, drug use came to be synonymous with deviance, lack-of-control, violence, and moral decay. As Goode (1984:218) points out, "By the 1920s the public image of the addict had become that of a criminal, a willful degenerate, a hedonistic thrill-seeker in need of imprisonment and stiff punishment." The result was the emergence of an underground illicit drug subculture, which continued until World War II. In the early 1940s, however, rates of drug addiction in the United States took a sudden drop. The decline, caused by the War's disruption of drug trafficking systems, was short-lived. Soldiers who had used drugs overseas began to bring their addictions and knowledge of drug use home with them. And it was in the ghettos and barrios along the East and West coasts that drug injection found a new home after the war, especially among young men whose hopes for equality, raised by a war against totalitarianism, were smashed by racism and the postwar economic downturn.

In addition to the press of social conditions, the postwar U.S. inner-city drug epidemic was the end result of several events, including: (1) the 1949 retreat of defeated Kuomintang Nationalist Chinese forces into eastern Burma and their takeover of opium production in the Golden Triangle poppy-growing region of Southeast Asia, (2) the emergence of Hong Kong and Marseilles as heroin-refining centers, and (3) the reestablishment of Mafia-controlled international drug trafficking networks (Inciardi 1986; Schultheis 1983; Singer et al. 1990). The individual responsible for the latter was none other than Lucky Luciano. Arrested in 1936 on drug charges, from his jail cell he sent messages to Sicily directing the Mafia to support the U.S. Army during World War II. It is widely believed that in return for helping the Allies during the invasion of Sicily, and for opposing communism in Italy after the war, the Mafia was made various promises by the U.S. government, including the return of weapons confiscated by Mussolini's Fascists (McCoy 1991). In addition, Luciano was able to build an unparalleled international narcotics syndicate soon after his arrival in Italy in 1946 (McCoy, Read, and Adams 1986:114). As Musto (1987:236) notes, a key factor in Lucky Luciano's "success" as a drug kingpin was "police collusion with drug suppliers in communities like Harlem."

In short, Nixon's War on Drugs, although launched with great fanfare and, in fact, accompanied by a significant expansion in the availability of drug treatment, followed a long tradition of contradictory motivations and actions that undercut the expressed goal of fighting illicit drug use. The same types of patterns also characterize America's continually renewed War on Drugs *since* the Nixon presidency. For example, after the fall of the Shah of Iran, the CIA developed a growing presence in Afghanistan—which had become one of the world's largest opium-producing areas—including developing supportive relationships with opium-growing Baluchi and Pashtun peoples. When the Soviet Union invaded Afghanistan in 1979, the CIA, on the authority of President Jimmy Carter, began supplying arms and logistic support to the northern tribes. As a result of "high-powered CIA largess" (Levins 1986:125) and a record poppy crop in the region, there appeared a new "monster source of opium production [that] . . . promise[d] to send a veritable hurricane of heroin swirling once again through the streets of Europe and America: Afghanistan" (Levins 1986:125).

That wave struck in the early 1980s. In response, Presidents Reagan and Bush resuscitated a somewhat indolent drug war (again without any real success), and Bill Clinton joined the battle by appointing a general, Barry McCaffrey, to lead America's charge. In the introduction to his 1996 National Drug Control Strategy, President Clinton (1996:3) claimed: "In the last few years our Nation has made significant progress against drug use and related crime. We have dealt serious blows to the international criminal networks that import drugs into America."

A street-level view of the drug scene, however, does not support these rosy pronouncements (Singer 1999). Drops in the levels of some kinds of drug use appear to be unrelated to supply issues and are offset by rises in other kinds of drug use (Community Epidemiological Work Group 1998). Cocaine use, for example, may be down, but use of heroin, methamphetamine, and designer drugs is up significantly. Indeed, data from the U.S. Substance Abuse and Mental Health Services Administration indicate that since 1988 there has been a significant drop in the mean age of first-time heroin users, from 27.4 years in 1988 to 17.6 years in 1997 (Dee 1999). Recent studies have shown that teenagers report that marijuana is readily available in high school and can be easily acquired within a short period of time. In fact, there has been little change in the level of adolescent access to marijuana in 25 years, with approximately 90 percent currently reporting that it is "very easy" or "fairly easy" to obtain (Johnson, Bachman, and O'Malley 1997).

Now in its fourth decade, the War on Drugs, in short, continues to fail at achieving its primary goal of significantly stemming the flow of illicit drugs into the United States (Guttman 1996). Indeed, as Bertram and Sharpe (1996:C-1), coauthors of the book *Drug War Politics: The Price of Denial,* argued, "Drug law-enforcement budgets increased from $1 billion to $9 billion annually during the past 15 years, but heroin and cocaine are cheaper and more available than ever." Notably, since 1996, the drug law enforcement price tag has jumped another $3 billion annually without any significant record of success.

Consequently, during the War on Drugs, the National Institute on Drug Abuse has reported a steady increase in the drug abuse cost to society. Indeed, in the thick of the recent War on Drugs years, from 1985 to 1992, there was a 50 percent increase in the estimated cost to society of illicit drug use in terms of the combined impact of drug-related crime, health care expenditures, and lost wages. In light of this reassessment of somewhat hidden features of the War on Drugs, a rationale appears for why the program has continued, year after year, decade after decade, at great cost and with little overt success. This rationale consists of the following secondary gains of the "war."

Global Designs

At the international level, the War on Drugs serves to further U.S. geopolitical and geo-economic interests (as some in power would define them) when overt actions toward serving those ends is illegal or embarrassing, or would prove unpopular with the American people. Repeatedly, as has been noted, behind the public face of the drug war has been a backstage effort to collude with (and hence foster) drug producers/distributors and the use of the drug war as a Trojan Horse for the achievement of other political economic aims. At the same time, while political enemies like Castro of Cuba or the Sandinistas of Nicaragua have been repeatedly publicly accused by U.S. government spokespersons of having deep involvement in drug trafficking (often without much evidence)—and this accusation has been used to demonstrate to the American people the immoral character of hated regimes—the clear involvement of U.S. clients and intelligence personnel in the drug trade has been hidden from public view. Exploiting the drug problem in the service of international political power in this way reflects the phenomenon that Chomsky (1988:169) has referred to as "the reality that must be effaced."

The Benefits of Blame

Secondly, by scapegoating drug users as the nefarious cause of contemporary urban suffering and decay—a practice that is even more common among government spokespersons than accusations made against foreign heads of state—attention is diverted from the role of class inequality as a source of social misery. Since the full implementation of federal laws banning the sale of some substances, and ever more so since the formal declaration of the War on Drugs, there has been an effort to paint the drug addict as the very essence of deviance and badness in U.S. society. Addicts are not simply socially devalued; they are portrayed as the reason why our streets and homes are unsafe, our inner cities are eyesores that must be avoided by suburbanites at all costs, and our ability to experience a traditional American feeling of community has been shattered. Lost in this interpretation is any assessment of the role of corporate policy—including rampant mergers, buyouts, restructuring, downsizing, hiring and training policies, shrinking public giving patterns, and factory closings—in reshaping American social life. The inner-city areas commonly identified in the popular imagination with drug use are the very areas that have been abandoned in corporate shifts, producing rampant unemployment, deteriorating services, failing schools, and the resulting short-term coping strategies for surviving social misery that come to be seen as the causes and not the consequences of pressing urban problems (Bourgois 1995; Singer 1994; Waterston 1993).

Racism and the Demonization of (Some) Drugs

Thirdly, by widely promoting the image of the drug user of color as a modern social bogey man, the War on Drugs effectively reinforces divisive racist stereotypes that contribute to a well-contained labor force with negligible working-class consciousness. Consistently, the demonized image of the drug user and drug dealer presented to society through all arms of the mass media is that of the African American male nationally and the Latino male internationally. At the neighborhood level, these threatening images are used to justify nightly police assaults in full battle gear on minority neighborhoods, a campaign that has telling social consequences. As Chambliss (1994:679) points out, "The war on drugs in the United States has produced another war as well: it is a war between the police and minority youth from the 'ghetto underclass,'" as reflected in rap song lyrics.

Indeed, whatever its failures, one of the things that the War on Drugs has done quite well is to arrest a lot of people and put them in prison. A profile of those incarcerated on drug-related charges, however, suggests that enforcement of drug policy is a better reflection of the "politics of race" than it is of a meaningful effort to stop the sale and use of illicit drugs. While studies show that 15 percent of the nation's cocaine users are African American, they account for approximately 40 percent of those charged with powder cocaine violations and 90 percent of those convicted on crack cocaine charges (Davidson 1999). Overall, African Americans, who comprise 12 percent of the U.S. population, make up 55 percent of those convicted for illicit drug possession. One in 15 African American males currently is incarcerated, primarily as a result of drug laws. Moreover, in 1995, approximately 30 percent of African American males between the ages of 20 and 29 years were under some form of criminal justice supervision, up from 23 percent in 1990.

The significantly higher proportion of African Americans charged with crack cocaine offenses has been found to be "the single most important difference accounting for the overall longer sentences imposed on blacks, relative to other groups" according to a 1993 Justice Department report (quoted in Muwakkil 1996:21). Ironically, while still clinging to patriotic slogans about the unparalleled freedoms of American society, compared to other industrialized countries on a per capita basis the United States is the most incarcerating nation in the world.

Lost in the "lock 'em up" drug war mentality is any systematic assessment of why socially marginalized working-class youth turn to drugs and the drug trade, including any examination of the direct contributions of structurally imposed inequality of access to socially valued statuses, avenues of social success, and coveted material wealth. As Bourgois (1995:320) notes, the drug trade is "the biggest equal opportunity employer" for inner-city youth. By hiding this painful reality behind demonized images of drug users of color, the War on Drugs blocks a full public consideration of reality.

The Wages of Sin

Fourth, by sustaining the existence of an exploitable pariah subcaste of low-cost, drug-dependent workers, and by allowing a revolving system for warehousing segments of this labor pool behind publicly funded prison walls, the War on Drugs slashes production costs and bolsters corporate profits. While street drug users often lack steady full-time employment, they do acquire shorter-term blue-collar jobs of various sorts in the formal economy. Sociologists of work have long recognized that an effective means of lowering salaries across the board in the working class is the existence of a sector of semi-employed workers at the bottom of the labor market. This desperate pool of workers who are resigned to accept socially marginal, low-status jobs at minimal wages functions to competitively pull down the wage levels of other strata of labor. As Waterston (1993:241) notes, "As a special category, addicts are politically weak and disconnected from organized labor, thereby becoming a source of cheap, easily expendable labor. Moreover, the costs of daily reproduction are absorbed by addict-workers themselves."

Moreover, the dramatic increase in the number of imprisoned Americans has created a large pool of potentially available superexploited workers, some of whom earn as little as 17 cents an hour. As Chien, Connors, and Fox (2000:319) point out, "[Prison] employers can freely dismiss and recall workers, need not deal with unions, and do not have to pay for benefits or even work facilities, as these costs are borne by taxpayers." The prison industry, they note, which has a number of subsectors, including the building and running of prisons and the leasing of prison labor, is but one arena in which the private sector directly profits from the War on Drugs.

Unfortunately, as the director of the National Institute on Drug Abuse has argued, there remains "a widespread misperception that drug abuse treatment is not effective. . . . [However] there are now extensive data showing that addiction is eminently treatable if the treatment is well delivered and tailored to the needs of the particular patient" (Leshner 1999:1314). Rates of success in drug treatment are comparable to those for other chronic diseases such as diabetes, hypertension, and asthma. Ironically, studies of the social benefits of drug treatment support the very kinds of changes that those who demonize drug users would most support. First, criminal activity among individuals in and after drug treatment is two-thirds of that of comparable out-of-treatment drug users (Gerstein et al. 1994). Rajkumar and French (1996), for example, calculated that the costs of crime averaged $47,971 per drug user per year prior to drug treatment, compared to $28,657 in the year following drug treatment. Second, French and Zarkin (1992) have found that even a 10 percent increase in the amount of time spent in a residential drug treatment program increases the subsequent legal earning of a drug user by 2.4 percent and decreases illegal earnings by 4.1 percent. Similar findings exist for methadone treatment (French and Zarkin 1992). Third, cost savings in terms of AIDS infection, tuberculosis, and other diseases that are much more common among drug users who are out of treatment compared to those in treatment significantly adds to the demonstrated cost and health benefits of drug treatment (French, Mauskopf, Teague, and Roland 1996). Injection drug users who are not in treatment have been found to be six times more likely to be infected with HIV than those who enroll and stay in drug treatment (Metzger et al. 1993). Further, there is a consistent finding indicating an association between duration of drug treatment and protection from HIV infection (Metzger, Navaline, and Woody 1998).

Currently, of the $18 billion in the federal drug budget, only one-third is directed toward prevention and treatment efforts. However, only 10 percent of the approximately $6 billion of federal money targeted to reduce the demand for drugs is earmarked for the treatment of the estimated 4 million hardcore drug users in the United States (Stocker 1998). Importantly, as a widely cited 1994 RAND study found, from a cost-benefits standpoint, drug treatment is seven times more cost-effective than domestic law enforcement and incarceration, ten times more effective than interdiction programs designed to stop drugs at the U.S. border, and 23 times more effective than efforts to attack the sources of illicit drug production abroad (cited in Massing 1999). In other words, the least funded aspect of the federal drug strategy—treatment—produces the greatest benefit in terms of lowering the use of illicit drugs.

While there are shortcomings to a fully medicalized model of drug treatment (Waterston 1993)—one that does not recognize and respond to the social origins of drug abuse—and sound concerns about the growing "commodification of treatment" (Murphy and Rosenbaum 1999), nonetheless a radical shift toward an emphasis on treatment would go a long way toward creating a healthy drug abuse policy orientation. Of special note, in her ethnographic study of cocaine-using women in Atlanta, the women Sterk (1999:209–210) interviewed emphasized the need for community-based programs that addressed all aspects of their lives. They proposed a harm-reduction approach, which included low-threshold programs that do not penalize drug users who have not quit totally or who relapse, that provide psychological services to help them cope with their past experiences as well as practical services such as basic education, life-skills training, job preparation, and employment opportunities. They yearned for large social changes as well, especially for an end to poverty and an increase in welfare benefits for the poor.

As this finding suggests, while U.S. policy makers haven't figured out how to effectively address our national drug crisis, drug users—those who bear the painful burden of their own addictions—often have a very clear sense of a healthy drug policy. Perhaps it is time that we listen.

References

Agar, M., and H. Schacht Reisinger. (2002). "A Tale of Two Policies: The French Connection, Methadone, and Heroin Epidemics." *Culture, Medicine and Psychiatry* 26, no. 3: 371–96.

Baer, H., M. Singer, and I. Susser. (2003). *Medical Anthropology and the World System*, 2nd ed. Westport, CT: Praeger.

Bertram, E., and K. Sharpe. (1996, September 26). "Drug Abuse: Is the Cure Worse than the Crime—Candidates Lack Answers to Questions." *Hartford Courant*, C–1, C–4.

Bourgois, P. (1995). *In Search of Respect: Selling Crack in El Barrio*. Cambridge: Cambridge University Press.

Browning, F., and B. Garrett. (1986). "The CIA and the New Opium War." In *Culture and Politics of Drugs*, edited by Peter Park and Wasyl Matveychuk, 118–24. Dubuque, Iowa: Kendall/Hunt.

Castillo, F. (1987). *Los Jinetes de la Cocaina*. Bogota: Editorial Documentos Periodisticos.

Chambers, C., and J. Inciardi. (1974). "Forecasts for the Future: Where We Are and Where We Are Going." In *Drugs and the Criminal Justice System*, edited by J. Inciardi and C. Chambers, pp. 218–34. Beverly Hills, CA: Sage.

Chambliss, W. (1994). "Why the U.S. Government Is Not Contributing to the Resolution of the Nation's Drug Problem." *International Journal of Health Services* 24, no. 4: 675–90.

Chien, A., M. Connors, and K. Fox. (2000). "The Drug War in Perspective." In *Dying for Growth*, edited by J. Y. Kim, J. Millen, A. Irwin, and J. Gershman, 293–327. Monroe, ME: Common Courage Press.

Chomsky, N. (1988). *The Culture of Terrorism*. Boston: South End Press.

Clinton, W. (1996). "Transmittal Letter from the President." In *The National Drug Control Strategy*, 3. Washington, DC: White House.

Coffin, P. (1999). *Safer Injection Rooms*. New York: Lindesmith Center.

Community Epidemiological Work Group. (1998). *Epidemiologic Trends in Drug Abuse, vol. 1: Highlights and Executive Summary.* Rockville, MD: National Institute on Drug Abuse.

Davidson, J. (1999). "The Drug War's Color Line: Black Leader's Shift Stances on Sentencing." The Nation 269, no. 8: 42–43.

Dee, J. (1999, November 15). "New Face of Heroin: First-Time Users Getting Younger." *Hartford Courant,* A1, A6.

Domestic Council Drug Abuse Task Force. (1975). *White Paper on Drug Abuse.* Washington, DC: U.S. Government Printing Office.

Drug Abuse Council. (1980). *The Facts about "Drug Abuse."* New York: Free Press.

Eaton, V. (1888). "How the Opium Habit Is Acquired." *Popular Science* 33: 665–66.

Egan, T. (1999). "The War on Drugs Retreats, Still Taking Prisons." *New York Times,* February 28, 1.

Epstein, E. (1977). *Agency of Fear.* New York: G. P. Putnam's.

Forero, J., and T. Weiner (2002, June 8). "Latin American Poppy Fields Undermine U.S. Drug Battle." *New York Times,* Sunday, 1.

French, M., and G. Zarkin. (1992). "Effects of Drug Abuse Treatment on Legal and Illegal Earnings." *Contemporary Policy Issues* 10: 98–110.

French, M., J. Mauskopf, J. Teague, and E. Roland. (1996). "Estimating the Dollar Value of Health Outcomes from Drug Abuse Interventions." *Medical Care* 34: 890–910.

Fresia, J. (1988). *Toward an American Revolution: Exposing the Constitution and Other Illusions.* Boston: South End Press.

Gerstein, D., R. Johnson, H. Harwood, D. Fountain, N. Suter, and K. Mallory. (1994). *Evaluating Recovery Services: The California Drug and Alcohol Treatment Assessment (CALDATA).* Contract No. 92–00110. Sacramento: State of California, Health and Welfare Agency, Department of Alcohol and Drug Programs.

Goode, E. (1984). *Drugs in American Society.* New York: Alfred A. Knopf.

Guttman, W. E. (1996, January). "The War No One Wants to Win." *Z Magazine,* 1–5.

Helmer, J. (1983). "Blacks and Cocaine." In *Drugs and Society,* edited by M. Kellcher, B. MacMurray, and T. Shapiro, 14–29. Dubuque, Iowa: Kendall/Hunt.

Inciardi, J. (1986). *The War on Drugs: Heroin, Cocaine, Crime, and Public Policy.* Mountain View, CA: Mayfield.

Johnson, L., J. Bachman, and P. O'Malley. (1997). *National Survey Results on Drug Use from the Monitoring the Future Study.* Rockville, MD: National Institute on Drug Abuse.

Kleber, H. (1996). "Outpatient Detoxification from Opiates." *Primary Psychiatry* 1: 42–52.

Kruger, H. (1976). *The Great Heroin Coup.* Boston: South End Press.

Leshner, A. (1999). "Science-Based Views of Drug Addiction and Its Treatment." *Journal of the American Medical Association* 282, no. 14: 1314–16.

Levins, H. (1986). "The Shifting Source of Opium." In *Culture and Politics of Drugs,* edited by P. Park and W. Matveychuk, 124–25. Dubuque, Iowa: Kendall/Hunt.

Massing, M. (1999, September 20). "It Is Time for Realism." *The Nation,* 11–15.

McCoy, A. (1991). *The Politics of Heroin.* Brooklyn: Lawrence Hill.

McCoy, A., C. Read, and L. Adams. (1986). "The Mafia Connection." In *Culture and Politics of Drugs,* edited by P. Park and W. Matveychuk, 110–18. Dubuque, Iowa: Kendall/Hunt.

Metzger, D., H. Navaline, and G. Woody. (1998). "Drug Abuse Treatment as AIDS Prevention." *Public Health Reports* 113, supp. 1: 97–106.

Metzger, D., G. Woody, A. McLellan, C. O'Brien, P. Druly, and H. Navaline. (1993). "Human Immunodeficiency Virus Seroconversion among in- and out-of-Treatment Intravenous Drug Users: An 18-Month Prospective Follow-Up." *Journal of Acquired Immune Deficiency Syndromes* 6: 1049–1056.

Murphy, S., and M. Rosenbaum. (1999). *Pregnant Women on Drugs.* New Brunswick, NJ: Rutgers University Press.

Musto, D. (1987). *The American Disease: Origins of Narcotic Control.* New York: Oxford University Press.

Muwakkil, S. (1996, March 18). "Politics by Other Means." *In These Times,* 20–21.

National Commission on Marijuana and Drug Abuse. (1972). *Marijuana: A Signal of Misunderstanding.* Washington, DC: U.S. Government Printing Office.

Rajkumar, A., and M. French. (1996). *Drug Abuse, Crime, Costs and the Economic Benefits of Treatment.* Unpublished manuscript, University of Maryland.

Schultheis, R. (1983). "Chinese Junk." In *Drugs and Society,* edited by M. Kellcher, B. MacMurray, and T. Shapiro, 234–41. Dubuque, Iowa: Kendall/Hunt.

Singer, M. (1994). "AIDS and the Health Crisis of the U.S. Urban Poor: The Perspective of Critical Medical Anthropology." *Social Science and Medicine* 39, no. 7: 931–48.

———. (1999). "The Ethnography of Street Drug Use before AIDS: A Historic Review." In *Cultural, Observational, and Epidemiological Approaches in the Prevention of Drug Abuse and HIV/AIDS,* edited by P. Marshall, M. Singer, and M. Clatts, 228–64. Bethesda, MD: National Institute on Drug Abuse.

Singer, M., C. Flores, L. Davison, G. Burke, Z. Castillo, K. Scanlon, and M. Rivera. (1990). "SIDA: The Sociocultural and Socioeconomic Context of AIDS among Latinos." *Medical Anthropology Quarterly* 4: 72–114.

Singer, M., T. Stopka, C. Siano, K. Springer, G. Barton, K. Khoshnood, et al. (2000). "The Social Geography of AIDS and Hepatitis Risk: Qualitative Approaches for Assessing Local Differences in Sterile Syringe Access among Injection Drug Users." *American Journal of Public Health* 90, no. 7: 1049–1056.

Singer, M., Z. He, and H. Salaheen. (2004). "Cross-border Trafficking in Women for Commercial Sex Work and the Spread of HIV." Presented at the Society for Applied Anthropology, Dallas, Texas.

Sterk, C. (1999). "Fast Lives: Women Who Use Crack Cocaine." Philadelphia: Temple University Press.

Stocker, S. (1998). "Drug Addiction Treatment Conference Emphasizes Combining Therapies." *NIDA Notes* 13, no. 3: 1, 13.

U.S. Congress, House, Select Committee on Narcotics Abuse and Control. (1977). *Southeast Asian Narcotics.* Hearings, 95th Congress, 1st Session. Washington, DC: U.S. Government Printing Office.

Waterston, A. (1993). "Street Addicts in the Political Economy." Philadelphia: Temple University Press.

U.S. Inner-City Apartheid and the War on Drugs: Crack among Homeless Heroin Addicts

20

PHILIPPE BOURGOIS

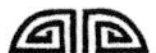

HISTORICALLY, DRUG EPIDEMICS have coursed through U.S. society and across the world with dramatic ebbs and flows (Morgan 1981; Musto 1973). During the last two decades of the twentieth century, for example, the United States cycled out of a heroin epidemic and into a cocaine hydrochloride epidemic that subsequently exploded into crack, only to be supplanted by marijuana and alcohol (Golub and Johnson 1999). Anthropologists, sociologists, and epidemiologists have offered explanations for these changing patterns of drug preferences that emphasize the importance of changes in supply and childhood socialization (Johnson and Gerstein 2000), the utility of ethnographic methods for documenting emerging drug-use practices that impact health (Singer 2000), the effect of drug stigmatization among youth (Furst, Johnson, Dunlap, and Curtis 1999), and the size and relative distress of socially marginalized population subgroups (Bourgois 2003a). A commonsensical understanding links the duration of a drug epidemic to the physical and emotional destructiveness of the particular substance involved as well as to the global and local supply lines affecting supply. Following Michael Agar's work (2003) on "trend theory," but from a political economy of health perspective within critical medical anthropology (cf. Singer and Baer 1995; Farmer 2003), I suggest that these kinds of patterns of drug preferences and addiction rates are linked to the larger historical and structural forces that create vulnerable social groups. Using the cocaine/crack epidemic as a case study, I draw on participant observation among homeless heroin addicts in San Francisco to examine how intimate preferences for drugs at the street level are shaped by macrostructural power relations. This relationship is not linear. The details of the outcomes and durations of drug epidemics change historically due to the catalyst dynamics noted in the literature, including cultural values, accessibility, cost, and pharmacological effects.

Dysfunctional government policies have often exacerbated the negative consequences of drug consumption and have even increased the availability of narcotics in poor, inner-city neighborhoods. Most notably, smuggling and organized crime thrive on counterinsurgency warfare. Throughout the world, drug flows tend to follow the same routes as arms trafficking. Consequently, historically, global Realpolitik has promoted the flow of drugs across international borders—whether it be opium from India to China in the nineteenth century, heroin from southeast Asia during and following the Vietnam War, hashish from Afghanistan during the Soviet occupation in the 1980s, cocaine via Central America during the civil wars in that region in the 1980s, and heroin from Afghanistan following the U.S. invasion in the early 2000s (*The Economist* 2001; McCoy 1991; Webb 1998). Inside the United States, the logics of law enforcement and public sector breakdown channel drugs to poorer neighborhoods where unemployment, discrimination, and a rachitic social welfare net ensure a ready market of unemployed youth eager to sell and consume narcotics (Bourgois 2003b). With respect to crack, for example, the congressional record and declassified law enforcement correspondence reveal that during the early 1980s U.S. officials promoting the overthrow of the Sandinistas protected Nicaraguan counterrevolutionaries when they smuggled cocaine into African American neighborhoods in Los Angeles in order to raise money to purchase guns (Hitz 1998; Scott and Marshall 1991; Webb 1998). The cocaine was subsequently processed into crack and distributed by local youth, fueling the epidemic on the West Coast and promoting gang violence.

Repressive law enforcement practices also frequently backfire. Once again, this was the case in the early 1980s with the cocaine epidemic, which followed a federal crackdown in 1981 on marijuana smugglers causing organized crime to diversify into shipping lower-volume, higher-value cocaine into the United States (Bourgois 2003b:350n77). According to the Drug Enforcement Agency, the price of wholesale cocaine dropped fivefold (Drug Enforcement Agency 1988) and the average retail price of grams dropped 2.25-fold while purity increased by over 160 percent between 1981 and 1988 (Office of National Drug Control Policy 1998:4). This prompted the marketing innovation of processing powder cocaine into its smokable base form known as crack, which efficiently releases the psychoactive molecules of cocaine when burned.

In fieldwork among a social network of middle-aged homeless heroin addicts in San Francisco, conducted with Jeff Schonberg, we have noted dramatic racial antagonisms and distinct ethnic patterns of drug consumption among African Americans and whites who often live side by side in the same shooting encampment. The concept of "habitus" developed by the sociologist Pierre Bourdieu is useful here to link on the level of theory the ways an individual's deepest likes and dislikes are shaped by macro power relations—in this case, race and class. Racially polarized logics organize identity formation consciously and unconsciously, creating distinct definitions of desire and different experiences of everyday social suffering. These "ethnicized habituses" emerge out of the apartheid-like relations that govern social life in the United States and become embodied in differential vulnerabilities to addiction, disease, violence, and incarceration (Bourgois and Schonberg, forthcoming). When applied to inner-city substance abuse, the term apartheid is particularly apt given the disproportional incarceration of Latinos and African Americans following the escalation of the War on Drugs during the late 1980s through the 1990s.

Epidemiological statistics confirm that there are relatively clearly demarcated patterns to drug consumption that follow socially relevant power categories such as ethnicity, gender, sexuality, class, age, and community. For example, with respect to crack, in 1997 the federal government's *National Household Survey on Drug Abuse* reported that African Americans over 35 years of age were 11 times more likely than whites to have used crack during the "past month" (Substance Abuse and Mental Health Services Administration 1997: 37). On the street, addicts take this for granted, as if it were common sense that certain ethnicities prefer one particular drug over another. Because this process operates at the level of habitus, it is generally understood in moral terms as an individual choice rather than as the product of structural forces and public policies that have been embodied by socially vulnerable sectors of society. Similarly, many epidemiological researchers in the United States treat race as an independent risk variable that predicts vulnerability to substance abuse and infectious disease as if that association needed no further explaining. There is an underlying racialized assumption in the United States—conscious or unconscious—that addiction might be genetically determined.

This ethnographic examination of the daily lives of two dozen homeless heroin addicts who we have befriended over the past decade, unpacks the ethnic patterns in drug statistics in the United States (Bourgois 1998). Most of the addicts also smoke at least some crack on occasion and have at least a psychological or even physical dependence on alcohol. They identify themselves with ambivalent pride as "dopefiends." Nevertheless, depending upon their ethnicity, they have very distinct ways of defining their identities and constructing their sense of moral worth and dignity. To overstate for the sake of brevity, the African Americans in the homeless encampments that we visit embrace an oppositional outlaw identity. They dress in color-coordinated outfits and strive to maintain a public appearance of being in control of their lives and relationships. In contrast, the whites present themselves to the public as broken-down winos who are down on their luck. They conceive of themselves as being in a state of chronic crisis and decrepitude. They usually dress in dirty, ripped clothes and talk as if they were depressed and ill. The African Americans supplement their heroin injections with crack smoking and occasional cocaine injection. They frequently stay up all night bingeing on these stimulants. The whites, in contrast, supplement their heroin with fortified wine. This accentuates their sedation, and they usually go to sleep just after sunset.

On any given day, members of these two ethnic groups who share the same street corners and shooting encampments will break these behavioral stereotypes. On occasion, an African American injector will express personal distress and make a contrite plea for help and rehabilitation. Similarly, a white heroin addict will go on a crack binge and celebrate an energized outlaw identity. However, when looked at closely, these transgressions across apartheid lines of behavior and polydrug consumption tend to confirm the racialized and gendered boundaries that define drug preferences on the street rather than contradict them. Hence, a particular African American male will lose status for spending time with "White bitches [effeminate males]" and will complain about their lack of hygiene and their body odor. White injectors in the midst of crack binges will often try to pretend shamefully that they only smoke when others treat them and that they would never waste their money on such a "nigger drug."

Most dramatically, these status hierarchies and differential subjectivities manifest themselves in distinct flesh-and-blood practices with respect to modes of drug administration (Bourgois, Lettiere, and Quesada 1997). This results in differential vulnerabilities to abscesses and HIV infection. For example, all of our network members, because of their advanced age and long careers of heroin injection, suffer from scarred veins and have a difficult time injecting themselves intravenously. The African Americans, however, usually persevere in searching for a suitable vein in order to "direct deposit" the heroin into their bloodstream. Following the logic of their oppositional outlaw identity, they are in pursuit of a successful, euphoric heroin high. This is expressed as a preference for the rush of exhilaration and relaxation that is provided by an intravenous rather than an intramuscular injection. In contrast, following the logic of their identity as depressed social failures, almost none of the whites regularly seek such euphoric highs. They do not even attempt to inject intravenously. Instead, they sink their needles perfunctorily into their fatty tissue or muscle mass, often injecting through their clothes. They claim to be resigning themselves to the boredom of staving off heroin withdrawal symptoms rather than getting high. The whites criticize the African Americans for "nodding out" in public and, conversely, the African Americans criticize the whites for being "lame no-hustles."

Relative preferences for injecting a mixture of heroin and cocaine known as a "speedball" offer a further dramatic contrast between white and African American polydrug preferences and modes of drug administration. The African Americans more frequently treat themselves to speedballs, which hold higher prestige in street drug hierarchies. In the process of injecting these mixtures, they sometimes engage in "booting and jacking" (i.e., drawing blood into the syringe chamber upon registering the needle in their vein and partially reinjecting that blood-drug mixture several times in order to have multiple experiences of the initial cocaine/heroin rush). Booting and jacking is dismissed in a racist idiom by the whites in our network as something "only niggers do." In other words, once again, congruent with their socially constructed identities, the African American heroin injectors are pursuing an ecstatic, active high, while the white addicts are passively staving off withdrawal symptoms.

The ethnic contrasts are not limited to substance abuse. They express themselves in distinct constructions of gender and sexuality. Most notably, the aging African American males present themselves as sexually active and strive to enter into romantic or casual relationships with women. In contrast, most of the older white male addicts openly discuss their lack of interest in sex and describe having erectile dysfunction with no special emotion or concern. Unlike the African Americans, who pursue a hegemonic hypermasculine street-based persona that is considered "cool" and even intimidating, there is no masculine role model for the street-based, middle-aged, white males except that of the Vietnam veteran suffering from post-traumatic stress syndrome. When they try to act tough and effective, they change the way they dress, and talk and move their bodies in order to imitate African American street style—hence the youth culture term "wigger," for whites who want to be black.

The contrast between white and black male identities within street culture is partially determined by differential access to income-generating options due to U.S. patterns of racial discrimination. The general public tends to pity the whites, who thereby become effective, subordinated panhandlers reinforcing the logic for appearing—and feeling—down and out. In contrast, even the oldest, most broken-down African Americans in our network inspire fear and distrust in much of the general public who otherwise contribute spare change to needy street people. The police also subject African Americans to more rigorous surveillance than whites. Consequently, the African American homeless cannot beg as effectively or as passively as white street people even if they wanted to. This helps explain why most of the African Americans experience passive begging as awkward and boring at best and as a racist humiliation at worst. Consequently, when they do panhandle or ask for help, they tend to be more oppositional and demanding, thereby minimizing the dishonor inherent to seeking alms. Unlike the whites who usually avert their eyes dejectedly when they ask for money, the African Americans catch the eye of passersby, sometimes offering to wash their car windows or trade a joke. An immediately visible indicator of this different relationship to passive requests for help and sympathy can be documented on the streets of San Francisco, where the majority of the homeless who display signs at traffic islands—"Vietnam vet-Need help-Will work for food-God bless"—are white.

The whites also obtain day jobs more easily from the primarily white-owned local business owners in their immediate panhandling neighborhood. They represent an extremely flexible and exploitable source of experienced, just-in-time labor for construction supply yards, moving van companies, holiday rush sales operations, and unloading delivery trucks. To ensure the stability and loyalty of their underpaid, off-the-books casual employees, many of the business owners establish patron/client or indentured servant relationships. They lend their favorite homeless person money in advance for their doses of heroin on days when they anticipate needing extra labor power. Several business owners who interacted with our network members limited the maximum daily wage they paid their favorite homeless day laborers to $20 because they have calculated that $20 was the amount of money the average addict in San Francisco required per day in the early 2000s to stave off withdrawal symptoms. They do not want them to have anything extra that might allow them to nod off euphorically on a heroin high or, worse yet, to binge erratically on crack and thereby interfere with their labor discipline.

The African American addicts do not have such fluid access to legal odd jobs during daylight hours. Local business owners generally express a racist distrust of them. The African Americans in turn resist accepting the subordinated status that the business owners demand of their casual employees. This resistance to exploitation and racism may be rooted in the historical labor migration experience of many of the African American addicts in San Francisco. Most of their parents migrated from Texas and Louisiana in the 1940s and 1950s to seek a better life in shipyard and heavy industrial employment in California. Some of their families were fleeing debt peonage relationships in the rural South, and they find it especially noxious to have to reenter that kind of a subordinated exploitative labor relationship two generations later at the turn of the twenty-first century. In other words, they suffer the humiliation that white business owners impose on homeless addicts more acutely than do their white counterparts.

The whites confirm that the abusive nature of their dependence on the local business owners is often personally humiliating. To quote one of the white heroin addicts limping into the encampment at the end of a day spent lifting heavy items at his boss's used furniture store, "It feels like he's got a collar around me. [Grabbing his neck.] I'm a dog on a leash and chain." This man was particularly angry at his employer, who had punished him for arriving late to work that morning by refusing to lend him $10 for an extra heroin injection to control his chronic back pain exacerbated by heavy lifting.

Instead of entering this kind of humiliating and often abusive arena of legal, but off-the-books, daytime employment, the African Americans in our network usually generate the bulk of their income in the evenings after dark in search of opportunities for petty burglary. The following ethnographic vignette depicts one afternoon in the life of an African American couple we befriended. It illustrates the practical dimensions of their professional gangster identity as well as the intimate emotional implications of their modes of substance abuse, their gendered identities, and the pride they take in their income-generating strategies:

JEFF SCHONBERG'S FIELD NOTES, AUGUST 1998. *Tina apologizes for the condition of the Chinook camper. She had planned on cleaning it up last night but she and James were out on a lick [a robbery] and "you know how it goes." James, too, apologizes, except he apologizes for Tina's negligence as a female homemaker. I push aside a pile of clothes and squeeze onto the back seat.*

As we chit-chat, Tina inserts her syringe into a vein that looks like a cord of tar coiled along the inside of her forearm. After two pokes, she registers blood inside her syringe chamber without difficulty and, in one fluid motion flushs the heroin into her bloodstream, withdraws the needle, and then licks clean a drop of blood oozing from the injection spot. She returns her syringe to her change purse after rinsing it once quickly with water.

James places his syringe between his teeth and rolls up his sleeve. He flexs his arm muscles several times, placing the needle point into a vein at his triceps (the brachial muscle just below his shoulder).

After almost 10 minutes of poking, angry cursing, and occasionally pausing to clear out new air bubbles, James asks Tina for help. She wraps a rag tourniquet above James's elbow to try to make one of his veins pop up, and he finally manages to make a direct deposit of heroin into his bloodstream. He thanks Tina for helping, hugging her head in both of his arms and kissing her on the forehead as she flutters her eyelids in an appreciative nod.

They sit nodding in one another's arms for several minutes, savoring the initial flood of sedation from their injections until we are startled by the sound of a beeper. James reaches into his black sweatsuit pants made of parachute material and pulls out a new, clear plastic beeper, explaining almost with pride, "It's my client, the contractor. He gave me this beeper so's to contact me for special orders." He then winks at Tina, "It's time for that lick I was tellin' you about."

We hop out of the Chinook camper into the front seat of a little, orange, banged-up Chevy Luv pickup truck parked next to us. It has old San Francisco Public Works lettering flaking off its sides.

James drives us rapidly through a residential neighborhood a few miles away and parks abruptly under a shady tree next to a block-long park. He and Tina put on traffic reflector vests that he is carrying in the back of the pickup.

Nonchalantly, they rearrange the barricades and traffic cones marking an excavation trench covered by two thick sheets of plywood. They wave to the stalled traffic to continue passing. Imitating public works employees paid by the hour, slowly and deliberately they lift the large sheets of plywood one by one onto the truck. James rearranges the barricades and cones, leaving things as they were minus the plywood covers.

Back in the pickup they seal the lick with a kiss before driving to a McDonald's parking lot where the contractor is waiting for them. We then drive directly to Hunter's Point (a predominantly African

American neighborhood) to buy crack with the $15 they have earned. Before smoking, they clink their glass crack pipes in a toast as if they were champagne glasses.

James and Tina's gendered and racialized versions of outlaw dignity and achievement as "righteous dopefiends" who burglarize effectively and find romance in their ecstatic substance abuse of both heroin and crack are criticized by the whites in our network who share encampments, drugs, and ancillary injecting equipment with them. When Tina and James spend windfall profits from successful burglaries on crack and celebrate late into the night, the whites complain that "the niggers be smoking that crack all night," keeping them awake and making them tired for work in the morning. Tina and James dismiss the whites as unresourceful, lazy individuals who lack self-respect.

It is easy to be drawn into the polarized contest of racialized moral judgments that frames street addicts as flawed individuals who make bad decisions and have weak willpower. Without a theoretical analysis, the structural forces of unequal opportunity remain largely invisible. Most dramatic from the perspective of race relations, however, is the way the escalation of the War on Drugs rendered these ethnicized habituses into an almost formal structure of apartheid by tripling the size of the incarcerated population between 1980 and 1994. The U.S. incarceration rate doubled during the 1990s and was 6–12 times higher than that of any of the nations in the European Union (Wacquant 1999:72). Between 1980 and 1999, incarceration for drugs increased more than thirteenfold (Sentencing Project 2003), and for most of that period the African American increase for drug offenses was over twice that of whites: 707 percent versus 306 percent from 1985 through 1995 (Human Rights Watch 2000). Although they constituted less than 13 percent of the U.S. population, African Americans represented 44 percent of the carceral population in 2002 (Human Rights Watch 2003), a 325 percent increase since 1974 (Bureau of Justice Statistics 2003), prompting sociologists analyzing social inequality in the United States to identify the penal state as the new emergent mode of managing race and class relations following the former state-sanctioned modalities of slavery, Jim Crow, and the inner-city ghetto (Wacquant 2000).

A close look at the technical details of how drug laws disproportionately incarcerated African Americans at the end of the twentieth century reveals that the federal laws passed by politicians in 1986 at the height of the moral panic over crack define five grams of crack to be a felony carrying an automatic five-year prison term. In contrast, 500 grams of powder cocaine were required to justify the same lengthy sentence. This represents a 1:100 punishment ratio, despite the fact that the active pharmacological ingredient is identical in powder cocaine hydrochloride and in crack cocaine base (American Civil Liberties Union 2002). As we have documented ethnographically, crack was disproportionately located in

African American communities—hence, 96 percent of the individuals prosecuted for violating the federal crack laws were African American in the late 1980s (Human Rights Watch 2000).

The future bodes ill. At the height of the War on Drugs during the early 2000s, heroin and cocaine were cheaper and purer on most U.S. streets than they had been two decades earlier (Ciccarone 2004). Through the luck of fashion and a rejection of the negative health consequences of chronic crack and heroin use, the drug of preference among inner-city youth during the 1990s and early 2000s remained marijuana, and the use of syringes was, for the most part, shunned. The United States continued to have the highest income inequality between rich and poor of any industrialized nation, and that gap was growing (Seelye 2001:A12). African American youth in the inner city continued to find themselves largely excluded from the legal labor market, and disproportionately high numbers were forced to seek careers in the underground economy, especially crack and marijuana sales, an occupation that often leads to chronic consumption. At the turn of the twenty-first century, African American youth were over seven times more likely to serve time in prison than their white counterparts (Mauer 1999). Arguably, the most noxious scourge of the crack epidemic in African American communities was the social effects of massive incarceration rates, which continued to relegate growing numbers of black males to outlaw status.

Acknowledgments

Participant-observation fieldwork for this study was initiated by contract N01DA-3-5201 from NIDA's Community Epidemiology Work Group and continued under Professional Services Contract 263-MD-519210 (from NIDA's Community Research Branch), which was subsequently expanded into R01-DA10164. Comparative data was also facilitated by NIDA R01-DA12803, NINR R01-NR08324, NIMH RO1-54907, Russell Sage Foundation 87-03-04, UARP R99-SF-052, Wenner-Gren Trustee Program, and National Endowment for the Humanities through the Institute for Advanced Study in Princeton, New Jersey. My colleague and friend Jeff Schonberg undertook dedicated fieldwork among the homeless. Ann Magruder typed and edited the first versions of this article, and Mimi Kirk completed the final drafts.

References

Agar, M. (2003). "The Story of Crack: Towards a Theory of Illicit Drug Trends." *Addiction Research & Theory* 11, no. 1: 3–29.

American Civil Liberties Union. (2002). "Interested Persons Memo on Crack/Powder Cocaine Sentencing Policy." Accessed at ww.aclu.org/news/NewsPrint.cfm?ID=10360&c=229, July 22, 2004.

Bourgois, P. (1998). "The Moral Economies of Homeless Heroin Addicts: Confronting Ethnography, HIV Risk and Everyday Violence in San Francisco Shooting Encampments." *Substance Use and Misuse* 33, no. 11: 2323–51.

———. (2003a). "Crack and the Political Economy of Social Suffering." *Addiction Research and Theory* 11, no. 1: 31–37.

———. (2003b). *In Search of Respect: Selling Crack in El Barrio*, 2nd ed. New York: Cambridge University Press.

Bourgois, P., M. Lettiere, and J. Quesada. (1997). "Social Misery and the Sanctions of Substance Abuse." *Social Problems* 44, no. 2: 155–73.

Bourgois, P. and J. Schonberg. (Forthcoming). *Righteous Dopefiend.* Berkeley: University of California Press.

Bureau of Justice Statistics. (2003). Prevalence of Imprisonment in the U.S. Population, 1974–2001. Accessed at www.ojp.usdoj.gov/bjs/abstract/piusp01.htm, September 11, 2003.

Ciccarone, D. (2004, November 17–21). "Paradoxics in the 'War on Drugs.'" Paper presented at the 103rd annual meetings of the American Anthropological Association, San Francisco.

Drug Enforcement Agency. (1988). "Crack Cocaine Availability and Trafficking in the United States." Washington, DC: U.S. Department of Justice, Drug Enforcement Administration.

The Economist. (2001). "War and Drugs: Another Powder Trail." 19–20.

Farmer, P. (2003). *Pathologies of Power.* Berkeley: University of California Press.

Furst, R. T., B. D. Johnson, E. Dunlap, and R. Curtis. (1999). "The Stigmatized Image of The 'Crack Head': A Sociocultural Exploration of a Barrier to Cocaine Smoking Among a Cohort of Youth in New York City." *Deviant Behavior* 20, no. 2: 153–81.

Golub, A., and B. Johnson. (1999). "Cohort Changes in Illegal Drug Use among Arrestees in Manhattan: From the Heroin Injection Generation to the Blunts Generation." *Substance Use and Misuse* 34, no. 13: 1733–63.

Hitz, F. (1998, March 16). "Regarding Investigation of Allegations of Connections between CIA and The Contras in Drug Trafficking to the United States, vol. I: The California Story. Statement of F. P. Hitz, Inspector General, Central Intelligence Agency, before the Permanent Select Committee on Intelligence, U.S. House of Representatives." Press Release. Accessed at www.cia.gov/cia/public_affairs/press_release/1998/ps031698.html, April 14, 2004.

Human Rights Watch. (2000). *Statement to the 56th Session of the UN Commission on Human Rights.* Accessed at www.hrw.org/campaigns/geneva/item6.htm, April 14, 2004.

———. (2003). *Incarcerated America.* Accessed at www.hrw.org/backgrounder/usa/incarceration/, April 14, 2004.

Johnson R. A., and D. R. Gerstein. (2000). "Age, Period, and Cohort Effects in Marijuana and Alcohol Incidence: United States Females and Males, 1961–1990." *Substance Use & Misuse* 35, nos. 6–8: 925–48.

Mauer, M. (1999). *The Crisis of the Young African-American Male and the Criminal Justice System.* Accessed at www.sentencingproject.org/pdfs/5022.pdf, April 14, 2004.

McCoy, A. (1991). *The Politics of Heroin: CIA Complicity in the Global Drug Trade.* New York: Lawrence Hill Books.

Morgan, H. (1981). *Drugs in America: A Social History, 1800–1980.* New York: Syracuse Press.

Musto, D. (1973). *The American Disease: Origins of Narcotic Control.* Oxford: Oxford University Press.

Office of National Drug Control Policy. (1998). "Fact Sheet Drug Data Summary." Rockville, MD: ONDPC Drug Policy Information Clearinghouse (February NCJ-167246). Accessed at http://www.marijuana.com/pdf/drugdata.pdf, April 13, 2004.

Scott, P., and J. Marshall. (1991). *Cocaine Politics: Drugs, Armies, and the CIA in Central America.* Berkeley: University of California Press.

Seelye, K. Q. (2001, September 26). "Poverty Rates Fell in 2000, but Income Was Stagnant." *New York Times,* A12.

Sentencing Project. (2003). *U.S. Prison Populations—Trends and Implications.* Accessed at www.sentencingproject.org/pdfs/1044.pdf, April 14, 2004.

Singer, M. (2000). "Drug-Use Patterns: An Ever-Whirling Wheel of Change." *Medical Anthropology* 18: 299–303.

Singer, M., and H. Baer. (1995). *Critical Medical Anthropology.* Amityville, NY: Baywood.

Substance Abuse and Mental Health Services Administration (SAMHSA). (1997). *National Household Survey on Drug Abuse.* Rockville, MD: U.S. Government Publishing Office.

Wacquant, L. (1999). *Les Prisons de la Misère.* Paris: Raisons d'agir/Éditions du Seuil. Reprint, *Prisons of Poverty* (Minneapolis: University of Minnesota Press, 2004).

———. (2000). "The New 'Peculiar Institution': On the Prison as Surrogate Ghetto." *Theoretical Criminology* 4, no. 3: 377–89.

Webb, G. (1998). *Dark Alliance: The CIA, the Contras, and the Crack Cocaine Explosion.* New York: Seven Stories Press.

III

IMPACT OF POLICY ON THE PRACTICE OF MEDICINE

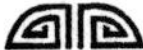

U.S. Health Policy on Alternative Medicine: A Case Study in the Co-optation of a Popular Movement

21

HANS A. BAER

PUBLIC INTEREST IN ALTERNATIVE MEDICINE has become a mass phenomenon as a result of widespread dissatisfaction with the bureaucratic and iatrogenic aspects of biomedicine. This interest initially emerged in the form of the holistic health movement, which came to incorporate an extremely variegated assortment of alternative therapies and practices and which contained a diverse cast of characters, including lay heterodox practitioners, psychic or spiritual healers, New Agers, holistic M.D.s, osteopathic physicians, chiropractors, naturopaths, acupuncturists, herbalists, and homeopaths (Baer 2001). While undoubtedly some biomedical physicians were genuinely sympathetic to alternative medicine, patients created the climate that prompted an increasing number of biomedical physicians to give serious consideration to holistic health and alternative therapies. Biomedical physicians increasingly faced the danger of losing many of their most affluent patients, namely white upper- and upper-middle-class individuals who had become disenchanted with biomedicine and who had disposable income that permitted them to seek alternatives to it.

This chapter examines how biomedical physicians and schools, the federal government, and various corporate bodies have responded to the growing public interest in alternative medicine. I argue that health policies promoted on the part of these parties have been transforming a popular health movement into what increasingly is being termed "complementary and alternative medicine" (CAM) or "integrative medicine." Whereas initially biomedical physicians interested in alternative therapies often tended to speak of holistic health, holistic medicine, or simply alternative medicine, these terms have increasingly been displaced by the terms "complementary and alternative medicine" and "integrative medicine." "Alternative medicine" often refers to the use of therapies as substitutes for biomedical treatment, and "complementary medicine" refers to the use of such therapies in conjunction with biomedicine. "Integrative medicine" refers to a system of medicine that integrates biomedicine with CAM. Furthermore, I argue that various corporate bodies, namely health insurance companies, HMOs, and hospitals, have come to express a growing interest in alternative medicine largely as a means of cost containment.

While the growing interest of biomedicine, the federal government, and corporate bodies in alternative therapies has some positive implications, one of the main drawbacks of present health policy relating to CAM or integrative medicine is that it tends to favor the more affluent social classes and by and large neglects the less affluent social classes, particularly those parties who do not have any health insurance coverage at all. Ultimately, I argue that the incorporation of alternative medicine into the larger U.S. health care system must be coupled with the creation of a universal health care system and a broader conception of health than that with which the holistic health movement or CAM/integrative medicine presently functions.

The Growing Interest of Biomedical Physicians and Schools in Alternative Medicine

Since the 1970s, an increasing number of biomedical physicians have turned their attention to alternative medicine. Some 220 physicians formed the American Holistic Medical Association (AMHA) in 1978. Andrew Weil, a Harvard-trained family physician at the University of Arizona medical center, has become the most prominent holistic M.D. in the United States and probably the world. He has written several holistically oriented bestsellers, including *The Natural Mind* (1972), *Health and Healing* (1983), *Natural Health, Natural Medicine: A Comprehensive Manual for Wellness and Self Care* (1990), and *Spontaneous Healing* (1995). Although he contends that alternative medicine is a mixed bag in terms of its efficacy, he advocates the integration of standard medicine and alternative medicine. Another well-known holistic M.D. is Deepak Chopra, the author *of Perfect Health: The Complete Mind-Body Guide* (1990) and some 25 other popular books. He initially played an important role in introducing the U.S. public to Ayurvedic medicine, but has more recently evolved into a New Age guru who promotes the gospels of self-improvement and financial prosperity. James Gordon, another Harvard-trained physician, authored *Holistic Medicine* (1988) and *Manifesto for a New Medicine: Your Guide to Healing Partnerships and the Wise Use of Alternative Medicines* (1996). He is a clinical professor in the Department of Psychiatry and Family Medicine at Georgetown University and the director of the Center for Mind-Body Medicine in Washington, DC, and has served as the chairperson of the Program Advisory Council of NIH's Office of Alternative Medicine.

In 2002, at least 81 out of the 125 U.S. biomedical schools offered instruction on CAM, either in required courses or electives or both (see www.healthwwweb.com/courses.html, which shows schools offering CAM courses). Andrew Weil, for example, directs the Program in Integrative Medicine at the University of Arizona, which provides continuing medical education (including quarterly mini-conferences) and a two-year fellowship for M.D.s and D.O.s who have completed residencies in primary care specialties. Many biomedical schools now conduct research on CAM, have started centers of integrative medicine, or both. David Eisenberg directs the Division of Research and Education in Complementary and Integrative Therapies at Harvard Medical School. Former Surgeon General C. Everett Koop has been developing a center at Dartmouth University that combines biomedicine and CAM. As Wolpe (2002:169) observes, "The conventionalization of CAM into the academic medical center is part of a long history of medicine containing control over modalities by co-opting them."

While specific biomedical physicians and biomedical schools have taken the lead in adopting alternative therapies, the rather conservative American Medical Association has shifted its stance from stanch antipathy to cautious openness toward them. In December 1995 the Resident Physician Section of the AMA passed a resolution encouraging its members to support the scientific evaluation of alternative therapies. The *Journal of the American Medical Association* devoted its November 11, 1998, issue to "Alternative Medicine."

Despite the growing interest of biomedical and osteopathic physicians in alternative medicine, as Alster (1989:161) so aptly observes, "It is important to recall that physicians were latecomers, arriving to find other groups already well established and claiming to offer different and even superior services than those available from physicians or physician-controlled agencies." Within the corridors of biomedicine itself, nurses, occupational therapists, and physical therapists expressed an interest in holistic health or alternative therapies well before physicians did. While undoubtedly some biomedical physicians are genuinely sympathetic to holistic and alternative approaches, patients and other health professionals appear to have created the climate that prompted an increasing number of biomedical physicians to give serious consideration to the holistic health movement. While some holistic M.D.s and D.O.s subscribe to the philosophical underpinnings of various heterodox medical systems, others adopt their techniques without wholeheartedly subscribing to the ideology of the holistic health movement. Contrary to the claim on the part of holistic health proponents that they wish to contribute to a process of demedicalization by shifting responsibility for health care from the physician to the patient, the growing emphasis on the holistic or CAM model within biomedicine may actually be contributing to further medicalization in U.S. society.

Growing Governmental and Corporate Interest in Alternative Medicine

Health services have become matters of public concern, particularly to third-party payers such as government, industry, business, insurance companies, and labor. In order to define and evaluate the "health care crisis" in the United States, numerous commissions and task forces have been formed over the past few decades and have made recommendations for health policy. Alford (1972:137) notes, "Predominant in all of these commissions are hospital administrators, health insurance executives, corporate executives and banks, medical school directors, and city and state public health administrator." A striking feature of these commissions is the relative absence of physicians, particularly those in private practice. Salmon (1985) argues that a "class-conscious corporate directorship" has come to wield considerably power over health policy decision making. According to Berliner and Salmon (1980),

> Because holistic health is generally provided on an ambulatory basis and stresses prevention and health maintenance, alternative modalities tend to be less expensive than scientific medicine interventions; thus, they may gain an advantage in policy discussions if their efficacy can be assured (538).

As a result of a congressional mandate, the National Institutes of Health (NIH) established an Office of Alternative Medicine (OAM) in 1992. The office reportedly was created "under pressure from Congress alarmed by the soaring costs of high-tech healing and the frustrating fact that so many ailments—AIDS, cancer, arthritis, back pain—have yet to yield to standard medicine"(Toufexis 1993:43). OAM received a mandate to explore the efficacy of various heterodox therapies. The funding for OAM and its successor body, the National Center for Complementary and Alternative Medicine, has increased in virtually each fiscal year. Whereas its budget was $2 million in fiscal year 1992, it grew to $3.5 million in FY 1993, $5.4 million in FY 1995, $7.4 million in FY 1996, $12 million in FY 1997, $20 million in FY 1998, and $50 million in FY 1999. Nevertheless, the OAM budget remains miniscule given the fact that the annual NIH budget was set at $13.648 billion for FY 1998.

OAM created advisory boards and sponsored conferences, publications, and newsletters, and it funded research on the efficacy of various alternative therapies. It had a series of directors—a pattern that reflects its rather tumultuous internal politics. Joseph Jacobs, a Yale-trained pediatrician, served as OAM's first director. Advocates of alternative medicine, including some on the OAM Advisory Council, regarded him to be too conventional and subservient to the larger NIH bureaucracy. Alan Trachtenberg, a biomedical physician with training in acupuncture and homeopathy, succeeded Jacobs as OAM director in October 1994, but served only until July 1995. Wayne Jonas, a biomedical physician who took a three-year leave from the Walter Reed Army Institute of Research, replaced Trachtenberg as director. As a medical research scientist in toxicology and immunology, the new director argued that research on alternative therapies should be "scientifically rigorous and contextually sensitive" (quoted in Goldstein 1999:179). The OAM Advisory Council consisted of 18 members—research scientists, health practitioners, and other interested parties, most of whom have a biomedical orientation.

OAM funded 13 Specialty Research Centers, 11 of which were situated at biomedical institutions. The two exceptions were Bastyr University—a naturopathic institution in Bothell, Washington—and the Palmer Center for Chiropractic Research in Davenport, Iowa. Each research site investigated the efficacy and safety of alternative therapies for various disease or health problems, such as asthma, AIDS, cancer, stroke, cardiovascular complications, and drug additions.

Congressperson Peter DeFazio (D-Oregon) introduced legislation in March 1997 that called for elevating OAM into a Natural Center for Integrative Medicine within NIH with funding of nearly $200 million. Twelve other Democratic congresspersons cosponsored the bill. Passage of a modified appropriations bill in 1999 resulted in the designation of OAM as the National Center for Complementary and Alternative Medicine (NCCAM). As a center rather than a NIH office, NCCAM can directly fund research grants that have undergone a NIH peer-review process. Its mission is to facilitate research on and evaluation of alternative therapies and to disseminate this information to the general public. Congress appropriated $68.7 million for FY 2000 and $89.1 million in FY 2001 to NCCAM. Stephen Straus, an M.D. and clinical researcher, became the first director of NCCAM on October 6, 1999, and continues to serve in that capacity. The National Advisory Council for Complementary and Alternative Medicine consists of 18 voting members. NCCAM's advisory council has more of an alternative complexion than did OAM's advisory council. The present advisory council includes six CAM practitioners—two chiropractors, a naturopathic physician, two Oriental Medicine physicians, and a massage therapist. NCCAM funds 12 centers for CAM, only two of which are located at alternative medical institutions (the Consortial Center for Chiropractic Research in Davenport, Iowa, and the Maharishi International University in Iowa). It also funds four Centers for Dietary Supplements Research, all of which are situated in biomedical settings. In addition to NCCAM, 17 other federal public health agencies fund research on alternative therapies (Goldstein 1999:9).

On March 7, 2000, President Bill Clinton created the White House Commission on Complementary and Alternative Medicine Policy in response to heavy political lobbying, including from Senator Tom Harkin (D-Iowa) and Senator

Orrin Hatch (R-Utah). Stephen Groft, Ph.D., served as the executive director of the commission that had been charged with making recommendations on various aspects of CAM, including training, licensure, and dissemination of information (Final Report of the White House Commission on Complementary and Alternative Medicine Policy 2002). James Gordon, M.D., served as the chairperson of the commission that had 19 other members, including seven other biomedical physicians, one of whom was a licensed acupuncturist. Other members of the commission included a dentist; Effie Poy Yew Chow, a well-known qigong grandmaster and the president of the East West Academy of Healing Arts; another licensed acupuncturist; Joseph E. Pizzorno, Jr., president emeritus of Bastyr University; and five laypersons. In addition to summarizing the status of CAM in the United States, the commission report makes 22 recommendations on topics such as increased funding for CAM training and research, guidelines for scientific research on CAM, the need for dialogue and collaboration between biomedicine and CAM practitioners, the incorporation of CAM into the biomedical curriculum, the provision of training in biomedical principles and practices to CAM practitioners, and the dissemination of information on CAM to the general public.

The demise of the Clinton managed-competition health care plan in the early 1990s provided a shot in the arm to an already-expanding managed health care industry. Various health insurance companies, health maintenance organizations (HMOs), and hospitals have expressed a willingness to provide coverage for CAM, not so much because it offers alternative paradigms and therapies but rather in order to satisfy upper- and upper-middle-class subscribers and patients and for cost containment. In 1996 Oxford Health Plan, which provides care to 1.4 million people in the eastern United States, announced that it would add alternative medicine to some of its health plans. Insurance companies have tended to select CAM therapies such as chiropractic, acupuncture, nutrition, and biofeedback as opposed to seemingly more controversial therapies such as herbal medicine, Ayurveda, and craniosacral manipulation. Indeed, Washington State requires health insurers to cover naturopathic medicine, acupuncture, massage therapy, and other types of licensed alternative health care.

Most of the large HMOs in California now offer chiropractic and acupuncture care (Rees 2001:4). HMOs in other parts of the country are also starting to reimburse CAM treatment. Various health care corporations and numerous group practices also offer CAM or integrative treatment. American WholeHealth provides integrative treatment, which includes family practice, internal medicine, Chinese medicine, chiropractic, and Reiki, in Boston, Chicago, Denver, and Washington, DC (Rees 2001:13).

An increasing number of hospitals have begun to incorporate CAM to differentiate themselves from their competition and satisfy consumer demand. The number of hospitals offering CAM therapies reportedly "doubled between 1998 and 2000 (topping 15 percent)" (Kapthuk, Eisenberg, and Komaroff 2002:48). Academic hospitals in particular have been prone to establish CAM or integrative medical centers.

Although health insurance companies, HMOs, and hospitals are expressing an increasing interest in CAM, Weeks (1999:108) argues that the extent of CAM incorporation into health insurance plans remains "extremely limited." Furthermore, based upon survey research on health insurance companies and managed care organizations, Pelletier and Astin (2002:42) state: "Like conventional therapies, CAM therapies are usually covered only if treatment is medically necessary for a specific diagnosis, and reimbursement is given only for a certain number of visits or dollar limit per year." Given that the United States is the only developed country that lacks some kind of health insurance system, it may be that the willingness on the part of corporations and the federal government to give some support to CAM may constitute a concession that deflects stronger demands on the part of the U.S. public for drastic health care reform. At the same time, incorporation of CAM therapies into health plans, managed care, and hospital care may serve to lower operating costs without necessarily lowering the price of insurance premiums and health care.

Toward an Authentically Holistic and Pluralistic Medical System

Most of the interest in alternative medicine on the part of biomedicine, corporations, and government agencies has been directed toward therapies that originally largely fell under the rubric of the holistic health/New Age movement. Adherents of this movement generally are white upper- and upper-middle-class people who are better positioned to receive a hearing from strategic elites than are working-class people, particularly ones of color, who rely, at least occasionally, upon various folk medical systems (Baer 2001). Nevertheless, various critical medical social scientists have argued that the holistic health movement contains the potential of serving as a form of medical counterhegemony or countersystem (Lyng 1990).

While the type of holistic and pluralistic medical system that Lyng proposes (1990) is an ideal worth striving for, it is important to reiterate that the holistic health or CAM movement by and large subscribes to a limited holism that stresses mind-body-spirit connections but fails to adequately make mind-body-spirit-society connections. The holistic health movement tends to leave out political, economic, and social structural factors in its search for the etiology of disease. It exhorts its adherents to make lifestyle changes, such as dieting, exercising, avoiding smoking and heavy drinking, and managing stress, but does not give adequate consideration to social forces that may induce people to engage in unhealthy behavior. Furthermore, the holistic health movement tends to downplay the role of poverty, low wages, unemployment and underemployment, alienation and stress in the workplace, excessive working hours, environmental pollution, occupational hazards, the culture of consumption, and the social isolation of modern life in illness. Indeed, its proponents all too often treat the notion of holistic health as a rhetorical device that serves their own ends, including professional and pecuniary ones, rather than as a substantive one that provides a critique of the existing U.S. political economy and its associated dominative medical system.

Despite the growing interest of biomedicine, various corporations (especially HMOs and insurance companies) and the federal government are providing alternative medicine with a long-sought legitimacy, it is being co-opted, if it has not already been co-opted, by political-economic forces that could even further erode the movement's concept of holism, limited as it is. In commenting upon the competitive and wary relationship that exists between biomedical and alternative practitioners, Loustaunau and Sobo make the following astute observation:

> Some biomedical practitioners may only be interested in a one-way process of cooptation. Sometimes, plans to bring competing systems under control may be initiated only in order to bring more people into the biomedical system proper with no real understanding of what other systems may offer in terms of care and treatment (Loustaunau and Sobo 1997:180).

Indeed, in a matter of a few decades, it appears that biomedicine, the federal government, and various corporate entities have tamed holistic health as a popular movement and transformed it into CAM, in which heterodox therapies of various sorts often function as adjuncts to the arsenal of high-tech approaches. As CAM therapies are increasingly incorporated into university-based and private integrative medicine care centers directed by biomedical physicians or operated by HMOs, health corporations, and hospitals, they run the risk of being adjuncts to the high-tech, capital-intense biomedical practices that have come more and more under corporate dominance. In essence, by usurping CAM therapies and retooling them in the image of biomedicine, governmental and corporate policies may be robbing heterodox medical systems of their tradition role as authentic alternatives to biomedicine. This transformation constitutes yet one more manifestation of the ability of capitalist institutions to co-opt progressive institutions.

Despite the fact that the notion of holistic health has been in large part eroded, perhaps critical medical anthropologists and other critical medical social scientists can play a role in resuscitating and expanding upon this concept. While this would be a monumental task, critical medical social scientists need to present lectures and even offer courses on the political economy of health in both CAM programs at biomedical schools and at schools of alternative medicine, as well as publish articles on a broader concept of holism in a growing number of CAM journals, which often publish articles by both holistic M.D.s, D.O.s, and nurses and alternative or heterodox health practitioners.

Along with this effort, critical medical social scientists can promote the creation of a universal health care system, particularly a Canadian-style single-payer or even a national health service in which health providers function as public servants (Baer, Singer, and Susser 1997; Waitzkin 2001). The creation of an authentically holistic and pluralistic medical system ultimately will have to be coupled with the demand for a universal health care system that treats health care as a human right rather than a privilege. While the Canadian single-payer system provides universal health care, by and large it is neither holistic nor pluralistic. According to Lyng, within the context of his medical "countersystem,"

> no one medical professional group enjoys a monopology over the right to practice medicine (a monopoly that is granted by social or legal sanction). All professional groups are granted the legal right to offer their knowledge and technique to those who need resources to attain their health care goals. Such a structure is believed to afford patients the best opportunity to attain the knowledge that is most appropriate to their own unique health care needs and to provide a truly comprehensive system of knowledge and technique (Lyng 1990:97).

Waitzkin (2000:204) argues that "because of the powerful economic and political interests that dominate the health-care system, the alternative health [or holistic health] movement cannot succeed unless it connects itself to broader political activism as well." The creation of a universal health care system in the United States could pave the way to provide alternative therapies not only to relatively affluent patients who presently pay for them out of pocket or have access to health plans that cover CAM therapies. Indeed, Waitzkin (2000:205) asserts that "components of alternative medicine ultimately may also be useful for people in low-income and minority communities."

Despite the fact that the plan for a managed-competition health care system failed early on in Clinton's first presidential term, growing dissatisfaction with managed care on the part of both health care personnel and patients, and the failure of the existing system to provide adequate health care to a significant portion of the population, health care reform has reentered the public discourse, particularly as various Democratic presidential hopefuls offered their health care plans. Opposition to a universal health care system in the United States does not for the most part emanate from the public, but rather from a narrow but powerful group consisting of insurance companies, pharmaceutical companies, health care corporations, some health care providers, and small businesses that provide minimal or no health care coverage for their employees. Whereas most corporate interest and physician groups have opposed the creation of a single-payer health care system, various other physician groups, grassroots organizations, and legislators have favored it. Progressive medical social scientists should urge their various professional associations to join with the National Medical Association, the American Public Health Association, and the National Association of Social Workers to endorse a single-payer health care system in the United States. Given their knowledge of both professionalized heterodox and folk medical systems, medical anthropologists could argue in favor of including them into a universal heath care plan. Rather than being divided as they were on the Clinton plan, grassroots groups, professional associations, and health activists may have a unique opportunity to rally behind a single-payer system and force it onto center stage in the health reform plan. As Flacks (1993:465) so aptly argues, "The demand for a universal health-care program . . . has the potential to unite very diverse movement constituencies and to link these with middle-class voters."

References

Alford, R. (1972). "The Political Economy of Health Care: Dynamics without Change." *Politics and Society* 2: 127–64.

Alster, K. B. (1989). *The Holistic Health Movement.* Tuscaloosa: University of Alabama Press.

Baer, H. A. (2001). *Biomedicine and Alternative Healing Systems in America: Issues of Class, Race, Ethnicity, and Gender.* Madison: University of Wisconsin Press.

Baer. H. A., M. Singer, and I. Susser. (1997). *Medical Anthropology and the World System: A Critical Perspective.* Westport, CT: Bergin & Garvey.

Berliner, H., and J. W. Salmon. (1980). "Health Policy Implications of the Holistic Health Movement." *Journal of Health Politics, Policy and Law* 5: 535–53.

Flacks, R. (1993). *The Party's Over—So What Is to Be Done? Social Research* 60: 445–70.

Goldstein, M. S. (1999). *Alternative Health Care: Medicine, Miracle, or Mirage?* Philadelphia: Temple University Press.

Kapthuk, T., D. Eisenberg, and A. Komaroff. (2002, December 2). "Health for Life: Inside the Science of Alternative Medicine." *Newsweek*, 45–73.

Loustaunau, M. O., and E. J. Sobo. (1997). *The Cultural Context of Health, Illness, and Medicine.* Westport, CT: Bergen & Garvey.

Lyng, S. (1990). *Holistic Health and Biomedical Medicine: A Countersystem Analysis.* Albany: State University of New York Press.

Pelletier, K. R., and J. A. Astin. (2002). "Integration and Reimbursement of Complementary and Alternative Medicine by Managed Care and Insurance Providers: 2000 Update and Cohort Analysis." *Alternative therapies* 8, no. 1: 38–48.

Rees, A. (2001). *The Complementary and Alternative Information Source Book.* Westport, CT: Oryx Press.

Salmon, J. W. (1985). "Profit and Health Care: Trends in Corporatization and Proprietarization." *International Journal of Health Services* 15: 395–418.

Toufexis, A. (1993, March 1). "Dr. Jacobs' Alternative Mission." *Time*, 43–44.

Waitzkin, H. (2000). *The Second Sickness: Contradictions of Capitalist Health Care.* Lanham, MD: Rowman & Littlefield.

______. (2001). *At the Frontlines of Medicine: How the Health Care System Alienates Doctors and Mistreats Patients . . . and What We Can Do about It.* Lanham, MD: Rowman & Littlefield.

Weeks, J. (1999). "Insurance Coverage for Alternative Therapies." In *Current Review of Complementary Medicine*, edited by M. S. Micozzi, 107–19. Philadelphia: Current Medicine.

White House Commission on Complementary and Alternative Medicine. (2002). *Final Report of the White House Commission on Complementary and Alternative Policy.* U.S. Government Printing Office. Accessed at www.whccamp.hhs.gov/.

Wolpe, P. R. (2002). "Medical Culture and CAM Culture: Science and Ritual in the Academic Medical Center." In *The Role of Complementary and Alternative Medicine: Accommodating Pluralism*, edited by D. Callahan, 163–71. Washington, DC: Georgetown University Press.

Home Birth Emergencies in the United States: The Trouble with Transport 22

ROBBIE E. DAVIS-FLOYD

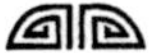

As proponents of the global Safe Motherhood Initiative have long stressed, in both the developing world where home birth is often a necessity and the developed world where it is a choice, primary keys to safe home birth include transport to the hospital in cases of need and effective care on arrival (Fullerton 2000). In this chapter, I examine what happens in the United States when transport occurs, how the outcomes of prior transports affect future decision making, and how the lessons derived from the transport experiences of U.S. birthing women and midwives could be translated into improvements in maternity care. In the developing world, two aspects are critical to the viability of transport: (1) Can the mother get there? In other words, is there a hospital within reach, and can a vehicle be found? And (2) What happens when she arrives? In the United States, where some form of transport is almost always available, the latter issue is by far the most salient. America's trouble with transport is not its lack, but rather what happens when it places the mother who had planned to give birth at home, and the midwife attending her, in interaction with biomedical personnel.

In the United States, as elsewhere, biomedicine and home birth midwifery exist in separate cultural domains and are based on overlapping but distinctively different knowledge systems. When a home birth midwife arrives in the hospital with her client, she brings with her the general ways of knowing and style of practice that characterize her cultural domain, and her specific prior knowledge about the woman's overall health, personality, desires, and labor process. This knowledge can be vital to the mother's successful treatment by the hospital system. But the culture of biomedicine in general tends not to understand or recognize as valid the knowledge of midwifery. Thus in the hospital, the midwife may have no authoritative status. Yet she must interface with medical personnel if she is to communicate information that the hospital staff may need to provide appropriate and effective care for her client. Smooth articulation of the medical and midwifery knowledge systems facilitates the safest transition for the woman and her baby, but, all too often, disjuncture and disarticulation occur. The tensions and dysfunctions that result are displayed in midwives' transport stories, which I here identify as a narrative genre. In this chapter, I unpack these stories for the collision of worlds they encapsulate and the points of fracture and permeability in the crusts of those worlds that they reveal.

I focus specifically on the transport stories told by American midwives with whom I have conducted extensive interviews. I narrate six of these stories, analyzing them as cultural terrains that reveal how childbirth can go unnecessarily awry when domains of knowledge conflict and existing power structures ensure that only one kind of knowledge counts. I describe such encounters as (1) *disarticulations* that occur when there is no correspondence of information or action between the midwife and the hospital staff, and (2) *fractured articulations* of biomedical and midwifery knowledge systems that result from partial and incomplete correspondences. I contrast these two kinds of disjuncture with the *smooth articulation* of systems that results when "mutual accommodation" (Jordan 1993) characterizes the interactions between midwife and medical personnel. In the conclusion, I link these U.S. transport stories to their international context, describing how they index some of the cross-cultural markers for "the trouble with transport."

Articulation and Authoritative Knowledge: Biopower Meets the Home Birth Midwife

> ***ar.ti.cu.late*** vt. *(1) to put together by joints; (2) to arrange in connected sequence, fit together, correlate.* vi. *to be jointed or connected.* n. *a joint in a stem or between two separable parts, as a branch and leaf [or] a node or space between two nodes*
>
> —WEBSTER'S NEW WORLD DICTIONARY, 2000

My use of the term "articulation" in this chapter comes from Gramsci through Lawrence Grossberg (1992:54), who notes that the concept of articulation "provides a useful starting place for describing the process of forging connections between practices and effects." His starting place will be my ending place, as most of the stories I recount below illustrate connections that could potentially have been forged, but instead were either never made or only partially constituted. These disjunctures in what could have been functional, smoothly bending joints stem from the dominance of biomedicine—a hierarchical system that has sought, in general, not to articulate with home birth midwifery, but rather to eliminate it through discounting its practices and knowledge base. In *Childbirth and Authoritative Knowledge: Cross-Cultural Perspectives,* Brigitte Jordan (1997:56) noted that

> for any particular domain several knowledge systems exist, some of which, by consensus, come to carry more weight than others, either because they explain the state of the world better for the purposes at hand (efficacy) or because they are associated with a stronger power base (structural superiority), and usually both. In many situations, equally legitimate parallel knowledge systems exist and people move easily between them, using them sequentially or in parallel fashion for particular purposes. But frequently, one kind of knowledge gains ascendance and legitimacy. A consequence of the legitimation of one kind of knowing as authoritative is the devaluation, often the dismissal of all other kinds of knowing.

Jordan (1997) maps out what happens when one kind of knowing does gain ascendancy, thus opening up the possibility of asking what happens when an ascendant knowledge system and a devalued one must interface. Why do adherents of a dominant knowledge system sometimes dismiss what adherents of a devalued system have to say, sometimes give them partial credence, and other times honor them, act promptly on their recommendations, and include them in the process? The stories I analyze below illustrate all of these possible scenarios.

In the process of describing how Western biomedicine gained its cultural ascendancy, Michel Foucault identified the cultural authority it carries as a form of "biopower," which he defined as "disciplines of the body" used as "numerous and diverse techniques for achieving the subjugation of bodies and the control of populations" (1978:140). This subjugation and control include the biomedicalization of bodily processes like childbirth and the development of institutions within which such processes are supposed to take place, along with formalized structures for managing them. Jordan augments Foucault's notion of biopower with her focus on the status of particular knowledge systems:

> It is important to realize that to identify a body of knowledge as authoritative speaks, for us as analysts, in no way to the correctness of that knowledge. Rather, the label "authoritative" is intended to draw attention to its status within a particular social group and to the work it does in maintaining the group's definition of morality and rationality. *The power of authoritative knowledge is not that it is correct but that it counts* (Jordan 1997:57; emphasis in original).

Although the American home birth midwives whom I have studied treat their own knowledge system as authoritative in the home context, they are acutely conscious of the larger and more valued authority carried by biomedicine not only inside the hospital but also in the culture at large. Much of the time, these midwives do not accept biomedical knowledge as truth or fact; many of their practices and much of their midwifery knowledge system constitute a radical critique of obstetrics, challenging its claims to the authority of fact and truth. But these midwives also understand that in the hospital as in the wider culture, including in courts of law, their radical critique goes largely unheard and their ways of knowing do not count. Faced with a formalized system of biopower that discounts their individualized approach to maternity care, during transport midwives nevertheless often seek to communicate what they know, in the interests of securing the care for which they brought the woman to the hospital—care that they deem to be necessary for their client's safety and well-being. So as they enter the hospital, they extend into that system what I identify as *fingers of articulation* in an effort to generate a productive interface. The following detailed examination of midwives' transport stories intends to illuminate what happens along a spectrum of possibilities from disarticulation to smooth articulation, from the dismissal of these outreaching fingers to their clasping by a biomedical hand. Through examining this spectrum of articulations between knowledge systems, I hope to augment Jordan's explanations of what happens when one system of knowledge discounts another with a more nuanced consideration of how, in specific situations, the dominant system can come to take the subaltern system into partial or fully accommodative account.

Methodology

This chapter is based on my continuing research on American midwives (begun in 1995).[1] The focus of much of this research has been midwifery education, praxis, politics, and status within the American technocracy (Benoit et al. 2001; Davis-Floyd 1998, 2003, 2004, in press; Davis-Floyd and Johnson in press). This research did not specifically focus on transport stories as a genre or on transport as a salient issue. But during its course, I heard many transport stories told. Over time, these transport stories began to emerge for me as a narrative genre that richly encapsulates clashes of power and ideology between the biomedical and midwifery systems and their potentially devastating consequences for mother and baby. The particular stories I present here embody the collision of worlds I seek to analyze. It is important to note that in the United States, there are approximately 200 nurse-midwives (out of over 5,000 Certified Nurse Midwives [CNMs] in practice) who attend both home and hospital births; their transport experiences are somewhat different, especially when they practice and carry authoritative status in both domains. I suggest them as potential subjects of a future study.[2] Because of the political problematics of midwifery practice and especially of transport, all names I utilize are pseudonyms.

Background and Context: Obstetrics and Midwifery in the United States

From an obstetrical point of view, every birth is a potential disaster and must be managed authoritatively and preventively to ensure the best possible outcome. Thus, most women laboring in American hospitals today are routinely hooked up to intravenous (IV) lines and electronic fetal monitors throughout labor. Their labors are often induced or augmented with a variety of pharmacologic agents, including pitocin and cytotec. Epidural anesthesia is commonly used to eliminate pain. Just under half of birthing women receive an episiotomy to enlarge the vaginal opening and speed delivery. Just under 30 percent of all babies in the United States are pulled out with forceps, vacuum extractors, or via cesarean section (Ventura, Martin, Curtin, Menacker, and Hamilton 2001). As various social scientists have previously described (Davis-Floyd 1992; Martin 1987; Rothman 1982, 1989), the performance of birth in American hospitals tells a cultural story about the female body as a defective machine in need of assistance by technical experts and other, more perfect machines; this has also been documented in Mexico (Castro 1999). It also enacts and displays the technocracy's supervaluation of speed, efficiency, control, high technology, and the flow of information through cybernetic systems. Technobirths are typical and normative in American hospitals through a consensual, biopowerful process jointly driven by physicians, who tend to be trained exclusively in that approach, and women, who tend to also to supervalue technology, control, and most especially the elimination of labor pain (Davis-Floyd 1994). For instance, the use of epidural anesthesia necessitates the use of many other technologies to monitor for and intervene in complications associated with the epidural. In other words, while some women might make other choices if they had more information, generally speaking the interventive American approach exists by mutual agreement between women and physicians steeped in the core values and overall approach to life characteristic of their technocratic culture. Both groups believe that this approach offers both comfort and safety in the face of an unpredictable natural process that proceeds more safely when carefully controlled, in the same way that a river subject to flooding seems improved when a series of dams and floodgates are installed.

To hospital-based practitioners, the choice for home birth appears to be a choice for danger, pain, and random chaos in contrast to order and control. Most hospital-based practitioners have never seen a home birth and know little about the knowledge base of home birth midwives, in part because of a near-total lack of contact. The many safe and woman-centered births that take place at home are invisible to the medical gaze; biomedical discourse tends to center around "botched home births." This phrase is often bandied about by medical practitioners who tend to assume that any home birth that ends up in the hospital must be "botched," even if it is the result of an appropriate transport.[3] The midwifery response is usually a sarcastic comment about enormous numbers of "botched hospital births"; women who have had "botched" hospital experiences and later choose home birth are an important source of such accounts. This trading of insults is an in-group phenomenon: hospital practitioners complain to other hospital practitioners about home birth and midwives; midwives complain to other midwives about hospital practitioners. Dialogue between these groups is rare. Mostly, their members inhabit separate worlds that only intersect when a home birth goes awry and a transport is the necessary result.

From an anthropological point of view, U.S. direct-entry midwives elide and confound the usual international distinctions between professional and traditional midwives: some of the American home birth midwives who are professionally licensed and certified were trained through apprenticeship or self-study (Benoit et al. 2001; Davis-Floyd 1998); others are nurse-midwives trained in university-based programs. Despite these differences, and because of their mutual dedication to the welfare of women and belief in the safety and efficacy of home birth, it is fair to say that all home birth midwives in the United States are inspired by a transnational ideology of home birth and "sisterhood" in midwifery. All home birth midwives critique the failures and limitations of biomedicine and have a strong sense of mission about preserving home birth in the face of biomedical hegemony. They believe in women's ability to give birth with little intervention most of the time, in the superiority of homes and birth centers as the sites of birth, and in the efficacy of their own knowledge systems and skills. They do not undertake transport unless they are convinced that the situation is truly in need of technomedical intervention, and when they do transport, their intent is to do all in their power to make the medical system respond in ways they consider appropriate. Thus, their transports usually involve at least two people from outside the biomedical realm: the mother who needs help, and the midwife who will not abandon her even when she is no longer in charge of her care.[4]

All midwives who practice out of hospital must occasionally transport. In the United States, home birth midwives have a transport rate of about 8 percent (Johnson and Daviss 2001).[5] In other words, 92 percent of their clients give birth safely at home, while 8 percent are transported to the hospital during or after labor for various reasons: 6 percent (six out of 100) are transported for precautionary reasons like failure to progress in labor, meconium staining in the amniotic fluid (possibly but not necessarily a sign of fetal distress), or a retained placenta after the birth. Approximately 2 percent (2 out of 100) are transported for potentially life-threatening emergencies (Johnson and Daviss 2001). The transport stories I have culled from my interview data and selected to recount below cluster inside that 2 percent; I urge my readers to keep in mind that the circumstances they recount are *quite rare* and not representative of the vast majority of births. These experiences are most likely to be encoded in narrative because they are so unusual and also because of their heavy emotional charge. Stories give meaning and coherence to experience; midwives who transport under frightening circumstances often need to find that coherence and to evaluate through narrative, with the benefit of hindsight, their own actions and those of the mother and the biomedical personnel.

In transport situations, there are various ways in which things can go wrong: (1) the fact that transport is indicated means that the natural process of birth has in some way gone awry, or seems likely to; (2) the midwife may wait too long to summon transport, usually because of prior bad experiences with transport; (3) the hospital staff taking the call may not understand the urgency of the mother's problems; (4) emergency medical technicians (EMTs) may fail to respond appropriately, or there may be disjunctive communication between the midwives and the EMTs; (5) arrival at the hospital can go awry for the mother and the midwife if either is ignored or mistreated; (6) even well-intended biomedical interventions can at times do more damage than they fix; and (7) not all natural disasters are fixable by biomedical means, so even with the very best of care, the death of the mother or baby can occur. Only some of these possible levels of awryness are illustrated in the stories I tell below. I selected these particular stories because they are typical: they represent the range of possible outcomes of transport and are emblematic of many other situations and possibilities I do not have room to treat here. Since I have no way of ascertaining the truth or untruth of these stories, for the purposes of this chapter I take them at face value and unpack them for what they reveal about midwives' perceptions of, and the meanings midwives attribute to, events as they unfold.

The Stories

In this section, the stories as the midwives recounted them to me are italicized; these stories are not direct quotes but my summarized retellings (unless otherwise indicated). Contextualizing information, my analyses and interpretations, and the midwives' additional comments appear in regular font.

Disarticulation

Carrie's First Story: Unnecessary Delay

Carrie Smiley is a certified professional midwife (CPM) who has practiced in Atlanta, Georgia, for over 18 years, attending during that time over 850 births. Her practice is "unlawful" (meaning that it is punishable in the misdemeanor category).

Most of the home births she attends are for white middle-class couples. She does prenatal care out of her own home, a two-story house at the edge of a small lake in an attractive Atlanta suburb. She began her birth career in the late 1960s working as a volunteer in labor and delivery, and then took training as a biomedical assistant, working in labor and delivery and for a pediatrician for several years. Starting in 1977 she began attending the home births of friends; in the early 1980s she undertook a year-and-a-half apprenticeship with another home birth midwife who later became her partner. The following episode took place in 1984, during the early years of Carrie's home birth midwifery practice. But it should not be regarded as dated, as it typifies many transports that presently occur, especially in "illegal" states.

Carrie and her partner are attending a mother pregnant with her first child, laboring at home and planning a home birth. After about eight hours of labor, the mother has reached ten centimeters dilation and is starting to feel the urge to push. Monitoring the baby's heart tones, the midwives detect strong decelerations, a sign of fetal distress. Hoping to get the baby out quickly, the midwives ask the mother to push a few times to see if the baby will come down. When they realize that the mother is not going to be able to get the baby out with sufficient expediency, they get her to kneel in a knee-chest position, put her on oxygen, and call the EMTs. When ten minutes pass and the EMTs have not yet arrived, the midwives help the mother into their car, planning on driving her to the hospital themselves. Just as they are ready to go, the ambulance pulls up and blocks the driveway. Announcing, "We're here now, we'll take it from here," the paramedics pull the mother out of the midwife's car and help her into the ambulance. But they refuse to heed the midwives, who are urging that they must rush the mother to the hospital, insisting that first they have to get a history. Asking questions like "Have you had any nausea during this pregnancy?" the EMTs are wasting precious time. Frantic at the delay, and knowing the baby might be suffering from oxygen deprivation, the midwives ask the paramedics to put the mother on oxygen. They refuse, wanting to continue with the history, so the midwives get their own oxygen tank out of the car, at which point the medics finally accede and hook the mother up to the ambulance oxygen tank. As the ambulance starts toward the hospital, the midwife riding with the mother asks her to get on her hands and knees to relieve any possible cord compression, but the paramedics get upset and turn the mother flat on her back. Knowing that this position will exacerbate cord compression and reduce blood and oxygen flow to the baby, the midwife compromises by turning the mother on her side, and continues to listen to the fetal heart tones.

Arriving at the hospital, the midwives are told that there are several obstetricians present in the hospital, but only the one on call is allowed to treat a "walk-in" and he is not in-house and will have to be called. Increasingly frantic, the midwives insist to the nurse in the emergency room (ER) that the baby is in distress. The nurse auscultates the heart tones, records them at 130, announcing this to the midwives and the mother, and tells the midwives, "Everything is fine; we will take over from here." She will not look at the records the midwives brought, which show the heart fluctuations, nor pay heed to their insistence that this is an emergency. The midwives are not allowed to remain with the mother in the ER or to accompany her to labor and delivery. Instead they are sent to the waiting room. Carrie says, "Every time we went outside the room, we noticed that everyone seemed to be looking at us and talking about us."

Terrified that they will be arrested and sent to jail, the midwives finally head home. Later they learn that it took the doctor on call one hour and 45 minutes to show up. In the meantime, the nurses caught the baby, who was stillborn. The cause of death was listed on the hospital record as "prolonged fetal distress." The EMT records said that the mother had been antagonistic and refused oxygen, which the midwives insist is untrue. The nurses said the mother refused the electronic fetal monitor. The hospital pushes the mother to file criminal charges against the midwives, but the mother tells the hospital personnel that this death is clearly the hospital's fault, that the midwives acted appropriately and bear no blame, and that if the hospital should try to harass the midwives in any way, she will sue the hospital, not the midwives.

In Carrie's view, she and her partner did their best. Trained to detect fetal heart rate decelerations and to recognize which ones are dangerous, they responded appropriately to the signs of fetal distress. But in retrospect, Carrie wishes that they had taken the woman to the hospital themselves. When I asked her why they called 911 in the first place, Carrie responded, "We were really dumb—we thought that was the appropriate thing to do."

From Carrie's point of view, blocking the driveway and announcing, "We'll take it from here," demonstrated the EMTs' arrogant and authoritative attitude, which at first glance seemed to leave no further role for the midwives to play. She feels that she and her partner demonstrated strength in their refusal to accept this dismissal. Rather, they flexibly and creatively tried to work with the EMTs to help the mother get what they felt she needed. Frustrated by their inability to convince the EMTs of the need for haste, they experienced their success in getting the mother back on oxygen as a small victory. They had good reason to believe that the baby was oxygen-deprived, so when the EMTs refused to act, the midwives resorted to the nonverbal but nonetheless eloquent strategy of getting their own oxygen tank out of the car, figuring that the EMTs would rather use their own oxygen than accept it from the midwives.

One possible reason for the baby's lack of oxygen might have been that the cord was compressed. Cord compression is usually exacerbated when a woman lies flat on her back, so the midwives wanted to put the mother on her hands and knees in the ambulance, as this is the position most likely to take the most pressure off the cord. (In addition, the flat on the back position can cause supine hypotension [low blood pressure] in women because it occludes the vena cava, resulting in inadequate circulation of blood [which carries oxygen] to the placenta and baby.) But a woman on her hands and knees in an ambulance is a strange and unsettling sight and most likely did not match the medic's internal maps of proper patient position or behavior, or of safety while driving. So the midwives had to give up on the most physiologic position; here again they creatively compromised, finding a position that minimizes both cord and vena cava compression while not challenging the medics' views of how a patient should be positioned. For Carrie and her partner, these stand as examples of midwives' ability to "think around" situations to get the system to meet the woman's needs. Such creativity has been demonstrated to be typical of subaltern groups, who must be as aware of the features of the dominant group as of their own in order to successfully navigate inside the dominant system (Schaef 1980).

Several obstetricians present in a hospital, but only the one on call is allowed to treat "walk-ins," and that one is not in the hospital: here Carrie's voice dripped with sarcasm. For her, this situation evidences hospitals' tendencies to be highly structured, category oriented, and rule-bound. Her outside gaze notes that people who have a place inside the biomedical system, having contracted with a private obstetrician, are more likely to get an immediate response than the anomalous, unplaced "walk-in." The fact that the nurses would not look at the midwives' records seems analogous to the medics' refusal to heed the midwives' insistence on haste. Instead, the EMTs wanted to take a history, which of course the midwives already had. But the information the midwives had obtained *did not count* for these biomedical personnel, who valued only the knowledge they themselves obtained. It seems to Carrie that reality as defined by biomedical categories (taking a history, allowing only one obstetrician to attend a walk-in, and counting only information obtained by biomedical personnel) was more salient here than reality as the midwives, the mother, and the stillborn baby experienced it.

Tragically, the mother's refusal to be put on the electronic monitor denied the biomedical system an indicator on which it might have acted. This refusal probably stemmed from the distrust of the biomedical system and its technology that led the mother to plan a home birth in the first place. When the ER nurse announced that the heart tones were at 130, the mother took this news to mean that the problem had resolved itself and "everything was fine." Carrie later learned that in the labor and delivery unit the fetal heart rate decelerations were noted and recorded by the nurses who were auscultating the mother, but for some reason they never told the mother that they could hear the decelerations, so she continued in the belief that the heart tones were still OK. Emphatically, Carrie stated that if the midwives had been allowed to remain with the mother, they would have convinced her to allow the monitor; she said, "We would have done everything from cutting a huge episiotomy to jumping on her tummy to get that baby out. But we were sent away."

Carrie's sarcasm extends to the "lie" that the EMTs told on their official records, a lie she is sure they told to cover themselves in case of lawsuit. It is likely that the paramedics assumed that as biomedically trained practitioners, their word carried more authority and cultural weight than the words of the midwives and the mother, so their notes were more likely to be seen as valid. Practicing inside a hegemonic cultural space can facilitate one's claim to truth. Practicing outside that space not only calls one's veracity automatically into question, but also puts one at risk of legal action: Carrie and her partner feared being sent to jail since their practice is unlawful in Georgia. They have dealt with this threat through their excellent outcomes, on which they keep careful statistics; through obtaining CPM certification, which is not recognized in Georgia but at least shows that they have been tested and have demonstrated the requisite competence; and through publicity: every few years, a local paper publishes a several-page spread on Carrie and her practice, showing pictures of her and of the happy couples she has attended. She feels that this high level of visibility affords her far more protection in the form of community support than would remaining underground.

Reality is as one perceives it, and the effects of any given event depend not on the actual circumstances of that event but on how they are narrated. On both sides of this particular biomedical/midwifery–biopower/counterpower fence, opinions were formed or reinforced by this experience. We can imagine that the story that circulated among hospital personnel about this birth was very different from the one the midwives tell: chances are it was a story about another botched home birth attended by irresponsible midwives. On the midwifery side, it was one more story about the absurdity of biomedical bureaucracies and the arrogance and narrow-mindedness of biomedical personnel—nurses, physicians, and EMTs alike. And it was a story about the dedication and loyalty of the midwives' clients: when I asked Carrie why the mother did not sue the hospital, she responded, "Because she knew that if she did, the hospital would come after us."

Later Carrie added, "Before this experience, I always thought that if you *have* a problem, you call the paramedics. Now I know that if you *want* a problem, you call the paramedics." She notes that this experience made her much savvier about the limitations of the biomedical system. Specifically, it taught her and her partner to always make sure they transported only to hospitals with on-call physicians in-house, and not to involve the paramedics if there was any way the midwives could transport the client on their own. And, as we will see below, it led Carrie over time to work to develop a network of relationships with individuals in the hospitals to which she now transports in order to enhance her ability to prevent this kind of disarticulation of systems, and to facilitate the kind of smooth articulation that can save lives.

Fractured Articulation

Lana's Story: An Inaudible Voice

Lana Lane, an American direct-entry midwife, learned midwifery through a two-year apprenticeship in Fairbanks, Alaska, during which, with her mentor, she attended over 100 births. Shortly after finishing her training in 1985, she moved to

Wasilla, Alaska, where she went into partnership with Susan Eakin. By then, the direct-entry midwives of Alaska had achieved their legislation and were practicing legally. This story, told to me by Lana's partner Susan, took place the following year.

Arriving at the home of a woman in early labor who lived less than five minutes away from a tertiary care center in Anchorage, Lana performed a vaginal exam to check the degree of cervical effacement, dilation, and station (the position of the baby's head), and suddenly found the umbilical cord in her hand. Susan said, "The cord was just below the baby's head. Lana tried to slip it up away from the vaginal opening, hoping the head would block it, which can sometimes be done if too much cord doesn't wash down. But the cord just kept slipping, so all Lana could do was keep the cord from being pinched (which would cut off the baby's blood and oxygen supply) by splinting it between her fingers and pushing the head off it." While the mother crouched on her knees and prayed, Lana maintained the head in place, telling her partners to administer oxygen to the mother and the father to call 911. He held the phone for Lana as she described the situation and begged them to have an operating room ready. At that point, the baby's heart tones were fine. The ambulance arrived in two minutes. The EMTs were cooperative and did not question the midwife's judgment. Lana straddled the stretcher below the mother, applying counterpressure to the baby's head with one hand and with the other using the Doppler to monitor heart tones that were steadily dropping. They were inside the hospital within minutes. But upon arrival, they found that nothing had been done to prepare for the cesarean. For thirty minutes, Lana knelt on the stretcher holding the head in place and listening to the heart tones drop—50, 40, 30. She lost her voice from screaming for the hospital staff to hurry. But by the time the cesarean was finally performed, the baby had died.

A prolapsed cord is life-threatening to the baby—when the cord is in front of the baby's head, it is compressed, thereby cutting off blood and oxygen circulation to the baby. Unless the baby can be birthed immediately or a cesarean quickly performed, the baby is likely to die. In this situation, wherever it occurs, the mother must get into the knee-chest position, which takes the pressure off the cord, while the practitioner kneels behind her and applies counterpressure to the baby's head so that the cord is not compressed between the head and the woman's pelvis. Keeping her hand inside the mother's vagina, the practitioner must hold up the baby's head until the baby is removed by cesarean—a dramatic scenario to say the least, the success of which depends on how quickly the cesarean is performed.

This story resonates with pain; indeed Lana's partner Susan, who first recounted it to me, was crying as she spoke. She did not know exactly why Lana's pleas for speed were ignored, but she felt sure that it had something to do with the hospital staff's disapproval of home birth. The worst-case scenario would interpret hospital personnel as deliberately ignoring this "walk-in" from outside to prioritize the women inside, to punish her for trying to give birth at home, or both. Prior and subsequent experiences have ensured that Susan holds this worst-case view. She said:

> In my opinion, the reason no one came to the rescue is because it was a planned home birth gone bad. I don't think they believed Lana knew a thing. More than once we've been forced to wait on circumstances they would normally be scam-

> pering to fix. I could tell you several stories in which the medical staff tried to hang us, instead of acknowledging that we transported appropriately.

In contrast, the scenario that attributes the best intentions to the hospital practitioners has to do with the logistics of hospital procedures. When a cord prolapse occurs in hospital, the practitioner who identifies it issues a crash call, the obstetrical team flies into action, and when all goes well the baby is delivered by cesarean within ten minutes. But getting everything in place for a cesarean is very expensive in terms of the personnel and equipment needed, and most hospitals have experiences of doctors, paramedics, nurses, and/or midwives telling them to prepare for a cesarean when one really isn't needed. Setting up unnecessarily ties up rooms, obstetricians, and anesthesiologists and may keep them from being available if needed elsewhere. Thus, it is logical that a hospital would want to assess the situation before taking action, especially on the word of a person unknown to them (which might include a private physician).

This transport took place in 1986 but is far from anachronistic—similar scenarios still play out around the country, especially in states where midwives practice illegally but also in states where they are legal but not well accepted by biomedical practitioners. It illustrates the dysfunctions generated by partial, fractured articulations between the biomedical and home birth midwifery systems. The biomedical system's first response was appropriate—the EMTs supported the midwife to continue her work and did not challenge the validity of her knowledge or approach. And on the phone the hospital promised a response. But somewhere between the promise and the mother and midwife kneeling on the stretcher in the hall, a fracture occurred in what had promised to be a system of smooth articulation, and it was the baby who fell through the crack. Both the worst-case scenario (that the hospital deliberately delayed action to punish the midwives and the mother for attempting a home birth) and the best-case scenario (that, given the expense and difficulty of preparing the operating room, hospital practitioners didn't feel they could risk taking these unknown midwives at their word) point up the importance of prior dialogue and relationship between the hospital and the midwives in order to establish mutual trust and systems of smooth articulation well in advance of this kind of emergency.

Dina's Story: Home Birth as Child Abuse?

Dina Farraw, an American CPM from Arkansas, transported a client after a home birth for a retained placenta. The doctor did remove the placenta, but only after sternly telling the woman and her husband that it was "child abuse" to give birth at home with midwives. This insulting remark was most likely made out of sincere beliefs that midwives are ignorant and that home birth is a highly risky enterprise. The statistics on the safety of home birth in the United States are not taught in medical school, and most obstetricians are simply unaware of the good outcomes home birth midwives generally achieve (Rooks 1997:345–384). Of course, it is ironic that the doctor's belief in the midwives' ignorance stems from his own. The hegemony of obstetrics has forced midwives to educate themselves in its ideology and assumptions, protocols, and lexicon to enhance their chances of successfully interfacing with it and of being able to defend their actions in its terms. In contrast, the marginality of midwifery has allowed obstetricians to remain ignorant about it. Obstetricians tend to be unilingual in the language and technologies of biopraxis, while midwives tend to be multilingual. They manipulate the lexicons of both obstetrics and midwifery, as well as of various folk systems of practice and belief that inform the lifeworlds of the clients they attend (such as Latinas in the Rio Grande Valley in Texas, or the Amish in Pennsylvania and Tennessee). Midwives thus transgress and elide professional boundaries on a daily basis, while obstetricians tend to reinforce them. Fractures in attempts at articulation (like this doctors' insulting remarks) often result from this kind of obstetrical boundary reinforcement.

A few U.S. physicians are willing to elide and transgress professional boundaries in order to support home birth midwives. Such support can be costly: in the United States, some physicians have lost their hospital privileges, their insurance, and their ability to practice in their communities as punishment for working with home birth midwives. Of course, the more physicians supportive of home birth midwifery are marginalized within biomedicine, the less ability they have to create needed structures for smooth articulation.

Smooth Articulation

It is important to remember that for all the transports that go awry, many others go smoothly and most do not result in anyone's death even when they are characterized by fractured articulations. Very few midwives in the United States ever lose a mother, but out of every 1,000 births, two or three babies will die no matter where they are born or who attends them. In the United States, home birth data indicate that babies whose births start out at home do not die at any higher rates than babies whose births start out in the hospital—there is no added risk to home birth (Rooks 1997; Macdorman and Singh 1998; Johnson and Daviss 2001). As I noted above, only 2 percent of transports are true emergencies; the same emergencies happen in hospitals. But clearly, transports that involve fracture or disarticulation between biomedicine and midwifery can amplify the problems already generated by the complication that motivated the transport; sometimes those disjunctures alone are enough to cause a death that would not otherwise have occurred. On the other hand, when a home birth transport is treated effectively, the chances for survival of mother and baby are greatly enhanced. This more positive scenario requires smooth articulation between the biomedical and home birth midwifery systems, which the following two stories will illustrate. They both come from Carrie Smiley, the aforementioned CPM from Atlanta, Georgia.

A mother pregnant with her second child started bleeding during mild early labor. Although the baby's heart tones were good, Carrie was concerned by the dark red color of the blood, which indicated that it was not from a superficial cause. She called the hospital and told the nurse-midwife that some kind of placental abruption might be occurring. Welcomed in the hospital, the mother labored for another three hours in the jacuzzi and on the birth ball. She pushed for about ten minutes, and delivered on her hands and knees while the nurse-midwife caught the baby. When Carrie and the nurse-midwife examined the placenta, they could see a five-centimeter clot on it—an indication that the placenta had partially detached in that area and had been bleeding from that place for a while. After the birth, the doctor told Carrie that she probably could have stayed at home for this one. And Carrie told him, "You have to realize that it's important for me to transport sooner rather than later when I have the option." And he said, "You are right—I don't always see it from your side."

A primary ingredient in Carrie's willingness to transport early rather than late was the excellent relationship she has established over time with this doctor and this particular hospital. Carrie's many positive experiences with the M.D. and the nurse-midwives who work with him illustrate how different kinds of articulations can happen in the same location as the actors come to know and develop trust in each other over time.

Brigitte Jordan's (1993) call for the replacement of top-down, culturally inappropriate obstetrical systems with models of mutual accommodation between biomedical and indigenous systems is equally significant for postmodern home birth midwifery systems. Nurse-midwives are especially well placed to achieve such mutual accommodation, as they inherently straddle and bridge (and occasionally fall into the fissures between) biomedicine and home birth midwifery. Establishing close relationships with home birth midwives who are not legal is simultaneously a transgressive and a boundary-spanning act. The prior communication and relationship between Carrie, the nurse-midwives, and the supportive physician certainly facilitated the smooth articulation of systems that this story illustrates. In fact, the articulation between Carrie's knowledge system and that of the hospital practitioners is *so* smooth that she is more than willing to transport even for situations that have nothing to do with risk:

A mother giving birth for the first time had pulled a muscle in her back. Carrie spent hours trying to relieve her back pain with showers and warm compresses and massage. She said,

> After a while we were running into brick walls as far as pain relief for the spasms, so we decided to go into the hospital where they have jacuzzis in the labor rooms. By the time we got there, she was 6 centimeters. The nurse-midwives who received us told her she was doing great. The jets did good counter-pressure on the back

> pain. They never started an IV and she had no pain medication. The baby's heart tones always sounded great. I was able to catch the baby as "the grandmother" on the chart—the nurse working with us had had her babies at home, and the nurse-midwife was very supportive and felt this mom really deserved the continuity. The baby was fine and the family went home twelve hours after the birth.

As these two stories illustrate, smooth articulation between knowledge systems proceeds through points of overlap, transition, and communication that facilitate the seamless flow of information and linked, imbricated decision making in which the actions taken by one person or group build on the information supplied by another. The relationships between Carrie and the hospital-based CNMs encompass such points. When this kind of decision making takes place within the top-down biomedical system, such imbrication requires a rejection of its tendency to discount or dismiss as irrelevant other ways of knowing. Such rejections can and do take place at the level of the individual even when the system as a whole remains dismissive.

What motivates or inspires a physician to reject the top-down system and give credence to home birth midwifery knowledge? My observations are that the ingredients key to an individual MD's predisposition to smooth articulation and mutual accommodation include (1) exposure to midwifery care, (2) exposure to midwives, and (3) attention to scientific evidence. I will briefly deal with each of these in turn.

Exposure to midwifery care. Some doctors train in hospitals where nurse-midwives practice and thus are able to observe firsthand the benefits of midwifery care, which can include birth in upright positions, without an episiotomy, and with a great deal of hands-on support. Nurturance and consideration tend to characterize the midwife's approach to the mother; shared decision making takes place in a context of mutual respect. These trainees often become imbued with a desire to incorporate this humanistic approach into their own practices, and will be more likely to work with nurse-midwives in the future from a partnership, rather than a hierarchical, perspective.

Occasionally a brave physician will venture outside hospital bounds and observe a midwife-attended home birth—an experience that tends to be emotionally evocative and ideologically transformative (e.g., Wagner 1997). Clinicians judge other clinicians as individuals, not just as members of a class or category; individual judgments can overcome prejudices based on subcultural differences. Does a specific practitioner give good care, make good decisions, and communicate accurately? Individual practitioners decide the answers on the basis of experience. All clinical practitioners constantly gather experience and information, and react differently to a comment, order, or action from someone they trust as opposed to someone whose judgment has been faulty in the past or whom they do not know. Midwives work best with the doctors they have come to trust as a result of experience, and vice versa. But most doctors have little or no experience of working with home birth midwives, and the experiences they do have may be skewed if they come only during emergency transports. It's a tautological circle: lack of experience with working together creates problems that exacerbate and perpetuate lack of experience with working together.

Exposure to midwives. It is accurate to say that in general, American home birth midwives have impressive personalities, a strong sense of commitment and dedication to serving women, a secure sense of their own self- and professional worth, and a large fund of knowledge about parturition that seamlessly permeates their conversation. Simply spending time with them can turn a hospital practitioner from an opponent to a supporter. In U.S. communities where smooth articulation characterizes transport, home and hospital midwives, and sometimes physicians, often participate in periodic potluck dinners where models of mutual accommodation begin to emerge over casseroles and drinks. Hospital midwives who develop respect for and good relationships with home birth midwives often transmit this trust to the physicians with whom they work, in a kind of spillover effect that paves the way for future smooth articulations during transport.

Attention to the scientific evidence. There is increasing emphasis these days on "evidence-based medicine" (Rooks 1999). As we have seen, midwifery tends to be more evidence-based than obstetrics because midwives are generally less interventive than physicians (Frye 1995; Davis 1997; Gaskin 1990; Rooks 1997), and the scientific evidence (Rooks 1997:345–384; Macdorman and Singh 1998; Goer 1999; Enkin et al. 2000) shows that many common interventions do more damage than good. Any doctor who actually looks at the evidence instead of relying solely on what he or she is taught by biomedical tradition will take note of the benefits of midwifery care, and will thus be less likely to assume a blanket superiority for tradition-based obstetrics.

Cross-Cultural Perspectives on Transport

Midwives transport in hopes of resolving a situation they feel they cannot or should not handle at home, with hopes and prayers for a good reception most especially for the mother, but also for themselves. A positive reception in the hospital reinforces midwives' sense of themselves as competent practitioners and elicits in them feelings both of pride in their good judgment and of gratitude toward the biomedical system for its efforts; a negative reception can leave the midwife (and the mother) emotionally scarred. Once burned, twice shy, they may in the future try too hard to avoid another transport, with potentially unfortunate results. Cross-cultural research provides multiple examples (e.g., Allen 2002; Barnes-Josiah, Myntti, and Augustin 1999; Davis-Floyd 2003; Iskandar, Atom, Hull, Dharmaputra, and Aswar 1996; Graham 1999; Kroeger 1996). For one brief example that stands for countless others, Deborah Barnes-Josiah and her colleagues have shown that, in Haiti, community midwives who have been badly treated in hospitals, or whose clients have received inadequate care after transport, try in the future to avoid transport by coping with emergencies at home as best they can, often until it is too late to seek help. If disaster befalls, the midwife is handed the blame, with no account taken of the prior experiences that generated her avoidance behavior (Barnes-Josiah, Myntti, and Augustin 1998).

The solution to the trouble with transport that the governments of developing countries have generally sought to implement usually involves the goal of eliminating home birth and traditional midwifery in favor of hospital or clinic birth attended by physicians and/or professional midwives trained in two-year, government-approved courses (Hsu 2002; Jenkins 2002; Sargent 1989). Yet for a variety of reasons (see Davis-Floyd 2000), women in many countries continue to choose their traditional attendants. Certainly, as Roger and Patricia Jeffrey pointed out in 1993, it is important not to romanticize indigenous midwifery and indigenous midwives: some indigenous customs are beneficial and some are not; some traditional midwives are competent practitioners within their own systems and some are not. Similar notes can be sounded about obstetricians: some intervene inappropriately, ignoring the evidence, while others exercise a more balanced and judicious approach. The transport stories I recount here should not be simplistically interpreted to indicate that all midwives are good and all biopowerful practitioners are bad or vice versa, but rather as ways of illuminating points of disjuncture and fracture, as well as models of smoothness, in the cross-boundary articulation of disparate knowledge systems.

Today in most developed countries, the home birth rate hovers around 1 percent. That home birth might be more widely chosen in the developed world if it were more readily available is indicated by the Netherlands, where the home birth rate has never dropped below 30 percent (Weigers 1997), and New Zealand, where in recent years it has risen to 12 percent as the result of a strong alliance between midwives and consumers that has generated active government support. These two countries stand as models of what I would name *seamless articulation*—their midwives practice, and their health care systems fully support birth in all settings, creating ease of choice and continuity of care across what in most other countries can only be seen as the home/hospital divide (DeVries, van Teijlingen, Wrede, and Benoit 2001). In Europe as in the United States, active movements seek to restore home birth as a viable option, with variable success. Meanwhile, in the developing world, home birth rates continue to decline in response to the pressures of modernization, yet millions of women still give birth at home, some because there is no other option, some out of active rejection of their region's biomedical system, and others out of philosophical choice.

Home birth was both normal and normative for most of human history. But with the advent of biomedicine in the industrialized West, hospital birth became normative and home birth for most women ceased to exist as a viable or even thinkable option. In the developing world, this process is still unfolding; in many Third World countries, it has already taken root to the extent that while home birth remains normative in rural areas, in the cities it has become an alternative and marginalized choice as it is in most of the developed world. Nevertheless, some women still make that choice, and traditional midwives continue to serve them; only now, like American midwives, some of these urbanized traditional midwives are developing hybrid techniques that reflect the multiple systems of knowledge that intersect in their practices (Davis-Floyd 2001b, 2003). They value the knowledge systems they are creating *and* the sometimes lifesaving knowledge system of biomedicine; yet the biomedical system, generally speaking, values only itself. Thus for home birth midwives everywhere, biomedicine stands at once as the ultimate recourse and the ultimate enemy, often with no guarantees in any given transport as to which aspect will manifest.

The transport stories I recounted and analyzed here are fractals for thousands of others that shed light on the trouble- and stress-full interface between the worlds of biomedicine and home birth midwifery. Spiraling beyond the bounds of the specific situations they recount, they index both the myriad possibilities for tragedy inherent in one knowledge system's closed dismissal of its marginalized competitor, and the enhanced possibilities for more positive outcomes when members of that system open its boundaries to admit the fingers of articulation extended by practitioners from the outside. When parallel fingers reach out from the inside, taking account of midwives' information, acting on their recommendations, and encouraging them to remain with the mother to provide ongoing support, the result can be what Grossberg (1992:57) terms "active structures . . . that cut across domains and planes." I encourage further studies by medical anthropologists of how such active structure of smooth articulation can develop between dominant and subaltern knowledge systems of all kinds. In this particular case of medicine versus midwifery, such studies could help practitioners to extend individualized links and notes across the home/hospital divide, and thereby to mend the fractures that generate much of the trouble with transport.

Acknowledgments

I express my appreciation to the Wenner-Gren Foundation for Anthropological Research for its support of my midwifery research through grants #6015 and #6427.

Notes

1. Much of this chapter is adapted from Davis-Floyd (2003).

2. Ideally, nurse-midwives' transport experiences should be seamless but often are not. While there are excellent data on the statistical *outcomes* of nurse-midwife-attended births in the United States, including home-hospital transports (Macdorman and Singh 1998), I know of no research on American nurse-midwives' transport *experiences*.

3. Medical practitioners who only see problematic home births that are transported to the hospital tend to think that all home births are "botched." The rate of problems derives as a function of a numerator (number of cases with problems) and a denominator (total number of cases—the majority—that have good outcomes). If one only sees the numerator, it is impossible to realize that the rate of transports is actually very low compared to the number of successful home births.

4. A caveat: to my knowledge, most home birth midwives who transport enter the hospital and stay with their clients for as long as they are allowed to stay. But some hospital practitioners criticize home birth midwives who "dump their clients at the hospital door and take off." Such midwives usually live in states where their practice is illegal or in places where local hospital personnel are known to be particularly negative and unreceptive. Leaving their clients at the door can be viewed as an extreme form of disarticulation stemming from midwives' fear that any interaction with the hospital system at best will result in serious harassment and at worst will send them to jail—a powerful argument for the legalization of midwifery, which certainly facilitates the development of systems of smooth articulation.

5. In the United States, there were 23,232 home births in 1998 and 23,518 in 1999—an increase of 1.2 percent. Midwives are not the only practitioners who attend home births. Of 23,518 home births reported on U.S. birth certificates in 1999, 2,476 (10.5 percent) were attended by a physician, 12,123 (51.5 percent) by a midwife, and 8,524 (36.2 percent) by someone else. Some but not all of the "other" attendants were probably midwives practicing without legal authority (Ventura et al. 2001).

References

Allen, D. R. (2002). *Managing Motherhood, Managing Risk: Fertility and Danger in Rural Tanzania.* Ann Arbor: University of Michigan Press.

Barnes-Josiah, D., C. Myntti, and A. Augustin. (1998). "The Three Delays as a Framework for Examining Maternal Mortality in Haiti." *Social Science and Medicine* 46: 981–993.

Benoit, C., R. Davis-Floyd, E. van Teijlingen, S. Wrede, J. Sandall, and J. Miller. (2001). "Designing Midwives: A Transnational Comparison of Educational Models." In *Birth by Design: Pregnancy, Maternity Care, and Midwifery in North America and Europe,* edited by R. DeVries, E. van Teijlingen, S. Wrede, and C. Benoit, 139–65. New York: Routledge.

Castro, A. (1999). "Commentary: Increase in Caesarean Sections May Reflect Biomedical Control Not Women's Choice." *British Medical Journal* 319: 1401–1402. Accessed at www.bmj.com/cgi/content/full/319/7222/1397#resp2.

Davis, E. (1997). *Heart and Hands: A Midwife's Guide to Pregnancy and Birth,* 3rd ed. Berkeley: Celestial Arts. (Originally published in 1983.)

Davis-Floyd, R. (1992). *Birth as an American Rite of Passage.* Berkeley: University of California Press.

———. (1994). "The Technocratic Body: American Childbirth as Cultural Expression." *Social Science and Medicine* 38, no. 8: 1125–40.

———. (1998). "The Ups, Downs, and Interlinkages of Nurse- and Direct-Entry Midwifery: Status, Practice, and Education." In *Paths to Becoming a Midwife: Getting an Education,* 4th ed., edited by J. Tritten and J. Southern, 67–118. Eugene, OR: Midwifery Today. Accessed at www.midwiferytoday.com/books/paths.asp, April 21, 2004.

———. (2000, March). "Global Issues in Midwifery: Mutual Accommodation or Biomedical Hegemony?" *Midwifery Today,* 12–17, 68–69.

———. (2001b, November). "Las parteras de Morelos: The Strategic Negotiation of Knowledge Systems by Postmodern Midwives in Mexico." Paper presented at the annual meetings of the American Anthropological Association.

———. (2003). "Home Birth Emergencies in the US and Mexico: The Trouble with Transport." In *Reproduction Gone Awry* (special issue), edited by Gwynne Jenkins and Marcia Inhorn. *Social Science and Medicine* 56, no. 9: 1913–31.

———. (2004). "Qualified Commodification: Consuming Midwifery Care." In *Consuming Motherhood,* edited by J. Taylor, D. Wozniack, and L. Layne. New Brunswick, NJ: Rutgers University Press.

———. (in press). "The History, Ideology, and Politics of American Midwifery." In Robbie Davis-Floyd and Christina Johnson, *Mainstreaming Midwives: The Politics of Professionalization.* New York: Routledge.

Davis-Floyd, R., S. Cosminsky, and S. L. Pigg, eds. (2001). *Daughters of Time: The Shifting Identities of Contemporary Midwives. Medical Anthropology* 20, no. 2–3/4 (special triple issue).

Davis-Floyd, R., and E. Davis. (1997). "Intuition as Authoritative Knowledge in Midwifery and Home Birth." In *Childbirth and Authoritative Knowledge: Cross-Cultural Perspectives,* edited by R. Davis-Floyd and C. Sargent, 315–349. Berkeley: University of California Press.

Davis-Floyd, R., and C. Johnson, eds. (in press). *Mainstreaming Midwives: The Politics of Professionalization.* New York: Routledge.

DeVries, R., E. van Teijlingen, S. Wrede, and C. Benoit, eds. (2001). *Birth by Design: Pregnancy, Maternity Care and Midwifery in North America and Europe.* New York: Routledge.

Enkin, M., M. J. N. C. Kierse, J. Neilson, C. Crowther, L. Duley, E. Hodnett, and J. Hofmeyr. (2000). *A Guide to Effective Care in Pregnancy and Childbirth,* 3rd ed. New York: Oxford University Press.

Foucault, M. (1978). *The History of Sexuality: An Introduction,* vol. 1. Translated by Robert Hurley. New York: Random House.

Frye, A. (1995). *Holistic Midwifery: A Comprehensive Textbook for Midwives in Home Birth Practice, vol. I: Care during Pregnancy.* Portland, Oregon: Labyrs Press.

Fullerton, J., ed. (2000). *Skilled Attendance at Delivery: A Review of the Evidence.* New York: Family Care International.

Gaskin I. M. (1990). *Spiritual Midwifery.* 3rd edition. Summertown, TN: The Book Publishing Company.

Goer, H. (1999). *The Thinking Woman's Guide to a Better Birth.* New York: Penguin Putnam/Perigree.

Graham, S. (1999). "Traditional Birth Attendants in Karamoja, Uganda." Ph.D. diss., South Bank University, London.

Grossberg, L. (1992). *We Gotta Get outa This Place: Popular Conservatism and Postmodern Culture.* New York: Routledge.

Hsu, C. (2002). "Making Midwives: The Logics of Midwifery Training in St. Lucia." In *Daughters of Time: The Shifting Identities of Contemporary Midwives* (special issue), edited by R. Davis-Floyd, S. Cosminsky, and S. L. Pigg. *Medical Anthropology* 20, nos. 2–3/4: 313–44.

Iskandar, M., B. Atom, T. Hull, N. Dharmaputra, and Y. Azwar. (1996). *Unraveling the Mysteries of Maternal Death in West Java: Reexamining the Witnesses.* Depok: Center for Health Research, Research Institute University of Indonesia.

Jenkins, G. (2002). "Modernization and Postmodernization in the Changing Roles and Identities of Midwives in Rural Costa Rica." In *Daughters of Time: The Shifting Identities of Contemporary Midwives* (special issue), edited by R. Davis-Floyd, S. Cosminsky, and S. L. Pigg. *Medical Anthropology* 20, nos. 2–3/4: 409–44.

Johnson, K. C., and B. A. Daviss. (2001, October). "Results of the CPM Statistics Project 2000: A prospective study of births by Certified Professional Midwives In North America (Abstract)." American Public Health Association Annual Meeting, Atlanta.

Jordan, B. (1993). *Birth in Four Cultures.* Revised and updated by R. Davis-Floyd. Prospect Heights, IL: Waveland Press.

Jordan, B. (1997). Authoritative Knowledge and Its Construction. In *Childbirth and Authoritative knowledge: Cross-cultural perspectives,* edited by R. Davis-Floyd and C. Sargent, 55–79. Berkeley: University of California Press.

Kolenda, P. (1998). "Fewer Deaths, Fewer Births." *Manushi* 105: 5–13.

Kroeger, M. (1996). *Final Consultant Report.* CHN III Project. Indonesia: Provincial Department of Health Central Java.

MacDorman, M., and G. Singh. (1998). "Midwifery Care, Social and Biomedical Risk Factors, and Birth Outcomes in the USA." *Journal of Epidemiology and Community Health* 52: 310–17.

Martin, E. (1987). *The Woman in the Body: A Cultural Analysis of Reproduction.* Boston: Beacon Press.

Rooks, J. P. (1997). *Midwifery and Childbirth in America.* Philadelphia: Temple University Press.

———. (1999). "Evidence-Based Practice and Its Applications to Childbirth Care for Low-Risk Women." *Journal of Nurse-Midwifery* 44, no. 4: 355–69.

Rothman, B. K. (1982). *In Labor: Women and Power in the Birthplace.* New York: W. W. Norton.

———. (1989). *Recreating Motherhood: Ideology and Technology in a Patriarchal Society.* New York: Norton.

Sargent, C. (1989). *Maternity, Medicine, and Power: Reproductive Decisions in Urban Benin.* Berkeley: University of California Press.

Schaef, A. W. (1981). *Women's Reality: An Emerging Female System in the White Male Society.* Minneapolis: Winston Press.

Ventura, S. J., J. A. Martin, S. C. Curtin, R. Menacker, and B. E. Hamilton. (2001). "Births: Final Data for 1999." *National Vital Statistics Reports* 49:1. Hyattsville, MD: National Center for Health Statistics.

Wagner, M. (1997). "Confessions of a Dissident." In *Childbirth and Authoritative Knowledge: Cross-Cultural Perspectives,* edited by R. Davis-Floyd and C. Sargent, 366–96. Berkeley: University of California Press.

Weigers, T. (1997). *Home or Hospital Birth: A Prospective Study of Midwifery Care in the Netherlands.* Ph.D. thesis, Leiden University, NIVEL, Utrecht.

Why Is Prevention Not the Focus for Breast Cancer Policy in the United States Rather than High-Tech Medical Solutions?

23

CATHERINE HODGE MCCOID

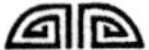

IN SPITE OF AN AGGRESSIVE HIGH-TECHNOLOGY "war on cancer," breast cancer has been increasing for the past 50 years, from one women in 20 in the 1950s to one women out of eight today. More women in the United States have died of breast cancer in the past two decades than all the Americans killed in World War I and II, the Korean War, and the Vietnam War combined. Similar patterns characterize other industrialized countries. And now the World Health Organization (WHO) identifies breast cancer as the highest cancer among women in the world (Davis, Axelrod, Bailey, Gaynor, and Sasco 1998), with about 1.2 million new cases of breast cancer worldwide and about 500,000 dying from the disease in 2000. Innumerable studies relate breast cancer and other cancers to environmental factors, including food, water, smoking, chemicals, and the use of drugs.[1] In spite of this environmental understanding, breast cancer policy tends to be directed toward "fixing up" the problem after it has occurred, rather than toward genuine environmental prevention. Why?

Money is a powerful factor inhibiting genuine breast cancer prevention. First, the supremacy of "bottom-line" thinking allows profits to be calculated in the short term, rather than in relation to long-term social and ecological consequences. Herbicides, pesticides, and other chemicals and toxins that cause breast cancer are profitable industries only because producers are not required to pay for the social costs (including those of cancer) of what they produce. Second, "fixing up" breast cancer at the individual level with the three "conventional" high-tech approaches of surgery, radiation, and chemotherapy also is an economically lucrative industry that often helps perpetuate the problem. As long as the focus is basically on "fixing up" the problem, individual by individual, breast cancer will remain unsolvable.

The Supremacy of the "Bottom-Line" Thinking

Eliminating breast cancer would require controlling the use of chemicals, such as pesticides, herbicides, and many drugs, as well as stricter regulation of foods. Such changes are strongly opposed by industry, especially pharmaceutical companies that produce carcinogenic pesticides and herbicides with one hand and "anti-cancer" drugs with the other. For example, the most widely prescribed breast cancer drug, tamoxifen citrate (Novadex), accounted for $500 million in sales in 1997 for the Zeneca Group (merged with Astra in 1999 and now called AstraZeneca), while the herbicide acefochlor, indicated as a probable carcinogen by the U.S. Environmental Protection Agency (EPA), accounted for $300 million in 1997 sales for them. At the time of their merger, the *Wall Street Journal* listed AstraZeneca as both the third largest pharmaceutical company and the third largest agrochemical company. According to Greenpeace's Bradley Angel, Breast Cancer Awareness Month is a "polluter-devised event" because it was created by Zeneca, which makes tamoxifen while also (with Monsanto) producing the pesticide acetychlor (Swissler 1997).

Another major anti–breast cancer drug, raloxifene, is produced by Eli Lilly and Co, which also produces the controversial bovine growth hormone Rumentin, a suspected carcinogen. Although legal in the United States, consumption of dairy products and meat treated with this hormone may alter estrogen levels and contribute to cancer risk. The pharmaceutical industry, therefore, has much at stake in promoting the use of drugs and other chemicals, and the Center for Responsible Politics indicates that the pharmaceutical industry is the second largest spender on lobbying and campaign contributions, with expenditures of $73.8 million in 1998, only surpassed by the insurance industry (Sloan 1999).

Out of the thousands of chemicals produced today by industrial societies, among the few of them that have been well studied for their carcinogenic effects are PCBs, DDT, and dioxin, organochlorines that mimic estrogen and are pervasive in the environment through pesticides, plastics, solvents, and even common household bleach (chlorine). Following Rachel Carson (1961, 1962), Colborn, Dumanoski, and Myers (1997), in an extensive review and synthesis of studies linking birth defects and reproductive difficulties in wildlife to synthetic chemicals (including organochlorines) that imitate natural hormones, show the implications for humans, including the global drop in sperm count for men and the rise in hormone-related cancers, endometriosis, and other problems among women. Several studies have found that some organochlorine compounds, including PCBs, act like estrogen and possibly could stimulate breast cancer (Hatakeyama and Matsumura 1999; Arcaro et al. 1999). While the link between these synthetic chemicals and breast cancer and other cancers is still debated, numerous studies support the link between organochlorines and breast cancer, especially when measured in breast tissue (Aronson et al. 2000; Guttes et al. 1998) or over time (Hoyer, Grandjean, Jorgensen, Brock, and Hartvig 1998; Hoyer, Jorgensen, Grandjean, and Hartvig 2000). However, there are enough studies that do not find a link to muddy the waters of debate, as occurred for years in the tobacco use and cancer debate in which industry was so influential. Industry is aided by major cancer institutions, such as the American Cancer Society, the National Cancer Institute, Sloan Kettering Cancer Center, and major universities in the United States, which have numerous ties to it through funding and exchange of personnel (Moss 1999).

Hormonal replacement therapy (HRT) is another area in which the pharmaceutical industry makes huge profits from controversial products implicated in breast cancer. Davis et al. (1998:523) suggest that the "cumulative exposure to estradiol and other hormones links many of the established risk factors for breast cancer." Increased risk of breast cancer is associated with the use of both estrogen (HRT) and estrogen plus progesterone (CHRT), with CHRT having an even higher risk (Ross, Paganini-Hill, Wan, and Pike 2000). In response, one doctor, John R. Lee, M.D., has communicated directly to women by writing such popular books as *What Your Doctor May Not Tell You about Breast Cancer* (Lee, Zama, and Hopkins 2002) to publicize what women can do to help themselves prevent this disease. Lee promotes the benefits of natural progesterone cream in preventing breast cancer and osteoporosis. He outlines critical differences between natural hormones and the synthetics produced and patented by the pharmaceutical industry, forcefully arguing that natural progesterone can help prevent breast cancer, including in women who have had it previously, and can help reverse osteoporosis.

Current Breast Cancer Policy and Practices

Current policy and practices in regard to breast cancer basically address the problem on the individual level (rather than on the social and ecological level), primarily either (1) through trying to encourage the modification of harmful lifestyle patterns, such as smoking, or through early diagnosis by self examination or frequent mammograms; or (2) though "treatment" by the three conventional methods of surgery, chemotherapy, or radiation. This is despite the fact that alternative medicine advocate Andrew Weil, a respected M.D., says that "only the first [i.e., surgery] makes sense" (1995:268). The treatment for the individual patient is an effort to "cure" them, which simply means helping them survive at least five years, a not very effective "cure."

Mammography is a technique emitting radiation, which is a known cancer cause, yet the procedure is touted as a method for "preventing" breast cancer. This seems driven more by convention and profit than scientific effectiveness. Gotzsche and Olsen (2000) argue that screening for breast cancer using mammograms is not justified. General Electric (GE) and DuPont, who are responsible for some of the most expensive Superfund toxic sites, combine to sell over $100 million in mammography machines every year (GE) and most of the film used in them (DuPont) (Paulsen 1994; Proctor 1995). The previously mentioned "polluter-devised" Breast Cancer Awareness Month also promotes mammography.

The conventional treatment of breast cancer tends to promote higher tech and more expensive rather than simpler approaches, with high resistance for decades to lumpectomy rather than mastectomy, although Harder (1978) suggested decades ago that survival rates were similar for both lumpectomy with radiation and for mastectomy. Today, even though long-term survival rates for lumpectomy with and without radiation are similar to each other and to mastectomy (60 percent for ten years; Nos et al. 1999), radiation is still promoted as the mode of preference using the rationale that recurrence rates are lower for lumpectomy followed by radiation. In fact, Fisher et al. (1992), finding at nine years of follow-up in the NSABP trial that patients treated with or without radiation had similar survival rates, suggested that recurrence is a marker for, not a cause of, distant disease. Whelan et al. (1997), also examining a number of studies, found that while radiation reduced local recurrence significantly, it had no effect on long-term survival, and most of the patients with local recurrence had undergone mastectomy.

The "conventional" approach to either mastectomy or lumpectomy involves lymph node dissection, used as a method of collecting information on staging the disease, not as treatment itself. Such lymph node dissection can result in painful lymphedema, or swelling of the arm—making the arm useless up to 25 percent of the time in older patients (Tengrup, Nittby, Christiansson, and Laurin 1999).

The effectiveness of the pharmaceutical industry's promotion of drugs in North America can be seen in the use of tamoxifen to treat breast cancer. Tamoxifen, the most popular "preventative" breast cancer drug, is surrounded by controversy and contradictory studies while its manufacturer heavily lobbies both the political and the medical establishments. Some studies show that tamoxifen increases endometrial cancer risk, while other studies suggest that it helps prevent new breast cancer tumor development (Radmacher and Simon 2000). Taylor, Adams-Campbell, and Wright (1999) caution that there still is no complete risk/benefit assessment of tamoxifen, including limited data on minority women. A heated debate continues on using tamoxifen and raloxifene, another popular drug, in healthy women to "prevent" breast cancer (Stephenson 1999; McNamee 1999).

Major cancer institutions stay focused on high-tech treatments like genetic experimentation, which could produce high profits, although genetic factors affect only a minority of cancers. Similarly, profit is implicated in conventional treatments. While conventional treatments like mastectomy, radiation after lumpectomy, axillary node dissection, and intensive follow-up seem to have little effect on long-term survival, these practices continue, as Beinfield and Beinfield (1997) argue, due to medical tradition and profitability rather than scientific proof.

A Personal Note

The medical establishment can be intimidating to a patient, even one well versed in the medical literature, and it can be difficult for an individual to chart an effective path. When I was diagnosed with breast cancer in 1999, I had been doing research on cancer for a few years and was familiar with much medical literature on breast cancer. As a political ecologist, I had been looking critically at the mainstream medical approaches to cancer, which tend to ignore or downplay the importance of broad environmental prevention in addressing cancer. In spite of my background, I still felt stressed trying to find a surgeon who would be willing to take the least invasive approach: a lumpectomy only, without radiation or lymph node dissection. Fortunately, I found empathetic women doctors who thought that the direction I wanted to go in was reasonable. However, my surgeon still required that I consult with a radiologist, another stressful experience because the radiologist was strongly convinced that only her approach was viable. While I rejected using radiation, for which my insurance company would have uncomplainingly paid thousands of dollars, I opted for a considerably cheaper and less invasive series of intravenous chelation treatments, for which I had to pay because most insurance companies and allopathic physicians find chelation "experimental." However, research suggested to me that chelation would increase my chances of not getting cancer again (Blumer and Cranton 1989). Fortunately, the physician who did my chelation therapy also introduced me to the benefits of regularly using a natural progesterone cream to help prevent cancer recurrence as well as osteoporosis and other problems.

Who Suffers as a Consequence of the Lack of Emphasis on Prevention, and in What Way?

While all the women who get breast cancer, along with their families and friends, suffer from the failure to emphasize real environmental prevention of cancer, minorities and the poor suffer disproportionately. African American women have a lower incidence of breast cancer but higher mortality than white women (Miller et al. 1996). These differences can be explained by differing socioeconomic status (Lannin et al. 1998), institutional racism, and the fact that many black cancer patients, and disproportionately those who are lower income, face obstacles such as transportation, poverty, and a distrust of doctors. Fewer black women's breast tumors are diagnosed when they are localized than white women's, another possible reason for black women's higher mortality rates (Roemer 2000). However, studies (Krieger et al. 1994; Schildkraut et al. 1999) finding higher concentrations of environmental contaminants, including organochlorines, in black women than white women may offer some broader explanations. For example, disposal of hazardous waste and harmful waste production are more likely to disproportionately hurt those with less economic and political leverage, including racial and ethnic groups, and have brought calls for "environmental justice." A 1987 study in the United States found that the highest concentrations of commercial hazardous waste sites were located in communities with the highest composition of racial and ethnic minority residents, and it found that three out of every five African Americans and Hispanic Americans were living in communities with uncontrolled waste sites (United Church of Christ Commission for Racial Justice 1987). Foster (1994) similarly outlines some of the destructive aspects of global capitalism as they have impacted the most vulnerable around the world.

Since the passage of the Occupational Safety and Health Act in 1970, manufacturers of asbestos, benzidine dyes, pesticides, plastics, and copper have increasingly moved those carcinogenic processes out of the United States to other countries (Moss 1999:346). Overconsuming industrial countries generate the majority of the more than 350 million metric tons of hazardous waste in the world each year and are increasingly transferring the effects of environmental damage to other countries, where there are lower wages and less effective protection of worker safety and the environment. This can be seen in the export of hazardous waste, a cancer catalyst, and particularly in the growing illegal and profitable export of it. While the actual numbers are unknown, the EPA estimates that illegal shipments outnumber legal ones by 8 to 1 (World Resources Institute et al. 1998:53).

Changing the Unhealthy Policies and Practices that Block Breast Cancer Prevention

Breast cancer prevention policy must be firmly grounded in both ecological and social justice principles. In the words of Baer, Singer, and Susser (1997:52), we need "to treat political economy and political ecology as inseparable." This means critically understanding how global capitalism destructively impacts both the social and the natural environment, and working to transform these forces. Through the pursuit of profit calculated in relation to the short-term bottom line rather than in relation to long-term social and ecological consequences, the world market is a major factor driving the growth of breast cancer and other cancers worldwide, as it is with infectious diseases. For example, half the antibiotics used in the

United States are used in livestock, aquaculture, and other biological industries to counter the effects of pesticide-intensive monocultural farming and agribusiness, in which a disease breakout can destroy a business with only one kind of animal or crop. And the use of synthetic pesticides (including organochlorines) and fertilizers imperils the lives of workers and consumers, increasing drug-resistant strains of bacteria, expanding infectious diseases (Robbins 1999:247–269), and enhancing the pharmaceutical and agrochemical industries and the growth of cancer.

If the short-term, bottom-line approach that focuses on treating individuals continues to prevail, we are faced with the prospect of a world in which, with one hand, industry perpetually produces carcinogens and, with the other hand, "fixes" the cancer caused, individual by individual, with genetic engineering or other high-tech "marvels."

To genuinely prevent breast cancer, health policy must promote ecological and social responsibility, rewarding producers with the most responsible products and helping to bring down the price of such products for everyone. For example, health care institutions could phase out their use of polyvinyl chloride (PVC) plastic, as called for by activists like Nancy Evans (1999) with the Breast Cancer Fund. PVC is the flexible plastic used in tubing, blood bags, and many other medical products. Since PVC is a carcinogen, it harms the workers who manufacture it and the patients who use it, and it creates dioxin when it is incinerated, a common method of medical waste disposal.

Health policy needs to promote the simplest and most effective and preventative approaches to solving health problems for patients and society, not the most profitable ones. Then, those effective approaches will also become profitable, whether this involves targeting chemical contaminants or fat in foods, or by promoting the least traumatic approaches, like lumpectomy, to "fix" cancer when it occurs. If there were no gender bias, it would be a puzzle as to why every woman in the United States who gets breast cancer is not being surveyed to help identify possible environmental factors, as people were in past health "epidemics," like polio or smallpox. Additionally, collecting breast tissue samples from those women could quickly target environmental factors being overlooked.

A preventative approach to health policy means integrating many "alternative" practices more into health policy to help prevent breast cancer and other diseases, and such an approach could help bring costs down. The growth of alternative medicine in the United States and other industrialized countries reflects a growing dissatisfaction with a nonpreventative approach to cancer and other diseases. For decades, studies have found links between cancer and food (including fat) and lifestyle (including exercise) (Gerson 1958; Stich 1982), with higher vegetable, fruit, fiber, and other nutrients associated with lower breast cancer risk (Ronco et al. 1999).

In both national and international contexts, health is a human rights issue that should include the right to a safe environment and the right to adequate and safe food and water for everyone. Adequate amounts of bacteriologically safe food and water are essential but are not enough, for unless food and water are also environmentally safe (i.e., also free of human contaminants, such as pesticides), people will not survive in good health in the long run. Similarly, national health systems that are open to everyone would help in addressing many of these problems, in the context of a focus on genuine prevention and equity. Such changes now are blocked in many countries, including the United States, by economic forces geared to short-term analyses. However, long-term ecological and social analyses could make such changes clearly more economic and humane choices.

Notes

This chapter is a revised version of a paper presented at the American Anthropological Association meetings in San Francisco, November 2000.

1. McCoid (2002) includes a summary of an analysis that I performed of cancer patterns in 23 countries from the 1950s through the 1980s. Like many other studies, that research found increasing rates of breast and other cancers associated with increasing industrialization, including fat, protein, and caloric consumption, as well as increased rates of smoking.

References

Arcaro, K. F., L. Yi, R. F. Seegal, D. D. Vakharia, Y. Yang, D. C. Spink, et al. (1999, January 1). "2,2,'6,6'-Tetrachlorobiphenyl Is Estrogenic in Vitro and in Vivo." *Journal of Cellular Biochemistry* 72, no. 1: 94–102.

Aronson, K. J., A. B. Miller, C. G. Woolcott, E. E. Sterns, D. R. McCready, L. A. Lickley, et al. (2000, January 1). "Breast Adipose Tissue Concentrations of Polychlorinated Biphenyls and Other Organochlorines and Breast Cancer Risk." *Cancer Epidemiology Biomarkers & Prevention* 9: 55–63.

Baer, H. A., M. Singer, and I. Susser. (1997). *Medical Anthropology and the World System: A Critical Perspective.* Westport, CT: Bergin & Garvey.

Beinfield, H., and M. S. Beinfield. (1997, September). "Revisiting Accepted Wisdom in the Management of Breast Cancer." *Alternative Therapies in Health and Medicine* 3, no. 5: 35–53.

Blumer, W., and E. M. Cranton. (1989). "Ninety Percent Reduction in Cancer Mortality after Chelation Therapy with EDTA." In *A Textbook on EDTA Chelation Therapy,* edited by E. M. Cranton, 183 pp. New York: Human Sciences Press.

Carson, R. (1961). *The Sea around Us.* Oxford: Oxford University Press.

———. *Silent Spring.* (1962). Oxford: Oxford University Press.

Colborn, T., D. Dumanoski, and J. Peterson Myers. (1997). *Our Stolen Future.* New York: Plume Books.

Davis, D.L., D. Axelrod, L. Bailey, M. Gaynor, and A. J. Sasco. (1998, September 9). "Rethinking Breast Cancer Risk and the Environment: The Case for the Precautionary Principle." *Environmental Health Perspectives* 109: 523–29.

Evans, N. (1999, July 30). Evening banquet special guest speech at the World Conference on Breast Cancer. Ottawa, Canada: Breast Cancer Prevention Coalition.

Fisher, B., D. L. Wickerham, M. Deutsch, S. Anderson, C. Redmond, and E. R. Fisher. (1992, May–June). "Breast Tumor Recurrence Following Lumpectomy with and without Breast Irradiation." *Semin Surg Oncol* 8, no. 3: 153–60.

Foster, J. B. (1994). *The Vulnerable Planet.* New York: Monthly Review Press.

Gerson, M. (1958). *A Cancer Therapy: Results of Fifty Cases.* Bonita, CA: Gerson Institute.

Gotzsche, P. C., and O. Olsen. (2000, January 8). "Is Screening for Breast Cancer with Mammography Justifiable?" *Lancet* 355, no. 9198: 129.

Guttes, S., K. Failing, K. Neumann, J. Kleinstein, S. Georgii, and H. Brunn. (1998, July). "Chlororganic Pesticides and Polychlorinated Biphenyls in Breast Tissue of Women with Benign and Malignant Breast Disease." *Arch Environ Contam Toxicol* 35, no. 1: 140–47.

Harder, F. (1978, July). "Therapy of Carcinoma of the Breast. Surgery: Present State of Knowledge and Problems" (in German). *Therapie Des. Rontgenblatter (TZP)* 31, no. 7: 412–16.

Hatakeyama, M., and F. Matsumura. (1999). "Correlation between the Activation of Neu Tyrosine Kinase and Promotion of Foci Formation Induced by Selected Organochlorine Compounds in the MCF-7 Model System." *Journal of Biochemical and Molecular Toxicology* 13, no. 6: 296–302.

Hoyer, A. P., P. Grandjean, T. Jorgensen, J. W. Brock, and H. B. Hartvig. (1998, December 5). "Organochlorine Exposure and Risk of Breast Cancer." *Lancet* 352, no. 9143: 1816–20.

Hoyer, A. P., T. Jorgensen, P. Grandjean, and H. B. Hartvig (2000, February). "Repeated Measurements of Organochlorine Exposure and Breast Cancer Risk (Denmark)." *Cancer Causes & Control* 11, no. 2: 177–84.

Krieger, N., M. S. Wolff, R. A. Hiatt, M. Rivera, J. Vogelman, and N. Orentreich. (1994). "Breast Cancer and Serum Organochlorines: A Prospective Study among White, Black, and Asian Women." *Journal of the National Cancer Institute* 86: 589–99.

Lannin, D. R., H. F. Mathews, J. Mitchell, M. S. Swanson, F. H. Swanson, and M. S. Edwards. (1998). "Influence of Socioeconomic and Cultural Factors on Racial Differences in Late-Stage Presentation of Breast Cancer." *Journal of the American Medical Association* 279: 1801–1807.

Lee, J. R., D. Zama, and V. Hopkins. (2002). *What Your Doctor May Not Tell You about Breast Cancer: How Hormone Balance Can Help Save Your Life.* New York: Warner Books.

McCoid, C. H. (2002). "Globalization and the Consumer Society." In *The Consumer Society,* edited by Emilio Federico Moran, in *Encyclopedia of Life Support Systems (EOLSS),* developed under the auspices of the UNESCO. Oxford: Eolss Publishers. Accessed at www.eolss.net.

McNamee, D. (1999, September 18). "Debate on Whether to Use Tamoxifen for Cancer Prevention Continues." *Lancet* 354, no. 9183: 1007.

Miller, B. A., I. N. Kolonel, L. Bernstein, J. L. Young, Jr., G. M. Swanson, D. West, et al. (1996). *Racial/Ethnic Patterns of Cancer in the United States, 1988–1992.* Report no. 96. Bethesda, MD: National Institutes of Health, National Cancer Institute, 4104.

Moss, R. W. (1999). *The Cancer Industry.* Brooklyn, NY: Equinox Press. (Originally published in 1980 as *The Cancer Syndrome* [New York: Grove Press].)

Nos, C., D. Bourgeois, C. Darles, B. Asselain, F. Campana, B. Zafrani, et al. (1999, February). "Conservative Treatment of Multifocal Breast Cancer: A Comparative Study." *Bulletin of Cancer* 86, no. 2: 184–88.

Paulsen, M. (1994, June). "The Cancer Business." *Mother Jones*: 41.

Proctor, R. (1995). *Cancer Wars.* New York: Basic Books.

Radmacher, M. D., and R. Simon. (2000). "Estimation of Tamoxifen's Efficacy for Preventing the Formation and Growth of Breast Tumors." *Journal of the National Cancer Institute* 92: 48–53.

Robbins, R. H. (1999). *Global Problems and the Culture of Capitalism.* Boston: Allyn & Bacon.

Roemer, J. (2000). "Inner-City Mammography Programs Aim to Make Breast Cancer 'A Visible Disease.'" *Journal of the National Cancer Institute* 92: 444–45.

Ronco, A., E. De Stefani, P. Boffetta, H. Deneo-Pellegrini, M. Mendilaharsu, and F. Leborgne. (1999). "Vegetables, Fruits, and Related Nutrients and Risk of Breast Cancer: A Case-Control Study in Uruguay." *Nutrition and Cancer* 35, no. 2: 111–19.

Ross, R. K., A. Paganini-Hill, P. C. Wan, and M. C. Pike. (2000). "Effect of Hormone Replacement Therapy on Breast Cancer Risk: Estrogen versus Estrogen Plus Progestin." *Journal of the National Cancer Institute* 92: 328–32.

Schildkraut, J. M., W. Demark-Wahnefried, E. DeVoto, C. Hughes, J. L. Laseter, and B. Newman. (1999, February). "Environmental Contaminants and Body Fat Distribution [See Comments]." *Cancer Epidemiology Biomarkers & Prevention* 8, no. 2: 179–83.

Sloan, A. (1999). "Profiting off of Breast Cancer: Are Treatment Drug Manufacturers Also Increasing Our Cancer Risk?" In *Censored 1999—The News That Didn't Make the News: The Year's Top 25 Censored Stories,* edited by Peter Phillips and Project Censored, 34–37. New York: Seven Stories Press.

Stephenson, J. (1999, July 2). "Experts Debate Drugs for Healthy Women with Breast Cancer Risk." *Journal of the American Medical Association* 282, no. 14: 117.

Stich, H. F. (1982). *Carcinogens and Mutagens in the Environment, vol. I: Food Products.* Boca Raton, FL: CRC Press.

Swissler, M. A. (1997, December 12). "Touring the Breast-Cancer Industry." *Progressive* 61: 14.

Taylor, A. L., L. L. Adams-Campbell, and J. T. Wright, Jr. (1999). "Risk/Benefit Assessment of Tamoxifen to Prevent Breast Cancer—Still a Work in Progress?" *Journal of the National Cancer Institute* 91: 1792–93.

Tengrup, I., L. T. Nittby, I. Christiansson, and M. Laurin. (1999, November 17). "Problems with Arms Are Common after Breast Surgery. Lymphedema Is a Frequent Complication in Elderly Women Treated for Breast Cancer." *Lakartidningen* 96, no. 46: 5089–5091.

United Church of Christ Commission for Racial Justice. (1987). *Toxic Waste and Race in the United States.* New York: Public Access.

Weil, A. (1995). *Spontaneous Healing.* New York: Fawcett Columbine.

Whelan, T. J., B. M. Lada, E. Laukkanen, F. E. Perera, W. E. Shelley, and M. N. Levine. (1997, August 3). "Breast Irradiation in Women with Early Stage Invasive Breast Cancer Following Breast Conservation Surgery." *Cancer Prevention Control* 1: 228–240.

World Resources Institute, United Nations Environment Programme, United Nations Development Programme, and World Bank. (1998). *World Resources 1998–99.* New York: Oxford University Press.

Index

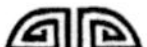

About the Editors and Contributors

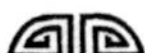

César E. Abadía-Barrero, D.M.D., D.M.Sc., received his degree in dentistry from the Universidad Nacional de Colombia in 1992. As a dentist in indigenous communities and in other poor sectors in Colombia, he provided clinical care and worked in various community development programs. He completed his doctoral studies in medical anthropology at Harvard University in June 2003, in which he studied the relationship between the social responses around AIDS in Brazil and the subjectivity of a group of children living with HIV. He received the Dean's Scholars Award from the Harvard School of Dental Medicine to conduct one year of postdoctoral training in which he is comparing the governmental and nongovernmental responses to AIDS between Colombia and Brazil. He is also investigating the political economy of oral health care. For the academic year 2003–2004, he holds appointments as a postdoctoral research fellow at both the Harvard School of Dental Medicine and the Department of Social Medicine at Harvard Medical School. He received the Student Rudolf Virchow Award 2003 of the Critical Anthropology of Health Caucus for his chapter in this book.

Francisco Armada, M.D., Ph.D., MPH, is a health officer at the Ministry of Health in Venezuela, where he works as general director of environmental health and health regulation. He was trained as a physician at the Universidad Central de Venezuela in Caracas; he received his M.P.H. and Ph.D. in social and health policy at the Johns Hopkins University in Baltimore. He conducts research in the area of social inequalities in health, welfare state, health sector reform in Latin America, and health politics. He has been involved in the formulation and implementation of public policy and health sector reform in Venezuela reverting neoliberal approaches and promoting universal health rights.

Hans A. Baer, Ph.D., is professor of anthropology and sociology at the University of Arkansas at Little Rock. He has been a visiting professor at Humboldt University in Berlin; University of California, Berkeley; Arizona State University; and George Washington University. Baer has conducted ethnographic research on the Hutterites in South Dakota; the Levites, a Mormon sect in Utah; African American Spiritual churches; osteopaths, chiropractors, and naturopaths in the United States and United Kingdom; sociopolitical and religious life in East Germany; and conventional and alternative HIV clinics. In medical anthropology, his books include *Encounters with Biomedicine: Case Studies in Medical Anthropology*; *Critical Medical Antropology* (with Merrill Singer); *Medical Anthropology and the World System: A Critical Perspective* (with Merrill Singer and Ida Susser); and *Biomedicine and Alternative Healing Systems in America: Issues of Class, Race, Ethnicity, and Gender*. Baer has served on the editorial board of the *Medical Anthropology Quarterly* since 1996. He presently is completing a book titled *The Taming of a Popular Health Movement in the United States: From Holistic Health to Complementary Medicine* that will be published by Altamira Press.

Katherine E. Bliss, Ph.D., is associate professor of history at the University of Massachusetts, Amherst. She has published articles in the *Hispanic American Historical Review* (1999), the *Journal of Family History* (1999), and the *Latin American Research Review* (2001). Her *Hispanic American Historical Review* essay, "The Science of Redemption: Syphilis, Sexual Promiscuity and Reformism in Revolutionary Mexico," received the Conference on Latin American History's James A. Robertson prize in 2000. Bliss's book, *Compromised Positions: Prostitution, Public Health and Gender Politics in Revolutionary Mexico City*, was published by the Pennsylvania State University Press in 2001. In 2000–2001, she was a David E. Bell Fellow at the Harvard Center for Population and Development Studies, where she began researching a new project on the intellectual history and cultural politics of health policy and programming in mid-twentieth century Latin America. As a Council on Foreign Relations International Affairs Fellow, she is currently working as regional advisor to the Office of International Health Affairs in the U.S. Department of State.

Philippe Bourgois, Ph.D., is a cultural anthropologist who is professor and chair of the Department of Anthropology, History, and Social Medicine at the University of California, San Francisco. He is best known for his fieldwork among drug dealers and addicts in U.S. inner cities. His most recent book, *In Search of Respect: Selling Crack in El Barrio* (1995, with an updated second edition in 2003), won the C. Wright Mills and the Margaret Mead prizes, among others. He is currently conducting fieldwork among homeless heroin injectors and crack smokers in San Francisco with photographer Jeff Schonberg to prepare a book for the University of California Press, *Righteous Dopefiend: Homeless Heroin Addicts in Black and White*. His website is www.ucsf.edu/dahsm/pages/faculty/bourgois.html.

David Buchanan, DrPH, was a co-principal investigator on the Syringe Access, Use, and Discard (SAUD) research project. He is a full professor of community health education at the School of Public Health and Health Sciences, University of Massachusetts, Amherst, and is founding director of the Office of Public Health Practice and Outreach. He earned both his master's and doctorate degrees from the School of Public Health at the University of California, Berkeley. His primary research interests include the epistemological foundations of the social sciences, the ethical implications of positivism, community-based participatory research, substance abuse, and AIDS. He has served as the principal investigator on the W. K. Kellogg Foundation Community-Based Public Health initiative, the SPH/DPH Interface project (a project designed to strengthen collaboration between academia and public health practitioners through providing training and technical assistance to community groups), and numerous substance abuse research projects funded by state and federal agencies. He is currently conducting a research fellowship on public health ethics at the National Cancer Institute. Among his many publications, he is the author of *An Ethic for Health Promotion: Rethinking the Sources of Human Well Being.*

Arachu Castro, Ph.D., MPH, is instructor in medical anthropology in the Department of Social Medicine at Harvard Medical School, director of the Institute for Health and Social Justice at Partners In Health, and medical anthropologist in the Division of Social Medicine and Health Inequalities at Brigham and Women's Hospital, all in Boston, Massachusetts. Her major interests are how social inequalities are embodied as differential risk for pathologies common among the poor and how health policies may alter the course of epidemic disease and other pathologies afflicting populations living in poverty. She has conducted public health research in Latin America and Europe in the areas of infectious disease, reproductive health, and nutrition, and has been actively involved in the design of several international health policy documents on tuberculosis and AIDS in conjunction with the World Health Organization and the Pan American Health Organization. From 1998 to 2000, Dr. Castro coordinated a reproductive health research project in Mexico aimed at improving the quality of obstetric services for poor women, as a consultant for the Population Council and the World Health Organization. She teaches social medicine at Harvard Medical School, where she serves as academic director of the Program in Infectious Disease and Social Change, and has previously taught at institutions in Spain, Argentina, France, Mexico, and Cuba. She has published several articles, as well as the book *Saber Bien: Cultura y Prácticas Alimentarias en la Rioja* (1998). She is currently writing the book *AIDS in the Pearls of the Antilles: Rethinking Public Health from Haiti and Cuba* for University of California Press. Dr. Castro is secretary-treasurer of the Society for Medical Anthropology, where she was chair of the Critical Anthropology of Health

Caucus from 1998 to 2002. She received her Ph.D. in ethnology and social anthropology from the École des Hautes Études en Sciences Sociales in Paris, her Ph.D. in sociology from the University of Barcelona, and her master's in public health from Harvard School of Public Health.

Claudia Chaufan, M.D., is a medical doctor specialized in diabetes and obesity, a diabetes educator, and a medical writer from Buenos Aires, Argentina. In her home country, she worked as a clinician while writing about health for the Argentine media and coauthoring several books on nutrition-related topics. She has been a speaker and has given papers on diabetes care and education, social ethics, and sociological aspects of diabetes care at several academic and professional conferences (American Diabetes Association, Society for the Study of Social Problems, American Sociological Association, International Diabetes Federation, and the University of British Columbia). Since moving to the United States, she has coordinated a diabetes education program for the Hispanic community in San Jose, California, and has done social research on diabetes. She later pursued a master's degree in sociology at the University of California, Santa Cruz, and is now completing her doctoral dissertation in sociology, with a parenthetical notation in philosophy, at the same university, where she teaches undergraduate sociology. She lives in Santa Cruz, California, with her husband and her 14-year-old son. She has lived with type 1 diabetes for 32 years.

Robbie Davis-Floyd, Ph.D., is a senior research fellow at the Department of Anthropology, University of Texas Austin. She is a cultural anthropologist specializing in the medical anthropology and the anthropology of reproduction. An international speaker, she is author of over 70 articles and of *Birth as an American Rite of Passage* (1992); coauthor of *From Doctor to Healer: The Transformative Journey* (1998), and *The Anatomy of Ritual* (forthcoming); and coeditor of eight collections, including *Childbirth and Authoritative Knowledge: Cross-Cultural Perspectives* (1997); *Cyborg Babies: From Techno-Sex to Techno-Tots* (1998); *Daughters of Time: The Shifting Identities of Contemporary Midwives* (a special triple issue of *Medical Anthropology* 20, nos. 2 and 3/4 [2001]), and *Mainstreaming Midwives: The Politics of Change* (forthcoming). Her research on global trends and transformations in health care, childbirth, obstetrics, and midwifery is ongoing. Her present projects address change in American, Mexican, and Brazilian midwifery and obstetrics.

Alice Desclaux, M.D., Ph.D. after some years of practice in public health, turned to medical anthropology, starting with a Ph.D. on the social treatment of AIDS in children by the health system in Burkina Faso. Since 1993, she has been working on AIDS mainly in Africa, on aspects such as social and cultural aspects of

HIV prevention in refugees camps; counseling provision in West Africa; cultural, political, and social construction of the relationship between HIV and breastfeeding in Burkina Faso and Ivory Coast; institutional management; and patients' experience of HAART treatment in Senegal. In France, she has worked on perceptions of risk among health professionals and HIV-positive women, and subsequent decisions about procreation. She is now teaching medical anthropology at Aix-en-Provence University and coordinating a research program on anthropological aspects of prevention of HIV transmission through breastfeeding in five African and Asian countries. She is the secretary of Anthropologie Médicale Appliquée au Développement et à la Santé (AMADES, www.amades.net), a French association promoting medical anthropology and working on the relationships between theoretical issues and applications.

Paul Farmer, M.D., Ph.D., has worked in infectious-disease control in the Americas for nearly two decades. He is the founding director of Partners In Health, an international charity organization that provides direct health care services and undertakes research and advocacy activities on behalf of those who are sick and living in poverty. Dr. Farmer is the Maude and Lillian Presley Professor of Medical Anthropology in the Department of Social Medicine at Harvard Medical School. He also trains medical students, residents, and fellows at the Brigham and Women's Hospital in Boston, where he is an attending physician in infectious diseases and chief of the Division of Social Medicine and Health Inequalities, and at the Clinique Bon Sauveur, in rural Haiti, where he serves as medical director. He has been a visiting professor at institutions throughout the United States as well as in France, Canada, Peru, the Netherlands, Russia, and Central Asia. Along with his colleagues at the Brigham and in the Program in Infectious Disease and Social Change at Harvard Medical School, Dr. Farmer has pioneered novel, community-based treatment strategies for infectious diseases (including AIDS and multidrug-resistant tuberculosis) in resource-poor settings. Author or coauthor of over 100 scholarly publications, his research and writing stem in large part from work in Haiti and Peru, and from clinical and teaching activities. He is the author of *Pathologies of Power* (University of California Press, 2003), *Infections and Inequalities* (University of California Press, 1998), *The Uses of Haiti* (Common Courage Press, 1994), and *AIDS and Accusation* (University of California Press, 1992). In addition, he is coeditor of *Women, Poverty, and AIDS* (Common Courage Press, 1996); and of *The Global Impact of Drug-Resistant Tuberculosis* (Harvard Medical School and Open Society Institute, 1999).

Didier Fassin, M.D., Ph.D., is a sociologist, anthropologist, and medical doctor. He practiced internal medicine in Paris, India, and Tunisia and simultaneously studied social sciences, doing his first fieldwork in Senegal on urban health and social change. He then coordinated a research program on reproductive health and structural violence in Ecuador. Back in France, he worked on health inequalities, local public health, immigration, and discrimination in France, as well as on the politics of AIDS in southern Africa. He is director of the Centre of Research on Public Health Issues (CRESP) of the University Paris North and INSERM. At the École des Hautes Études en Sciences Sociales, he is director of studies in political anthropology of health. His recent books are *L'espace politique de la santé* (Presses Universitaires de France, 1996) and *Les enjeux politiques de la santé* (Karthala, 2000). He edited *Les figures urbaines de la santé publique* (La Découverte, 1997) and *La question sociale en souffrance* (Syros, 2003). He coedited *Les inégalités sociales de santé* (La découverte, 2000) and *Critique de la santé publique* (Balland, 2002). He contributes to scientific forums as well as public debates on contemporary biopolitics in France and the Third World.

Robert Heimer, Ph.D., received his B.A. from Columbia College and his Ph.D. in pharmacology from Yale University. Dr. Heimer's major research efforts include scientific evaluation of HIV prevention programs for drug injectors, virological assessment of the risk of drug injection behaviors, and analysis of the contributions of hepatitis virus infections and injection drug use to chronic liver disease. His laboratory has developed molecular and virological methods to test syringes for the presence of HIV-1 and hepatitis B and C viruses. Dr. Heimer, in collaboration with Dr. Edward H. Kaplan at the Yale School of Management, evaluated the New Haven Needle Exchange Program relying on the tracking and testing of syringes. These analyses determined that the New Haven Needle Exchange Program reduced the transmission of HIV-1 and hepatitis B by at least one-third. He has collaborated in the study of syringe exchange programs in other cities in the United States. Dr. Heimer's laboratory has demonstrated how long HIV-1 remains viable within used syringes and which drug injection practices can increase the risk or protection of injectors from HIV-1 infection. Dr. Heimer is the director of the Yale Emerging Infections Program and a member of the Yale Center for Interdisciplinary Research on AIDS and of the Substance Use Working Group, HIV Prevention Trials Network, NIAID.

Sarah Horton, Ph.D., received her Ph.D. in cultural anthropology from the University of New Mexico (UNM) in 2003. From 1997 to 1999, she was a researcher on a UNM team led by Louise Lamphere and Howard Waitzkin on the effects of Medicaid managed care on the safety net in New Mexico. This research project culminated in the team's coauthoring an article on their findings in *American Anthropologist* (2000). Her interests include minorities' access to health care, the effect of privatization on the safety net, ethnomedicine, ritual symbolism, and religious healing systems. She received the Student Rudolf Virchow Award 2002 of the Critical Anthropology of Health Caucus for a paper on the effect of neoliberal health care policies on immigrants' health status. She joined the Department of Social Medicine at Harvard University as a postdoctoral fellow in the fall of 2003.

Kristen Jacklin, M.A., is a Ph.D. candidate in the Department of Anthropology at McMaster University, where she studies applied medical anthropology. Her dissertation research examines First Nations community health and development. Her work includes a critical examination of Aboriginal health policy in Canada and its ability to provide needed and appropriate services to Aboriginal people at the community level. In addition, her dissertation examines the use of participatory action research in a First Nations community. Jacklin is also a practicing anthropologist, working as a consultant to First Nations organizations and Tribal Councils. Her practical applications are mainly concentrated in the area of needs-based research and planning, and evaluation research with First Nations communities. Her most recent work includes the design, implementation, and analysis of a community youth needs assessment using participatory action research; and the development of culturally appropriate policies and procedures for a First Nation Health Centre.

Salmaan Keshavjee, M.D., Ph.D., is a researcher in the Department of Social Medicine at Harvard Medical School, the Center for Middle Eastern Studies at Harvard University, and the Division of Social Medicine and Health Inequalities at the Brigham and Women's Hospital in Boston. He is also a resident in the Department of Medicine at the Brigham and Women's Hospital. Dr. Keshavjee received a Ph.D. in anthropology and Middle Eastern studies from Harvard University in 1998, and an M.D. from Stanford University in 2001. He lived in Badakhshan, Tajikistan, in 1996–1997 while conducting dissertation research. Dr. Keshavjee's current research involves the implementation of an ambulatory treatment program for patients with multidrug-resistant tuberculosis in Tomsk, Siberia, Russia. His research interests include the role of NGOs as agents of globalization and transnational civil society, and the anthropology of institution building and social change in societies in transition.

Kaveh Khoshnood, Ph.D., is an assistant professor at Yale School of Public Health, an investigator at the Yale Center for Interdisciplinary Research on AIDS (CIRA), and the deputy director of its International Summer Research Institute. Trained as an infectious disease epidemiologist, Dr. Khoshnood's primary research interests are the epidemiology, prevention, and control of HIV/AIDS and tuberculosis among drug users, prisoners, and other at-risk populations in the United States and in resource-poor countries. Khoshnood is an advocate for the relentless use of scientific knowledge and resources to instigate the development of public policy aimed at improving human health and well-being. Khoshnood mentors researchers from China, India, Russia, and South Africa in HIV/AIDS and tuberculosis, and directs research projects in China and the Russian Federation. In addition, Khoshnood teaches courses on HIV/AIDS and infectious disease epidemiology to graduate students at Yale, and was the recipient of the "excellence in teaching award" by the graduating class of 2003. Khoshnood's other interests are in the examination of the ethical dilemmas in conducting research involving vulnerable populations. Khoshnood serves on a number of advisory boards for domestic and international organizations and is the reviewer for several scientific journals.

Catherine Hodge McCoid is a political ecologist and ecofeminist whose publications include "Globalization and the Consumer Society" and "Equity" in *The Encyclopedia of Life Support Systems* (Geneva: UNESCO, 2000); and "Towards Decolonizing Gender: Female Vision in the European Upper Paleolithic" (with LeRoy D. McDermott, June 1996, *American Anthropologist* 98, no. 2, 319–26). Her June 1989 "Dowry Deaths in India: A Materialist Analysis" was based on fieldwork working with activists on dowry deaths in India in 1987 (Working Paper #188, *Women in International Development Publication* series, Michigan State University). Most of her work, including the book *Carrying Capacities of Nation-States* (New Haven, CT: HRAFlex Books, 1984), has involved doing macroecological analyses of the world system. Articles published before 1982, such as in the *Journal of Anthropological Research* in 1977 ("Carrying Capacities and Low Population Growth" 32, no. 4: 474–92) and 1976 ("Factors Affecting Carrying Capacities of Nation-States" 32, no. 3: 255–75), were under her married name, Catherine H. Maserang. She is a professor of anthropology who has taught at Central Missouri State University since 1971. She is working on a collected volume on violence against women.

Carles Muntaner, M.D., Ph.D., a native of Barcelona, Spain, is professor at the Department of Family and Community Health, University of Maryland; the Department of Mental Health, Bloomberg School of Public Health; and the University of Toronto's Institute for Work and Health. He has conducted research on social inequalities in health since the mid-1980s in the European Union, Latin America, the United States, and West Africa. His main research focus is the study of the health effects of social class, race, and politics in workplaces, neighborhoods, states, and countries. His workplace research is devoted to the study of the mental health effects of work organization among low-wage health care workers in collaboration with unions.

Joan E. Paluzzi, Ph.D., R.N., is a medical anthropologist who received her Ph.D. in anthropology from the University of Pittsburgh and was the 2002–2003 Post-Doctoral Fellow at the Institute for Health and Social Justice, the research, training, and advocacy branch of the NGO Partners In Health (PIH). Her past research has included a detailed study of the experience of tuberculosis among individuals diagnosed with the disease in the Ninth Region of southern Chile. She is currently employed at PIH working on special projects including the development and administrative coordination of Task Force Five: Infectious Diseases and Access to Essential Medicines within the United Nations Millennium Development Goals Project.

James Pfeiffer, Ph.D., MPH, is currently an assistant professor in the Department of Anthropology, Case Western Reserve University, in Cleveland, Ohio. He received his Ph.D. in anthropology and his MPH from UCLA, and has conducted fieldwork in Mozambique, Nicaragua, and Iran. Dr. Pfeiffer was country coordinator for Health Alliance International in Mozambique for nearly four years during the 1990s. His research interests include medical anthropology, the political economy of health in southern Africa, the aid industry in Africa, and the impact of structural adjustment on health. Dr. Pfeiffer's current research centers on the spread of Pentecostal and African Independent Churches in southern Africa, and their relationship to growing inequality, structural adjustment, and the AIDS epidemic in Mozambique.

Imrana Qadeer, Ph.D., is a professor of Public Health at the Center of Social Medicine and Community Health, Jawaharlal Nehru University, New Delhi, India. Her areas of interest include the organization of public health services, political economy of health, the health of workers and women in India, research methodology, and applications of systems thinking in health. Currently, Professor Qadeer is working on the health implications of structural reforms and policy issues arising out of it. She has critiqued both the National Population Policy as well as the National Health Policies. She has also been involved with the planning efforts at the national level of both the government and grassroots organizations. She is involved with the work of grassroots organizations that are taking up issues of health and health services. The health of women and children is of particular interest to her.

Susan Shaw, Ph.D., was an ethnographer on the Syringe Access, Use, and Discard (SAUD) project and now works for the Hispanic Health Council. Shaw received her Ph.D. in medical anthropology from the University of North Carolina at Chapel Hill in 2001. She is currently principal investigator on two projects related to community, culture, and health. The Community Attitudes study grew out of the SAUD project and looks at factors in community opposition to syringe exchange programs. Evaluating culturally appropriate primary health care is a formative research study investigating cultural beliefs and practices related to health care among four ethnic groups in Springfield, Massachusetts, and Hartford, Connecticut. Her research interests include community organizing around health issues, the relationship between community and identity, and access to health care.

Merrill Singer, Ph.D., is the associate director of the Hispanic Health Council (HHC) and director of the HHC's Center for Community Health Research in Hartford, Connecticut. Additionally, he is a research affiliate of the Center for Interdisciplinary Research on AIDS at Yale University. Dr. Singer has been the principal investigator on a continuous series of federally funded community health studies since 1984, and currently is the principal investigator on two NIH-funded studies: (1) the intersection of violence, substance abuse, and AIDS risk among women drug users; and (2) social environmental factors in sterile syringe availability and HIV risk among IDUs in three U.S. cities and the Virgin Islands. Additionally, he is the PI on a CDC-funded study designed to monitor emergent drug use trends and a U.S. Department of Health and Human Services rapid assessment study of late-night AIDS risk. Singer also serves as the co-principal investigator on two NIDA-funded studies: (1) syringe sharing among IDUs in Guangdong, China; and (2) hepatitis B vaccination of IDUs; he is also a co-principal investigator for a CDC-funded study of barriers to condom use among inner-city young adults. Singer serves as consultant to the Office of HIV/AIDS Policy in the U.S. Department of Health and Human Services, the NIH Office of AIDS Research's Priorities Planning Group, and the CDC's Global AIDS Program. Singer has over 150 published articles and book chapters, and is coauthor or editor of eight books.

Tom Stopka, MHS, is a research scientist with the HIV Prevention Research and Evaluation Section of the California State Office of AIDS in Sacramento. His research with the Office of AIDS focuses on surveillance of statewide HIV/AIDS and hepatitis infection rates and related risk behaviors among injection drug users (IDUs), MSM/IDUs, Latinos, and other high-risk populations. He also contributes as a member of the Office of AIDS' harm reduction working group, serves as the evaluator of the California HIV Planning Group, and provides technical assistance on research design and research methodologies to a number state- and federal-funded studies. Prior to his work in California, Tom worked at the Hispanic Health Council in Hartford, Connecticut, where he served as a project coordinator for the Access, Use, and Discard (SAUD) Study and Pharmacy Access to Syringes Study, and as a research associate. His research focused on

HIV/AIDS risk among IDUs, infant nutrition, migration, and childrearing behaviors. He has worked on a number of international public health interventions and research studies in the United States, Latin America, and East Africa and obtained his master's of health science degree in international health from the Johns Hopkins School of Hygiene and Public Health in 1999.

Wei Teng, Ph.D., was the statistician on the Access, Use, and Discard (SAUD) project and is now a senior statistical analyst at Center for Outcomes Research and Evaluation, Yale New Haven Health System, New Haven, Connecticut. She formerly worked as a research scientist on several research projects funded by the National Institute on Drug Abuse at the Center of Community Health Research of the Hispanic Health Council, Hartford, Connecticut. She received her Ph.D. in 1999 from Auburn University, Alabama. Her research interests focus mainly on women's health, including women's drug use and related health consequences. She is coauthor of multiple publications on drug use and HIV infection.

Graham A. Tobin, Ph.D. (University of Strathclyde, 1978), is professor of geography at the University of South Florida (USF). His research specialties include natural hazards, especially flooding; water resources management and policy; and environmental contamination. He has published eight books and monographs, eight book chapters, over 55 refereed articles and proceedings, 22 technical reports and working papers, and 22 book reviews, and has received nearly $1 million in grant funding. He has been department chair at two universities; has served on many committees at the national, university, college, and department levels; and has held office in various professional organizations. He has received the Research Honors Award from the Southeastern Division of the Association of American Geographers and a Presidential Award for Excellence at USF. His current research activities are concerned with evacuation strategies and health problems associated with volcanic eruptions, environmental impacts of flooding, and pollution reduction strategies in urban areas.

Fouzieyha Towghi, MPH, is a Ph.D. candidate in the Department of Anthropology, History, and Social Medicine with the joint program of medical anthropology at the Universities of California in San Francisco and in Berkeley. Her research focuses on women's reproductive health issues and the roles and practices of local community midwives. She is concerned with the impact of allopathic and establishment medicine on midwives and the women they serve, as well as the colonial and postcolonial development policy discourses and practices related to the health of rural populations in Pakistan. In her dissertation project, she will investigate the extensive use of plant medicine by women and midwives in district Panjgur, Balochistan. From 1996 to

1998, she was the co-investigator for the NIH-funded Balochistan Safe Motherhood Initiative project in Khuzdar, Balochistan, implemented to identify appropriate interventions and as a model to reduce maternal mortality. As a fellow at the Harvard Center for Population and Development studies in 1999, she wrote about Khuzdari women's perceptions of causes of obstetric bleeding.

Nalini Visvanathan, Ph.D., MPH, is on the faculty of the College of Public and Community Service at the University of Massachusetts Boston, where she teaches in the Asian American Studies Program. Her teaching and research interests include international development, transnational migration, women's health, and community development. She is active in movements for social change and immigrant rights.

William G. Wagner, M.A., received his master's degree in clinical social work from the University of Chicago, School of Social Service Administration, in 1994. Since then, he has worked as a clinical social worker with refugees and underserved populations. He is affiliated with the Anthropology Department at the University of New Mexico and is currently completing his dissertation on mental health, memory, and human rights in Guatemala. His ethnographic research on Medicaid and managed care is backed by years of working as a health care provider and as an advocate for Medicaid recipients.

Howard Waitzkin, M.D., Ph.D., is professor of Family and Community Medicine, Internal Medicine, and Sociology at the University of New Mexico. His award-winning research has focused on health policy in comparative international perspective and on psychosocial issues in primary care. He has been involved in advocacy for improved health access and currently is conducting studies of Medicaid managed care in New Mexico and the diffusion of managed care to Latin America.

Wayne Warry, Ph.D., is an applied medical anthropologist and associate professor, Department of Anthropology, McMaster University. He has over 17 years' experience working with and for various Aboriginal organizations, First Nations, Tribal Councils, and government ministries. He has been involved in the design, development, and evaluation of Aboriginal health systems and of culturally appropriate health care interventions and health promotions. His research has contributed to our understanding of the relationship between individual health and community well being in Aboriginal First Nations. This research led to a broader exploration of the relationship between community health and the self-government movement, issues that are explored in *Unfinished Dreams: Community Healing and the Reality of Aboriginal Self-Government* (1998, University of Toronto Press). Professor Warry has also contributed to our knowledge and understanding of culturally appropriate research methodologies, including approaches that combine praxis and participatory action research methods. With colleagues at McMaster University and the University of Toronto, he is developing a Centre for Aboriginal Health Research in Ontario, an initiative funded by the Institute of Aboriginal Peoples' Health, the Canadian Institutes of Health Research.

Linda Whiteford, Ph.D., MPH, is a professor of anthropology and chair of the Anthropology Department at the University of South Florida (USF). She is an applied medical anthropologist who is actively involved in teaching, research, and consulting. Dr. Whiteford received her doctorate in anthropology and her master's in public health from the Universities of Wisconsin and Texas, respectively. Her MPH training was in both epidemiology and international health: her doctoral research focused on economic decisions and reproductive choices among migrant farm workers in the Lower Rio Grande Valley. Since then, she has conducted research in Cuba, the Dominican Republic, Nicaragua, Costa Rica, Ecuador, and Bolivia through grants from the Rockefeller Foundation, the Center for Disaster Mitigation and Humanitarian Assistance; and as a consultant for the U.S. Agency for International Development and the World Bank. Maternal and child health were the original focus of her research, but for the last ten years, Dr. Whiteford has been in working on infectious/communicable diseases, such as cholera, dengue fever, and diarrhea, and on health system policy and analysis. Currently she is combining her interest in vector- and water-borne diseases with health consequences of forced evacuation or other population movements. Whiteford's most recent book (with Lenore Manderson) is *Global Health Policy, Local Realities: The Fallacy of the Level Playing Field*, published by Lynne Rienner Press. In March 2002 she became the president-elect of the Society for Applied Anthropology and received the George and Mary Foster Distinguished Lecture Award, and in 2003 she was awarded the USF Presidential Award for Excellence and was the Santa Clara University Visiting Scholar of the Year.

Cathleen E. Willging, Ph.D., is a scientist at the Behavioral Health Research Center of the Southwest and teaches in the Masters of Public Health Program at the University of New Mexico. Her current work centers on community-based, participatory research, mental health and substance use issues, and the influence of public policies and health care delivery systems on disparities among rural and ethnically diverse populations in New Mexico. She also is actively engaged in evaluation projects and qualitative studies concerning research ethics in cross-cultural settings.